Pandemic Planning in Pediatrics

Editors

YVONNE A. MALDONADO
STEVEN E. KRUG
ERICA Y. POPOVSKY

PEDIATRIC CLINICS
OF NORTH AMERICA

www.pediatric.theclinics.com

Consulting Editor
TINA L. CHENG

June 2024 • Volume 71 • Number 3

ELSEVIER

1600 John F. Kennedy Boulevard • Suite 1800 • Philadelphia, Pennsylvania, 19103-2899

http://www.theclinics.com

**THE PEDIATRIC CLINICS OF NORTH AMERICA Volume 71, Number 3
June 2024 ISSN 0031-3955, ISBN-13: 978-0-443-12971-1**

Editor: Kerry Holland
Developmental Editor: Saswoti Nath

The Pediatric Clinics of North America (ISSN 0031-3955) is published bimonthly by Elsevier Inc., 360 Park Avenue South, New York, NY 10010-1710. Months of issue are February, April, June, August, October, and December. Periodicals postage paid at New York, NY and additional mailing offices. Subscription prices are $290.00 per year (US individuals), $368.00 per year (Canadian individuals), $440.00 per year (international individuals), $100.00 per year (US students and residents), $100.00 per year (Canadian students and residents), and $165.00 per year (international residents and students). For institutional access pricing please contact Customer Service via the contact information below. To receive students/resident rare, orders must be accompanied by name of affiliated institution, date of term, and the signature of program/residency coordinator on institution letterhead. Orders will be billed at individual rate until proof of status is received. Foreign air speed delivery is included in all *Clinics* subscription prices. All prices are subject to change without notice. **POSTMASTER: Send address changes to *The Pediatric Clinics of North America*, Elsevier Health Sciences Division, Subscription Customer Service, 3251 Riverport Lane, Maryland Heights, MO 63043. Customer Service: 1-800-654-2452 (US and Canada). From outside of the US and Canada: 1-314-447-8871. Fax: 1-314-447-8029. For print support, E-mail: JournalsCustomerService-usa@elsevier.com. For online support, E-mail: JournalsOnlineSupport-usa@elsevier.com.**

Reprints. For copies of 100 or more, of articles in this publication, please contact the Commercial Reprints Department, Elsevier Inc., 360 Park Avenue South, New York, NY 10010-1710. Tel.: 212-633-3874; Fax: 212-633-3820; E-mail: reprints@elsevier.com.

The Pediatric Clinics of North America is also published in Spanish by McGraw-Hill Inter-americana Editores S.A., Mexico City, Mexico; in Portuguese by Riechmann and Affonso Editores, Rua Comandante Coelho 1085, CEP 21250, Rio de Janeiro, Brazil; and in Greek by Althayia SA, Athens, Greece.

The Pediatric Clinics of North America is covered in *MEDLINE/PubMed (Index Medicus), Excerpta Medica, Current Contents, Current Contents/Clinical Medicine, Science Citation Index, ASCA, ISI/BIOMED,* and *BIOSIS.*

Contributors

CONSULTING EDITOR

TINA L. CHENG, MD, MPH
BK Rachford Professor and Chair of Pediatrics, University of Cincinnati, Director, Cincinnati Children's Research Foundation, Chief Medical Officer, Cincinnati Children's Hospital Medical Center, Cincinnati, Ohio

EDITORS

YVONNE A. MALDONADO, MD
Taube Endowed Professor, Global Health and Infectious Diseases, Professor, Pediatrics, and Epidemiology and Population Health, Senior Associate Dean for Faculty Development and Diversity, Stanford University School of Medicine, Stanford, California

STEVEN E. KRUG, MD
Professor of Pediatrics, Northwestern University Feinberg School of Medicine, Chicago, Illinois

ERICA Y. POPOVSKY, MD
Assistant Professor of Pediatrics, Northwestern University Feinberg School of Medicine, Division of Emergency Medicine, Ann & Robert H. Lurie Children's Hospital, Chicago, Illinois

AUTHORS

BERNADETTE A. ALBANESE, MD, MPH
Medical Officer, Adams County Health Department, Brighton; Adjunct Assistant Professor, Department of Epidemiology, Colorado School of Public Health, Aurora, Colorado

SHANNON H. BAUMER-MOURADIAN, MD
Associate Professor, Department of Pediatrics, Director of Quality Improvement, Section of Emergency Medicine, Medical College of Wisconsin, Milwaukee, Wisconsin

JAMES D. CAMPBELL, MD, MS
Professor and Interim Division Head, Division of Infectious Diseases and Tropical Pediatrics, Department of Pediatrics, Center for Vaccine Development and Global Health, University of Maryland School of Medicine, Baltimore, Maryland

LISA J. CHAMBERLAIN, MD, MPH
Professor of Pediatrics (General Pediatrics) and, by courtesy, of Education, Stanford University School of Medicine, Center for Academic Medicine, Palo Alto, California

SARITA CHUNG, MD
Director, Disaster Preparedness, Division of Emergency Medicine, Boston Children's Hospital, Associate Professor, Pediatrics and Emergency Medicine, Harvard Medical School, Boston

WENDY M. CHUNG, MD, MS
Consultant, Texas Medical Association, Dallas, Texas

DEANNA DAHL-GROVE, MD
Professor of Pediatrics, Senior Pediatric Emergency Medicine Physician, UH Rainbow Babies and Children's Hospital, Cleveland, Ohio

HERBERT DELE DAVIES, MD, MSc, MHCM
Professor of Pediatrics, Infectious Diseases and Public Health, Senior Vice Chancellor for Academic Affairs, Dean for Graduate Studies, University of Nebraska Medical Center, Omaha, Nebraska

THOMAS DEMARIA, PhD
Clinical Psychologist, Advisor, National Center for School Crisis and Bereavement, Children's Hospital Los Angeles, Los Angeles, California

SANYUKTA DESAI, MD, MSc
Assistant Professor, Department of Pediatrics, Dell Medical School, University of Texas at Austin, Austin, Texas

ELIZABETH M. DUFORT, MD
Albany Medical College, Albany, New York

ZANAH K. FRANCIS, PhD
ORISE Fellow, United States Department of Health and Human Services, Washington, DC

LESLEY A. GARDINER, MD, PhD
Assistant Professor of Pediatrics, Department of Primary Care and Clinical Medicine, College of Osteopathic Medicine - Sam Houston State University, Conroe, Texas

SHANA GODFRED-CATO, DO
Assistant Professor, Division of Pediatric Emergency Medicine, Department of Pediatrics, Spencer Fox Eccles School of Medicine, University of Utah, Salt Lake, City, Utah

ELIZABETH A.D. HAMMERSHAIMB, MD, MS
Assistant Professor, Division of Infectious Diseases and Tropical Pediatrics, Department of Pediatrics, Center for Vaccine Development and Global Health, University of Maryland School of Medicine, Baltimore, Maryland

ANNIKA M. HOFSTETTER, MD, PhD, MPH
Department of Pediatrics, University of Washington School of Medicine, Center for Clinical and Translational Research, Seattle Children's Research Institute, Seattle, Washington

LARRY K. KOCIOLEK, MD, MSCI
Department of Pediatrics, Northwestern University Feinberg School of Medicine, Ann & Robert H. Lurie Children's Hospital of Chicago, Chicago, Illinois

ELLEN H. LEE, MD, MPH
Consultant, New York City Department of Health and Mental Hygiene, Long Island City, New York

ANNA LIN, MD
Assistant Medical Director, Division of Pediatric Hospital Medicine, Stanford Medicine Children's Health, Clinical Associate Professor, Department of Pediatrics, Stanford School of Medicine, Stanford, California

LAURENE MASCOLA, MD, MPH
Consultant, Los Angeles County Department of Public Health, Los Angeles, California

HILARY MCCLAFFERTY, MD, FAAP
Section Chief, Pediatric Emergency Medicine, Tucson Medical Center, Tucson, Arizona

ZACK MOORE, MD, MPH
State Epidemiologist, Division of Public Health, Epidemiology Section, Department of Health and Human Services, Raleigh, North Carolina

SCOTT NEEDLE, MD
Woodland Clinic Medical Group, Woodland, California

SEAN T. O'LEARY, MD, MPH
Director, Colorado Pediatric Practice-Based Research Network (PBRN), also known as COCONet (Colorado Children's Outcomes Network); Professor, Pediatrics-Infectious Diseases, Department of Pediatrics, Adult and Child Center for Health Outcomes Research and Delivery Science, University of Colorado Anschutz Medical Campus, Aurora, Colorado

DOUGLAS J. OPEL, MD, MPH
Professor, Department of Pediatrics, University of Washington School of Medicine, Director, Treuman Katz Center for Pediatric Bioethics and Palliative Care, Center for Clinical and Translational Research, Seattle Children's Research Institute, Seattle, Washington

ERICA PAN, MD, MPH, FAAP, FIDSA
State Epidemiologist, Deputy Director, California Department of Public Health, Richmond; Clinical Professor, Pediatric Infectious Diseases, University of California, San Francisco, San Francisco, California

SARAH Y. PARK, MD
Assistant Clinical Professor, Department of Pediatrics, John A. Burns School of Medicine, Kapiolani Medical Center for Women & Children, University of Hawaii at Manoa, Honolulu, Hawaii

CAITLIN PEDATI, MD, MPH
Virginia Beach Health District Director, Virginia Beach Department of Public Health, Virginia Beach, Virginia

KATHERINE E. REMICK, MD
Associate Chair of Quality, Innovation, and Outreach, Co-Director, EMS for Children Innovation and Improvement Center, Medical Director, San Marcos Hays County EMS System, Associate Professor, Department of Pediatrics, Dell Medical School, University of Texas at Austin, Austin, Texas

ALICE SATO, MD, PhD
Associate Professor, Department of Pediatrics, Division of Pediatric Infectious Disease, University of Nebraska Medical Center, Hospital Epidemiologist for Children's Nebraska, Omaha, Nebraska

LAUREN SAUER, MSc
Associate Director of Research, GCHS, Director, Special Pathogen Research Network, Associate Professor, Department of Environmental, Agricultural and Occupational Health, UNMC College of Public Health, Omaha, Nebraska

DAVID J. SCHONFELD, MD, FAAP
Professor of Clinical Pediatrics, Keck School of Medicine of the University of Southern California, Director, National Center for School Crisis and Bereavement, Children's Hospital Los Angeles, Los Angeles, California

ANDI L. SHANE, MD, MPH, MSc
Division Chief, Infectious Diseases, Marcus Professor of Hospital Epidemiology and Infection Control, Emory University School of Medicine, Medical Director of Hospital Epidemiology, Children's Healthcare of Atlanta, Emory Children's Center, Atlanta, Georgia

KARI A. SIMONSEN, MD, MBA
Carol Remmer Angle, MD, Presidential Chair of Pediatrics, Professor, Department of Pediatrics, Division of Infectious Diseases, UNMC College of Medicine, Associate Dean for Pediatric Affairs, College of Medicine, University of Nebraska Medical Center, Omaha, Nebraska

JOELLE N. SIMPSON, MD, MPH
Associate Professor, Departments of Pediatrics and Emergency Medicine, George Washington University School of Medicine, Chief of Emergency Medicine, Children's National Hospital, Washington, DC

SHAZEEN SULEMAN, MD, MPH
Clinical Associate Professor, Department of Pediatrics, Stanford University School of Medicine, Center for Academic Medicine, Palo Alto, California

GEORGE TURABELIDZE, MD, PhD
State Epidemiologist, Missouri Department of Health and Senior Services, St Louis, Missouri

JOSEPH L. WRIGHT, MD, MPH
Professor, Department of Pediatrics and Emergency Medicine, George Washington University School of Medicine, Washington, DC

REGINA YASKEY, MD
Assistant Professor of Pediatrics, Case Western Reserve School of Medicine, Pediatric Emergency Medicine Physician, Pediatric EMS Medical Director, UH Rainbow Babies and Children's Hospital, Cleveland, Ohio

DANIELLE M. ZERR, MD, MPH
Division Chief, Professor, Department of Pediatrics, University of Washington, Seattle Children's Hospital, Seattle, Washington

Contents

> Children make up approximately 25% of the population in the United States and are particularly vulnerable to the impact of disasters. The creation of federally-funded programs and advisory committees has had a positive impact on addressing the needs of children and families in disasters by identifying best practices, disseminating information, identifying gaps, and providing information with future investments that will contribute to expanding disaster science for children and their families.

> Although children account for 20% of all emergency department (ED) visits, the majority of children seek emergency care in hospitals that see fewer than 10 children per day. The National Pediatric Readiness Project has defined key system-level standards for all EDs to safely care for ill and injured children. High pediatric readiness is associated with improvement in mortality for critically ill and injured children. However, to improve readiness and sustain system-level changes, hospitals must invest in pediatric champions and empower them to engage in continuous quality improvement. Finally, incorporating pediatric readiness into policy is crucial for its long-term sustainability.

> Pediatric clinic preparedness is essential to improve the care and health outcomes for children during a pandemic and to decrease the burden on hospital systems. Clinic preparedness is a process that involves a well thought out plan that includes coordination with staff, open communication between the clinic and patient families, and collaboration with community partners. Planning for disasters can decrease some of the risks for our most vulnerable patients, including children and youth with special health care needs. There are plans, coalitions, and community partners that can help clinics in their preparedness journey.

The concepts of pediatric surge in the United States continue to evolve from a theoretical framework to practical implementation. As disasters become more frequent, ranging from natural to human-caused, children remain a vulnerable population. The coronavirus disease 2019 pandemic and the 2022 to 2023 tripledemic respiratory surge revealed advances and continued challenges in our ability to care for a large influx of pediatric patients. Understanding pediatric surge through the framework of the 4 S's (space, staff, stuff, and systems/structures) can identify gaps at multiple levels.

Physician burnout is pervasive and takes a heavy toll on individuals and the healthcare system. Post-coronavirus disease 2019 the negative impact of organizational culture on physician burnout has been highlighted. Substantial research has accrued identifying steps organizations can take to pivot and develop leaders committed to physician well-being. Physicians can also proactively explore research in sleep, nutrition, physical activity, stress management, and social connections. Positive mindset has a powerful protective effect in medicine, especially in the emerging areas of self-valuation, self-compassion, and positive psychology. Physician coaching can accelerate positive behavior change. Committed physician leaders are needed for sustained culture change to occur.

Special pathogens are broadly defined as highly transmissible organisms capable of causing severe disease in humans. Children's hospital healthcare personnel (HCP) should be prepared to identify patients possibly infected with a special pathogen, isolate the patient to minimize transmission, and inform key infection prevention, clinical, and public health stakeholders. Effective preparedness requires resources and practice with attention to education, policies and procedures, drills and training, and supplies. Successfully preparing for special pathogens is an important measure toward keeping communities, HCP, and patients and families safe in this global age that brings pathogens from across the world to our doorstep.

Pediatric health care providers can provide universal support to children and families to mitigate potential risk factors to adjustment while fostering protective factors to promote resiliency in children and families. They can educate caregivers about ways to enhance recovery of their children by modifying expectations and addressing the special emotional and social needs of their children. Most public health emergencies evolve through stages across an extended time period, often taxing the personal resources of health care providers. This underscores the need for pediatric health care providers to integrate self-care strategies in their personal and professional practice routines.

Zanah K. Francis, Elizabeth M. Dufort, Bernadette A. Albanese, Wendy M. Chung, Ellen H. Lee, Zack Moore, Laurene Mascola, Erica Pan, Caitlin Pedati, George Turabelidze, and Sarah Y. Park

This article examines lessons learned from previous pandemics, including the 2009 H1N1 influenza and the coronavirus disease 2019 pandemic. Pediatric providers have a unique and important role and strategies to improve collaboration and communication between public health and pediatric providers are essential during public health emergencies. A robust network of communication channels, effective public health messaging, and pediatric-focused disease related, and program outcome data are key to supporting a coordinated response to future pandemics. Critical issues include real-time communication with and engagement of pediatric providers as well as optimizing best evidence approaches for pediatric care while considering the distinct challenges facing children and their families.

Lauren Sauer, Alice Sato, and Herbert Dele Davies

Children have unique physiologic, developmental, and psychosocial needs and unique vulnerabilities, making them a challenging population for which to develop therapeutics. This is particularly apparent in the urgent and chaotic environment of a pandemic or outbreak. Advances in the development of medical countermeasures (MCMs) for pediatric populations have grown substantially over the last decade, and the coronavirus disease 2019 pandemic forced advancements in how we approach pediatric MCM development. Consequently, a MCMs pipeline targeting the pediatric population is essential. This article addresses the challenges inherent in these differences that must be taken into account.

Shannon H. Baumer-Mouradian, Annika M. Hofstetter, Sean T. O'Leary, and Douglas J. Opel

Vaccine confidence is a belief that vaccines work, are safe, and are part of a trustworthy medical system. The COVID-19 pandemic exposed the fragility of the public's confidence in vaccines and the vaccine enterprise, limiting the public health impact of vaccination. In this review, we examine the critical nature of vaccine confidence to pandemic preparedness and response.

Joelle N. Simpson and Joseph L. Wright

This article summarizes how pediatricians may be uniquely positioned to mitigate the long-term trajectory of COVID-19 on the health and wellness of pediatric patients especially with regard to screening for social determinants of health that are recognized drivers of disparate health outcomes. Health inequities, that is, disproportionately deleterious health outcomes that affect marginalized populations, have been a major source of vulnerability in past public health emergencies and natural disasters. Recommendations are provided for pediatricians to collaborate with disaster planning networks and lead strategies for public health communication and community engagement in pediatric pandemic and disaster planning, response, and recovery efforts.

This article considers ethical considerations surrounding pediatric vaccine development for pandemic preparedness, examines some historical cases of pediatric vaccines developed during past smallpox, influenza, and 2019 coronavirus disease pandemics, and discusses the current state of vaccine development for pandemic preparedness, including vaccines against smallpox/mpox, influenza, anthrax, and Ebola that are included in the US Strategic National Stockpile and vaccines being developed against priority pathogens identified by the World Health Organization.

In this article, the authors provide an overview how the COVID-19 pandemic impacted the health and wellbeing of migrant children in conflict zones, in transit and post-settlement in the United States. In particular, the authors explore how policies implemented during the pandemic directly and indirectly affected migrant children and led to widening disparities in the aftermath of the pandemic. Given these circumstances, the authors provide recommendations for child health care providers caring for migrant children to mitigate and bolster resilience and health.

PROGRAM OBJECTIVE

The goal of the *Pediatric Clinics of North America* is to keep practicing physicians and residents up to date with current clinical practice in pediatrics by providing timely articles reviewing the state-of-the-art in patient care.

TARGET AUDIENCE

All practicing pediatricians, physicians, and healthcare professionals who provide patient care to pediatric patients.

LEARNING OBJECTIVES

Upon completion of this activity, participants will be able to:

1. Review advances in the development of medical countermeasures (MCM) for pediatric populations and how it has grown substantially over the years.
2. Discuss the importance of pediatric clinic preparedness during a pandemic and the impact on pediatric populations when care is disrupted.
3. Recognize the impact of the COVID-19 pandemic on the health and wellness of pediatric patients especially concerning screening for social determinants of health that are recognized drivers of disparate health outcomes.

ACCREDITATIONS

Physician Credit

The Elsevier Office of Continuing Medical Education (EOCME) is accredited by the Accreditation Council for Continuing Medical Education (ACCME) to provide continuing medical education for physicians.

The EOCME designates this journal-based activity for a maximum of 13 *AMA PRA Category 1 Credit*(s)™. Physicians should claim only the credit commensurate with the extent of their participation in the activity.

All other healthcare professionals requesting continuing education credit for this journal-based activity will be issued a certificate of participation.

ABP Maintenance of Certification Credit

Successful completion of this CME activity, which includes participation in the activity and individual assessment of and feedback to the learner, enables the learner to earn up to 13 MOC points in the American Board of Pediatrics' (ABP) Maintenance of Certification (MOC) program. It is the CME activity provider's responsibility to submit learner completion information to ACCME for the purpose of granting ABP MOC credit.

DISCLOSURE OF CONFLICTS OF INTEREST

The EOCME assesses conflict of interest with its instructors, faculty, planners, and other individuals who are in a position to control the content of CME activities. All relevant conflicts of interest that are identified are thoroughly vetted by EOCME for fair balance, scientific objectivity, and patient care recommendations. EOCME is committed to providing its learners with CME activities that promote improvements or quality in healthcare and not a specific proprietary business or a commercial interest.

The planning committee, staff, authors, and editors listed below have identified no financial relationships or relationships to products or devices they or their spouse/life partner have with commercial interest related to the content of this CME activity:

Bernadette A. Albanese, MD, MPH; Shannon H. Baumer-Mouradian, MD; Tina L. Cheng, MD, MPH; Sarita Chung, MD; Wendy M. Chung, MD, MS; Deanna Dahl-Grove, MD; H. Dele Davies, MD, MSc, MHCM; Thomas Demaria, PhD; Sanyukta Desai, MD, MSc; Zanah K. Francis, PhD; Lesley A. Gardiner, MD, PhD; Shana Godfred-Cato, DO; Annika M. Hofstetter, MD, PhD, MPH; Shyamala Kavikumaran; Steven E. Krug, MD; Ellen H. Lee, MD, MPH; Anna Lin, MD; Michelle Littlejohn; Yvonne A. Maldonado, MD; Laurene Mascola, MD, MPH; Hilary McClafferty, MD, FAAP; Zack Moore, MD, MPH; Saswoti Nath; Scott Needle, MD; Sean T. O'Leary, MD, MPH; Douglas J. Opel, MD, MPH; Erica Pan, MD, MPH, FAAP, FIDSA; Caitlin Pedati, MD, MPH; Erica Y. Popovsky, MD; Katherine E. Remick, MD; Alice Sato, MD, PhD; Lauren Sauer, MSc; David J. Schonfeld, MD, FAAP; Andi L. Shane, MD, MPH, MSc; Joelle N. Simpson, MD, MPH; George Turabelidze, MD, PhD; Joseph L. Wright, MD, MPH; Regina Yaskey, MD

The planning committee, staff, authors, and editors listed below have identified financial relationships or relationships to products or devices they or their spouse/life partner have with commercial interest related to the content of this CME activity:

James D. Campbell, MD, MSa: *Researcher*: Moderna, Inc., Novavax, Emergent

Elizabeth M. Dufort, MD: *Independent Contractor*: Hutton Health Consulting

E. Adrianne Hammershaimb, MD, MS: *Researcher*: Moderna, Inc., Novavax, Emergent

Larry K. Kociolek, MD, MSCI: *Researcher*: Merck

Sarah Y. Park, MD: *Employee*: Karius

Kari A. Simonsen, MD, MBA: *Researcher*: Merck, Alinta

Danielle M. Zerr, MD, MPH: *Researcher*: Merck; *Consultant*: Allovir

UNAPPROVED/OFF-LABEL USE DISCLOSURE
The EOCME requires CME faculty to disclose to the participants:
1. When products or procedures being discussed are off-label, unlabelled, experimental, and/or investigational (not US Food and Drug Administration [FDA] approved); and
2. Any limitations on the information presented, such as data that are preliminary or that represent ongoing research, interim analyses, and/or unsupported opinions. Faculty may discuss information about pharmaceutical agents that is outside of FDA-approved labelling. This information is intended solely for CME and is not intended to promote off-label use of these medications. If you have any questions, contact the medical affairs department of the manufacturer for the most recent prescribing information.

TO ENROLL
To enroll in the *Pediatric Clinics of North America* Continuing Medical Education program, call customer service at 1-800-654-2452 or sign up online at http://www.theclinics.com/home/cme. The CME program is available to subscribers for an additional annual fee of USD 313.00.

METHOD OF PARTICIPATION
In order to claim credit, participants must complete the following:
1. Complete enrolment as indicated above.
2. Read the activity.
3. Complete the CME Test and Evaluation. Participants must achieve a score of 70% on the test. All CME Tests and Evaluations must be completed online.

In order to claim MOC points, participants must complete the following:
1. Complete steps listed above for claiming CME credit
2. Provide your specialty board ID#, birth date (MM/DD), and attestation.
3. Online MOC submission is only available for the American Board of pediatrics' (ABP) Maintenance of Certification (MOC) program

CME INQUIRIES/SPECIAL NEEDS
For all CME inquiries or special needs, please contact elsevierCME@elsevier.com.

PEDIATRIC CLINICS OF NORTH AMERICA

Foreword

Pandemic—Proofing for the Future

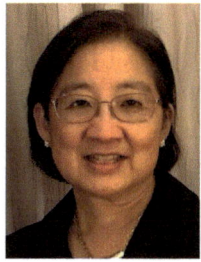

Tina L. Cheng, MD, MPH
Consulting Editor

For years, infectious disease experts warned that we were overdue for a pandemic. They were right. When COVID-19 struck, I recalled the Great Influenza Pandemic of 1918 (often mislabeled as the "Spanish flu"). There were four waves of recurrence through 1920, and it wasn't until the mid-1920s that the pandemic was felt to be "over." Naively, I assumed the COVID-19 pandemic wouldn't last that long because we are smarter now and science has progressed! But we repeated many of the struggles faced during that historical episode, including denials about the seriousness of the situation and misinformation about causes, preventive measures, and treatments. During both pandemics, low-income and minoritized communities suffered disproportionately. Clearly, we didn't learn the lessons of history. Luckily, the rapid development of effective vaccines and therapeutics were defining scientific successes this time. But misinformation and suspicion about science remained a central feature of society's reaction.

While we've been quick to shed our masks and we all wish for COVID-19 to be in the rearview mirror, it is now critical to understand and address the long-lasting impact of the pandemic on children, adolescents, families, and low-income and marginalized communities and pandemic-proof for the future. I was fortunate to be on the National Academies of Science, Engineering, and Medicine Committee on The Long Term Effects of the COVID-19 Pandemic on Children and Families (Chair, Tumaini Coker, https://nap.nationalacademies.org/catalog/26809/addressing-the-long-term-effects-of-the-covid-19-pandemic-on-children-and-families). The consensus report published last year recognized key lessons about the pandemic's effects within a context of pre-existing and ongoing social inequities. Both the disease and the response triggered direct effects of illness among family members and children, as well as secondary effects of learning loss, mental stress, and obesity. The pandemic is a major adverse

Pediatr Clin N Am 71 (2024) xv–xvi
https://doi.org/10.1016/j.pcl.2024.03.004
pediatric.theclinics.com

childhood and family experience with long-lasting life course impact, greatest among low-income and minoritized communities. Children are often the last protected and the longest affected. Along with the committee's recommendations, this issue of *Pediatric Clinics of North America* moves us forward in defining lessons learned, making those lessons stick, communicating science effectively, and preparing for the inevitable pandemics of the future.

Tina L. Cheng, MD, MPH
Cincinnati Children's Hospital Medical Center
University of Cincinnati
3333 Burnet Avenue MLC 3016
Cincinnati, OH 45229-3026, USA

E-mail address:
Tina.cheng@cchmc.org

Preface

Preparing the Pediatric Workforce for Future Pandemics and Disasters

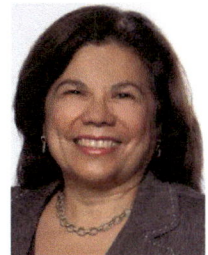
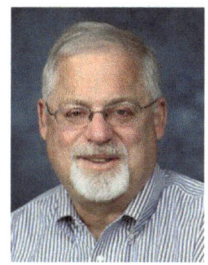
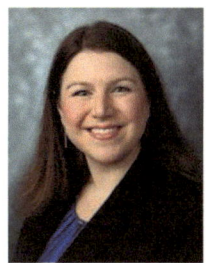

Yvonne A. Maldonado, MD   Steven E. Krug, MD   Erica Y. Popovsky, MD
Editors

As we emerge from addressing the historical challenges of the global COVID-19 pandemic, it is imperative that we take stock of our successes and failures, so that we can prepare for the next global crisis. In particular, it is critical to focus on the lessons that we learned in preparing our pediatric workforce to care for the youngest and most vulnerable members of our population. It is in this spirit that this issue was conceived and written. While major advances in biology and medicine have contributed greatly to our understanding of infants and children, there is an unfortunate dearth of scientific literature to guide effective and efficient pediatric pandemic and disaster responses. As the medical, psychological, social, and economic impact of past and impending pandemics becomes more fully appreciated, the time is appropriate for a brief overview of existing information on this subject.

Our goal for this issue is to provide a focused, critical, and contemporary review of available information, written by experts in the fields of pediatric emergency and disaster response, surge management, infectious diseases and infection control, mental health, workforce readiness, and vaccines and therapeutics. We also thought it was important to underscore critical considerations of social determinants of health in developing and disseminating principles of pediatric pandemic and disaster preparedness.

We hope this issue is of interest to all students of medicine interested in the care and well-being of children and hope to include among our readers medical students, residents and fellows, pediatricians, infection control professionals, emergency medicine physicians, emergency managers, first responders, and allied health care workers. We believe the issue to be of particular importance for infectious disease and infection control specialists; obstetricians and physicians who are responsible for the pregnant

Pediatr Clin N Am 71 (2024) xvii–xviii
https://doi.org/10.1016/j.pcl.2024.03.005
0031-3955/24/

woman and her developing fetus; office- and hospital-based pediatricians and family physicians who care for children; and psychologists, laboratorians, and other specialists who are responsible for children who may require urgent and emergent care in the wake of future pandemic or disaster situations.

We are indebted to our many colleagues who volunteered to share their tremendous expertise with us in writing this publication and sharing their lessons-learned from the pandemic. We also wish to express our appreciation to Dr Tina Cheng, Rachford Professor and Chair of Pediatrics, Director, Cincinnati Children's Research Foundation and Chief Medical Officer, Cincinnati Children's Hospital Medical Center, for suggesting and guiding this project to a successful conclusion; and to Ms Nancy Wilkening for her editorial assistance.

DISCLOSURES

The authors have no conflicts of interest to disclose.

Yvonne A. Maldonado, MD
Stanford University School of Medicine
Stanford, CA, USA

Steven E. Krug, MD
Feinberg School of Medicine
Northwestern University
Chicago, IL, USA

Erica Y. Popovsky, MD
Feinberg School of Medicine
Northwestern University
Chicago, IL, USA

E-mail addresses:
BonnieM@stanford.edu (Y.A. Maldonado)
skrug@luriechildrens.org (S.E. Krug)
epopovsky@luriechildrens.org (E.Y. Popovsky)

Pediatric Pandemics and Disasters - A Summary

Regina Yaskey, MD*, Deanna Dahl-Grove, MD

KEYWORDS

- Pandemics • Children • Disaster preparedness • Infectious disease
- Healthcare preparedness • Crisis standards of care

KEY POINTS

- Understand how children are vulnerable in disasters through the lens of epidemics and pandemics and other disasters.
- Review governmental initiatives/infrastructure to support children and families in the disaster cycle.
- Understand existing gaps and how developments in disaster science may impact further improvement in the care of children during the disaster cycle.

INTRODUCTION

A disaster is an event that overwhelms community resources to meet the needs of the impacted populations. The Federal Emergency Management Agency (FEMA) further defines a disaster as an "occurrence of a natural catastrophe, technological accident, or human-caused event that has resulted in severe property damage, deaths and/or major injury".[1] Disasters can be natural (hurricanes, tornados, wildfires, drought, earthquake, or infectious outbreaks) or man-made (bioterrorism, chemical/hazardous material spills, weapons of mass destruction, explosives, or active shooter). They may occur rapidly and without notice or may be prolonged in duration.[2] Each type of event creates unique strains on the emergency response resources needed. Understanding mitigation strategies before an event occurs, and the additional resources available through mutual aid can help a community achieve FEMA preparedness goals to plan for events. The Federal Emergency Management Agencydefines their national preparedness goal as: "A secure and resilient nation with the capabilities required across the whole community to prevent, protect against, mitigate, respond to, and recover from the threats and hazards that pose the greatest risk.".[3] Within this goal are 5 mission areas: Prevention, Protection, Mitigation, Response, and Recovery (**Fig. 1**).

UH Rainbow Babies and Children's Hospital, 11100 Euclid Avenue, Cleveland, OH 44106, USA
* Corresponding author.
E-mail address: regina.yaskey@uhhospitals.org

Pediatr Clin N Am 71 (2024) 353–370
https://doi.org/10.1016/j.pcl.2024.03.003
0031-3955/24/© 2024 Elsevier Inc. All rights reserved.

pediatric.theclinics.com

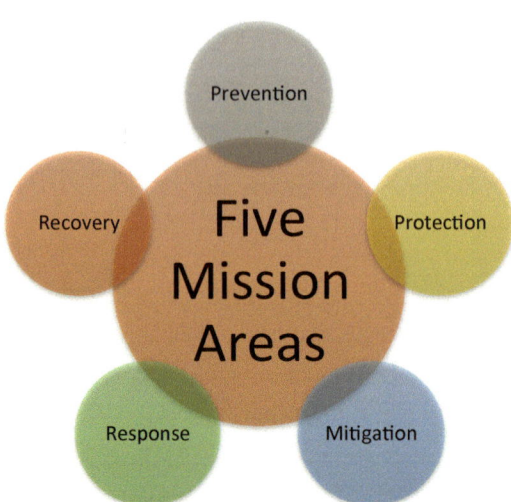

Fig. 1. The 5 mission areas from the national preparedness goal.

Prevention: The work that is done to avoid or stop an imminent or known threat or an act of terrorism.

Protection: Shielding our communities and keeping our citizens safe from threats and hazards.

Mitigation: The work done to reduce the number of lives lost from unpredictable events while also aiming to lessen the impact of future disasters.

Response: The efforts done to minimize the pain, destruction, and chaos caused by disasters.

Recovery: Restoring our communities and its citizens back to the way they once were.

CHILDREN AND DISASTERS

Children make up approximately 25% of the United States (US) population. They have unique needs and are more vulnerable than adults during and after disasters. They differ from adults in their physiology, developing organ systems, emotional response to stress and traumatic events, and their behavior and dependence on others for basic needs. This therefore creates unique considerations to meet their needs in the disaster cycle. Due to their increased surface area to body mass ratio, more permeable skin, less visceral fat, smaller size, increased respiratory rate, metabolism, and smaller circulatory volume, they are more susceptible to and can succumb quickly to biological/chemical threats (airborne and droplets) or explosions. Developmental and behavioral differences should also be taken into consideration when caring for children in a disaster, especially children and youth with special health care needs (CYSHCN). Many children are pre-verbal or nonverbal; therefore, it is difficult to accurately determine if they are injured or in pain. In addition, children may run toward a threat rather than away from it and may have difficulty following instructions from first responders.[2] Each specific disaster has its own unique ramifications and its direct effects on children. For example, wildfires expose them to numerous environmental hazards, highlighting their respiratory vulnerabilities, especially those children with asthma, allergies, or chronic health issues.[3] Floods highlight their vulnerability to unusual infectious agents (eg, cholera, malaria) or mold as families re-occupy formerly flooded dwellings.[4–6]

Prolonged disasters such as epidemics (infectious disease spread in a limited region) and pandemics (infectious outbreak on global scale) have affected humanity for centuries. The 1347 Black Death (Plague), 1520s Smallpox outbreak, 1918 Spanish Flu pandemic, 2009 H1N1/swine flu/influenza pandemic, and most recently the 2019 coronavirus disease (COVID-19) pandemic, caused millions of deaths and wreaked havoc on people's health, the global economy, and society.[7] The 1918 Spanish Flu and the 2019 COVID pandemics are among the most disastrous infectious disease emergencies of modern times. In addition to the countless lives lost, mitigation strategies for both included social isolation, which in itself may have precipitated a mental health crisis as was observed from the recent COVID pandemic.[8] Prior research shows that whenever there are infectious disease outbreaks, there are increases in depression, anxiety, post-traumatic stress disorder (PTSD), substance use disorders, domestic violence, and child maltreatment.[9]

PEDIATRICS, CORONAVIRUS DISEASE PANDEMIC, CRISIS STANDARDS OF CARE

The first suspected cases of COVID in the US appeared in Washington in February 2020. By March 2020, the US President had declared a national emergency and a stay-at-home order was issued in an attempt to decrease the rapid transmission and significant mortality of the virus. Within weeks, there was a noted 42% decrease in emergency department (ED) visits compared with the same time the year prior, with even greater volume reductions among children compared to adults.[10] Unanticipated consequences of decreased pediatric presentations to both primary care and the ED included delayed presentations of pediatric illnesses such as appendicitis,[11] and delayed diagnosis of new onset diabetes leading to increased cases of diabetic ketoacidosis.[12] Overall inpatient admissions for pediatric patients decreased by 35.1% during the COVID-19 period with the largest reductions seen in respiratory diseases such as asthma, bronchiolitis, pneumonia, and upper respiratory tract infections.[13] Unlike prior respiratory outbreaks, such as influenza, the COVID-19 virus disproportionately impacted adults as compared to children (**Fig. 2**). Children appeared to be less susceptible to severe infection and mortality rates were substantially lower compared to those in adults, particularly the elderly.[13] In 2020, there had already been 384,536 COVID-19 related deaths. Mortality rates were lowest amongst children aged 1 to 4 years (25 deaths) and 5–14 years (68 deaths) and highest amongst adults aged greater than or equal to 85 years (122,707 deaths).[14]

Hospitals across the country were forced to implement crisis standards of care due to the huge surge of adult patients with severe illness requiring inpatient admission.[15] These altered care standards are considered when healthcare systems operations are overwhelmed. They can be further classified into 3 levels of operations ranging from conventional care (usual day to day operations), contingent care (surge of patients but operations are adapted to maintain usual standards of care), and crisis care (unable to maintain usual standards of care due to insufficient resources in the face of an overwhelming surge).[16,17] The Institute of Medicine (IOM) published guidelines for state level implementation of crisis standards of care (CSC) in 2009.[16] Due to the low pediatric volumes, some adult patients were strategically redistributed to pediatric hospitals and many community hospitals closed their pediatric units, converting those beds, and staff, for adult care. This offers an example of how adaptability to crisis standards were applied to address the surge of adult patients during the pandemic. The COVID-19 pandemic highlighted the continued lack of surge guidelines among many locations in the US,[16] particularly guidelines addressing the needs of children. Minnesota is one state that has created a CSC guideline that takes children into

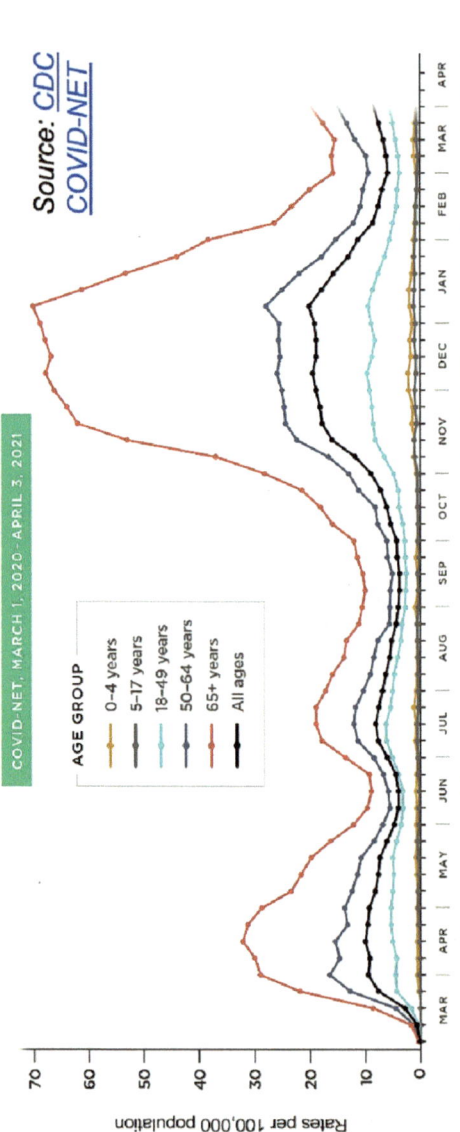

Fig. 2. Confirmed coronavirus disease 2019 associated hospitalizations by age group. COVID-NET Interactive Dashboard. URL: https://www.cdc.gov/coronavirus/2019-ncov/your-health/covid-net.html, Accessed September 17, 2023

account.[17] Basic ethical principles for all individuals within a society are important to consider when developing crisis standards of care, in particular the consideration of vulnerable populations, with their physical, ethnic, cultural, and societal perspectives that exist within the community at large.[15,18]

CHILDREN AND YOUTH WITH SPECIAL HEALTH CARE NEEDS

Children with underlying medical conditions and chronic illnesses are disproportionately impacted by public health emergencies and disasters and they are at increased risk for negative outcomes during and after disasters. This population is also at greater risk for abuse and neglect most likely secondary to their dependence on others, social isolation, and family stress.[19] While the COVID-19 pandemic resulted in a notable decrease in ED visits by children, the proportion of visits by CYSHCN increased. Children with co-morbidities and chronic illnesses were also at increased risk for severe COVID-19 disease. Due to the national stay at home mandate, social distancing, fear of COVID exposure, delays and cancellation in medical care, home health services and therapies, these patients experienced barriers to care access, and gaps in their treatments and therapies. One distinct positive of COVID-19 was that the pandemic ushered in a new era for providers to use telemedicine. Telehealth access was an important means by which caregivers of CYSHCN could access healthcare providers without leaving their homes and subsequently risking potential exposure to the virus in public.[19,20]

Future disaster planning should focus on incorporating disaster planning into routine anticipatory guidance provided by a patient's medical home. Physicians should work with all families toward the creation of a disaster emergency plan and should their regular care be disrupted. Disaster plans for CYSHCN should be prioritized and should include input from all multidisciplinary care providers involved in the child's treatment. It is also recommended for parents to have a surplus of critical medications and supplies on hand in case of shortages or other unforeseen needs.[20] Emergency Information Forms (EIF) aid in communicating key clinical information about CYSHCN and the goal is to have the EIF regularly up-dated. These forms summarize the child's medical history, medications, allergies, and recommendations for management for providers unfamiliar with the patient.[21]

TRIPLEDEMIC 2022

Near the end of the COVID pandemic, the pediatric population was impacted by the convergence of 3 viral epidemics nicknamed "The Tripledemic," in Fall 2022 leading to increased rates of viral respiratory illnesses and demand for emergency care and inpatient beds.[22] Case rates were the highest they had been in the preceding 5 years and hospital admissions increased exponentially.[23,24] Approximately 40% of homes had a family member infected with 1 of the 3 viruses.[25] Hospitalizations of children reached record levels throughout the respiratory season, resulting in long ED wait times, and a pediatric inpatient bed shortage, particularly pediatric critical care beds. At its peak, the CDC dashboard estimated 64.3 RSV associated hospitalizations per 100,000 in the 2022 to 2023 season seen in children aged 0 to 4 years.[23] Supply chains for medical products were impacted due to the surge in respiratory illness, further increasing hospitalization rates amongst the pediatric population. Common medications such as amoxicillin, albuterol, oseltamivir, and many others appeared on the Food and Drug Administration's (FDA) and American Society of Health System Pharmacists' (ASHP) drug shortage list.[26] The Department of Health and Human Services released oseltamivir through the Strategic National Stockpile to help combat supply issues.[27] Overall, the healthcare system was not well prepared for this surge and shortages in the pediatric space were severe. This emphasized to us that supply chain preparedness has ongoing gaps that have not been addressed, such as the yearly recurring oseltamivir supply shortages during influenza season.[28] All these impacts have magnified the fragility of the US healthcare system to care for children in a manner that the system had cared for adults during the COVID pandemic.

It has been well documented that pediatric inpatient hospital capacity has steadily declined over the past decade. Compelling evidence suggests that the COVID pandemic led many hospitals to further de-emphasize pediatric services. A 2021 study evaluating trends in pediatric inpatient unit capacity showed that US pediatric inpatient beds had decreased by 19.1% (34 units/year; 95% confidence interval (CI) 31–37) nationwide. Rural areas were noted to be most impacted by this trend, due in part to their distance from pediatric tertiary centers. This reduction was also driven by a decrease in pediatric inpatient bed utilization prior to the pandemic.[29] While proving to be an opportunistic tactic to optimize adult inpatient capacity this ultimately further added to the steady decline in hospital capacity to care for ill and injured children.[30,31]

LOCAL AND FEDERAL RESPONSE TO DISASTERS

During disasters or infectious disease outbreaks, public health entities work together with multiple national, state, and local health, and environmental systems to prevent spread and mitigate morbidity and mortality. All disasters begin locally with the scope changing depending on the event. The local government is responsible for organizing and managing the initial emergency response. When disasters overwhelm local resources leading to inability to manage the scale and magnitude of the event, local jurisdictions will seek mutual aid within the state. If these regional and state resources are unable to meet the demand for response in the disaster, the governor can then request resources at the federal level. The federal government includes organizational frameworks, response resources, and legal authorities that can aid local, state, or regional jurisdictions after a disaster. The larger and more complex the emergency, the greater are the number of organizations that are expected to respond. The Secretary of Health and Human Services (HHS), through the Administration for Strategic Preparedness and Response (ASPR) and the ASPR Office of Emergency Management and Medical Operations, oversees the preparedness, response, and recovery activities for healthcare and public health.

For disasters requiring medical response, requests for assistance are made through the local emergency management agency. The governor determines if the state possesses the necessary resources, and if not, they can activate the Emergency Management Assistance Compact (EMAC) and request assistance from other regional entities (**Fig. 3**). Only a governor, or his or her designee, can make a formal request to the President for a disaster declaration. Once a federal disaster is declared, the Robert T. Stafford Act is engaged. This act allows both presidential emergency and major disaster declarations for federal assistance to disasters.[32]

In December 2006, Congress passed, and the President signed the Pandemic and All Hazards Preparedness Act (PAHPA). Under this act, the Assistant Secretary for Preparedness and Response (now known as Administration for Strategic Preparedness and Response) and the Department of Health and Human Services (DHHS) have further expanded their role in administering the Health Care Readiness and Response (HCRR), formerly known as Hospital Preparedness Program, which addresses/enhances medical surge capacity and authorized funding for critical public health and medical necessities.[33] (**Table 1**)

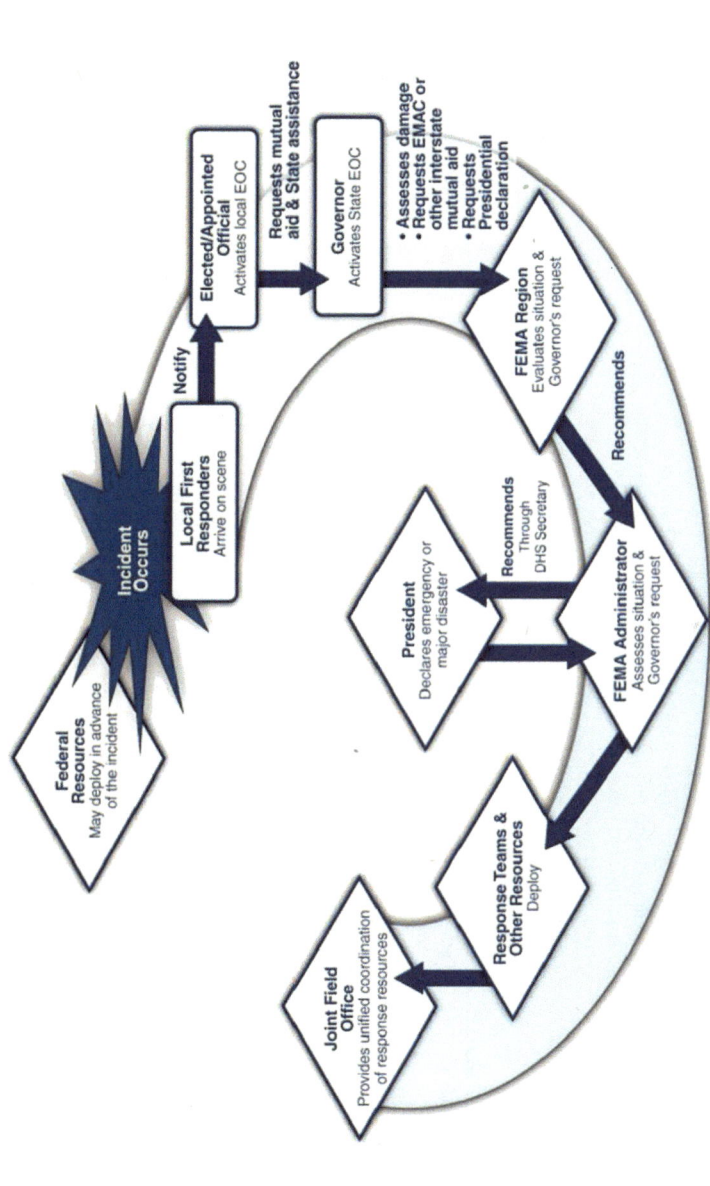

Fig. 3. FEMA, National Response Framework. URL: https://www.fema.gov/emergency-managers/national-preparedness/frameworks/response. Accessed February 6, 2024

Table 1
Resources that aid with disaster response

Name	Description	
Disaster Medical Assistance Team (DMAT)	Federal team composed of medical personnel that respond as a unit to a disaster and provide medical care. They are part of the National Disaster Medical System (NDMS) and are equipped with providing care for up to 72 hours. Federally appropriated resources are available from the DMAT if requested by the state office of emergency management.	https://aspr.hhs.gov/NDMS/Pages/dmat.aspx
Voluntary Organizations Active in Disaster (VOAD)	Organization composed of 55 states and territory of non-governmental organizations (NGOs) and other volunteers that exchange knowledge and resources in preparing for a disaster.	https://www.nvoad.org
Medical Reserve Corps (MRC)	Federally-funded network of volunteers that include medical and public health professionals. They are screened, trained, and organized to improve preparedness and response.	https://aspr.hhs.gov/MRC/Pages/index.aspx
Community Emergency Response Team (CERT)	Local volunteers organized by FEMA that train the civilian public in self-sufficient disaster preparedness and response under the Presidential Policy Directive's (PPD-8) goals of creating a resilient nation.	https://www.fema.gov/emergency-managers/individuals-communities/preparedness-activities-webinars/community-emergency-response-team
Emergency Support Functions (ESF)	Emergency Support Functions (ESF) are groupings of governmental and certain private sector capabilities into an organizational structure to provide support, resources, program implementation, and services that are most likely needed to save lives, protect property and the environment, restore essential services and critical infrastructure, and help victims and communities return to normal following domestic incidents.	https://aspr.hhs.gov/legal/Pages/Emergency-Support-Functions.aspx
Incident Command System (ICS)	Incident Command System provides an organizational structure for how personnel work together during an incident, using common terminology and vocabulary, processes, and systems to respond.	https://www.ready.gov/business/resources/incident-management and https://www.fema.gov/emergency-managers/nims

The COVID pandemic response utilized public health laws for mass vaccination campaigns to mitigate severe disease for high-risk individuals and healthcare personnel. Due to the public health emergency, many states approved prehospital providers (paramedics and emergency medical technicians) to administer the COVID vaccine in the out-of-hospital setting, something they were not authorized to do before[34] emphasizing how emergency laws could be implemented to support public health (**Table 2**).

FEDERAL FOCUS ON PEDIATRIC DISASTER PREPAREDNESS

Hurricane Katrina, one of the most devastating environmental disasters to ever occur in the United States, forced thousands of children to be evacuated from their homes, some without accompanying family. Estimates of the number of children evacuated and relocated, either temporarily or permanently, ranged between 200,000 and 370,000.[35] Immediately post-Katrina, it became clear to disaster response experts that the unique needs of children had been largely overlooked in federal and state disaster planning. Major gaps were also noted with the FEMA response, particularly reunification efforts, and stressed implications for future planning. More than 5000 children were reported missing to the National Center for Missing and Exploited Children (NCMEC).[35,36] Due to the many shortcomings noted post-Katrina that affected children, efforts commenced to assess the gaps in federal planning that put children at risk, and to formulate recommendations that could guide a national movement to close those gaps and help states better protect children. Thus, the National Commission on Children in Disasters (NCCD) was created in 2007 under President George Bush. The NCCD was charged with conducting a comprehensive study of the needs of children in the disaster cycle and provided specific findings, conclusions and a thorough list of recommendations to the President and Congress to improve the care of children before, during and after disasters.[36] The commission's comprehensive assessment found that "children were more often an afterthought than a priority" across 11 functional areas of US disaster planning. In 2010, the commission issued its final report, with 81 recommendations aimed at ensuring the unique needs of children would be accounted for in disaster preparedness, response, and recovery. Following the sunset of the NCCD, a federal advisory committee focused on pediatric readiness was formed. The National Advisory Commission on Children in Disasters (NACCD) was established in 2013 as a provision under the Pandemic and All-Hazards Preparedness Reauthorization Act of 2013. This federal advisory committee was active until 2018 when funding was not granted for reauthorization.[37] The NACCD generated many recommendations including strategies to improve readiness for pediatric surge[38] and healthcare preparedness[39](**Fig. 4**). Ten years after Hurricane Katrina, a 2015 National Report Card issued by Save the Children observed that 79% of the NCCD recommendations remained partially or fully unfulfilled, emphasizing that there was still a lot of work left to be done.[40] The current NACCD advisory committee established in 2023 is focusing recommendations on the mental health crisis for children and youth that has been amplified by the COVID pandemic and other items in the aftermath of disasters.[41]

NATIONAL ADVISORY COMMISSION ON CHILDREN IN DISASTERS APRIL 2015 SURGE CAPACITY
Recommendations Summary

A. The NACCD recommends that the ASPR develop a national network of stakeholders to examine issues and address barriers, and ultimately, implement solutions to family (child and adult caregiver) transport needs during infectious disease crises.

Table 2
Laws and presidential directives guiding federal medical response to disasters

Name	Year Enacted	Description
Federal Disaster Relief Act	1950	One of the earliest disaster legislation passed by Congress, allowing the federal government to "supplement the efforts and available resources of the state and local governments." This meant that the federal government was not the first-line provider of emergency assistance but would offer their assistance once the state and local government's resources were spent.
National Flood Insurance Act	1968	This act established the National Flood Insurance Program (NFIP) to provide insurance protection against flood losses and to encourage sound land use in flood prone areas. The act gave "individuals and communities a way to reduce their reliance on the federal government and take personal responsibility for their own recovery." This act was further strengthened in 1972 when Hurricane Agnes, the most devastating and costly disaster to hit the United States at the time, caused disastrous floods to spread across the country.
Disaster Relief Act	1974	On April 3rd, 1974, tornadoes struck communities across 10 states, naming the day "Terrible Tuesday." As a result, this act was passed, consolidating many changes that had been initiated in the period following Hurricane Agnes. It also provided the legislation to establish the Federal Emergency Management Agency (FEMA) to coordinate federal disaster response and recovery efforts.
Robert T. Stafford Disaster Relief and Emergency Assistance Act	1978	Presidential declaration that outlines the federal government's role in aiding state and local governments during major disasters and emergencies
Emergency Management Assistance Compacts (EMAC)	1996	A national mutual aid agreement that enables states to share resources during times of disasters. This can include medical professionals and their certifications and license across state lines are upheld
Homeland Security Act	2002	Following the September 11 attacks, this act was signed by the president and was responsible for the creation of the Department of Homeland Security (DHS). It addresses Emergency Preparedness and Response. FEMA and several other Executive branch components and functions are now housed under DHS.

(continued on next page)

	Year	
Name	**Enacted**	**Description**
Post-Katrina Emergency Management Reform Act (PKEMRA)	2006	Enacted after Hurricane Katrina, this law aimed to improve the nation's disaster response and recovery capabilities, including the establishment of the National Integration Center.
Pandemic and All-Hazards Preparedness Act (PAHPA)	2006	The purpose of this act is "to improve the nation's public health and medical preparedness and response capabilities for emergencies, whether deliberate, accidental or natural."
National Response Framework (NRF)	2008	While not a law, the NRF is a guide that establishes a comprehensive approach to national response to disasters and emergencies. It is often referenced in conjunction with the Stafford Act. The NRF is composed of a base document, Emergency Support Functions (ESF), and Support Annexes.
Presidential Policy Directive 8	2011	This directive is aimed at strengthening the security and resilience of the nation from acts of terrorism, cyber-attacks, pandemics and natural disasters.

Table 2
(continued)

B. That ASPR develops a national-level, real-time system to monitor pediatric resources, usage, and surge capacity, including pediatric primary and specialty care practitioners, pediatric transport, pediatric hospitals, network communications, and pediatric medical equipment and pharmaceutical caches.

C. Without data to quantifiably assess surge readiness of children's hospitals, the NACCD recommends that the ASPR bring together key stakeholders from children's hospitals to discuss current readiness, define the role of children's hospitals, and determine next steps for improving the capacity of all hospitals to quickly respond in an infectious disease crisis with national safety implications.

D. That the HHS Secretary takes steps to mitigate the gaps identified in the HRSA EMSC Readiness Study.

E. That the ASPR facilitate an ongoing workgroup of subject matter experts (SMEs) to develop pediatric surge strategies and guidelines to address staff, supplies, space, and systems that are flexible to be imposed at a local, state, regional, or national level.

F. That an ongoing HHS-guided, national discussion and review of potential future challenges and strategies and determine a regular means to disseminate what is developed and current to streamline efforts during infectious disease crises. A range of perspectives and expertise is needed to uncover gaps and to develop and share strategies.

G. Urges the ASPR to ensure constant and reliable funding of health care coalitions.

H. Calls on the ASPR to support convening pediatric health care coalition and preparedness stakeholders annually to assess strategic planning, gap analysis, and mitigation tactics for addressing pandemic and emerging infectious disease threats with national implications.

NACCD April 2015 Surge Capacity

VIII. Recommendations Summary

A. The NACCD recommends that the ASPR develop a national network of stakeholders to examine issues and address barriers, and, ultimately, implement solutions to family (child and adult caregiver) transport needs during infectious disease crises.

B. That ASPR develops a national-level, real-time system to monitor pediatric resources, usage, and surge capacity, including pediatric primary and specialty care practitioners, pediatric transport, pediatric hospitals, network communications, and pediatric medical equipment and pharmaceutical caches.

C. Without data to quantifiably assess surge readiness of children's hospitals, the NACCD recommends that the ASPR bring together key stakeholders from children's hospitals to discuss current readiness, define the role of children's hospitals, and determine next steps for improving the capacity of all hospitals to quickly respond in an infectious disease crisis with national safety implications.

D. That the HHS Secretary take steps to mitigate the gaps identified in the HRSA EMSC Readiness Study.

E. That the ASPR facilitate an ongoing workgroup of SMEs to develop pediatric surge strategies and guidelines to address staff, supplies, space, and systems that are flexible to be imposed at a local, state, regional, or national level.

F. That an ongoing HHS-guided, national discussion and review of potential future challenges and strategies and determine a regular means to disseminate what is developed and current to streamline efforts during infectious disease crises. A range of perspectives and expertise is needed to uncover gaps and to develop and share strategies.

G. Urges the ASPR to ensure constant and reliable funding of health care coalitions.

H. Calls on the ASPR to support convening pediatric health care coalition and preparedness stakeholders annually to assess strategic planning, gap analysis, and mitigation tactics for addressing pandemic and emerging infectious disease threats with national implications.

I. That the ASPR guide a national conversation among pediatric SMEs and health care coalition stakeholders on pediatric surge capacity during infectious disease outbreaks.

Fig. 4. Recommendations by the national advisory commission on children in disasters. NACCD April 2015 Surge Capacity - VIII. Recommendations Summary. National Advisory Commission on Children in Disasters (NACCD)

I. That the ASPR guide a national conversation among pediatric SMEs and health care coalition stakeholders on pediatric surge capacity during infectious disease outbreaks.

More recently, ASPR has funded 3 Pediatric Disaster Care Centers of Excellence (CoE). They are Region V for Kids, Western Region Alliance for Pediatric Emergency Medicine (WRAP-EM) (https://wrap-em.org), and most recently, Gulf-7 Pediatric Disaster Network (**Fig. 5**). These networks are tasked with bringing regional disaster response capabilities and developing coordinated pediatric disaster care capabilities for pediatric care in disasters.[42,43]

Established in 1984, and funded by the HHS Health Resources and Services Administration (HRSA), healthcare readiness is also a focus of the Emergency Medical Services for Children (EMSC) program. EMSC funds a state-partnership in all 50 states and in 7 territories. With an initial focus on day-to-day pediatric emergency readiness, EMSC has also become active in the realm of pediatric disaster readiness. Their focus areas include prehospital care, hospital and trauma care, disaster preparedness, research, and advocacy. Hospital readiness for acutely ill and injured

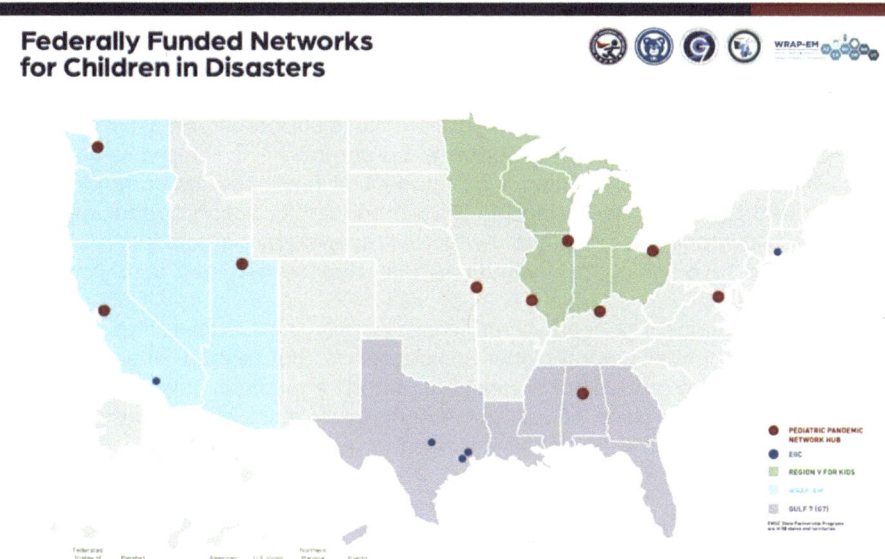

Fig. 5. Disaster care centers of excellence: Pediatric pandemic network, region V for kids, Gulf-7, Western Region Alliance for Pediatric Emergency Medicine, Emergency Medical Services for Children innovation, and improvement center. From Region V for Kids, The EMSC Innovation and Improvement Center.

children (eg, pediatric triage, provision of care, appropriate-sized equipment, medication dosing, and vaccinations) could be considered a proxy and a reasonable baseline for disaster readiness considering at least 80% of children receive emergency care in general EDs.[44] The National Pediatric Readiness Project (NPRP) was developed as a multidisciplinary, longitudinal quality initiative designed to identify gaps and improve the pediatric readiness and emergency care delivery within US hospitals.[45] With 10 pediatric centers, the Pediatric Pandemic Network (PPN) is the largest disaster network that includes subject matter experts in the field of pediatrics, and disaster and pandemic preparedness. Through its participants and partners, PPN touches institutions in nearly every US state and territory. As a network, it promotes readiness and seeks to improve health outcomes, and resiliency of children and their families affected by disasters and pandemics. The PPN is also funded by the Health Resources and Services Administration (HRSA) of the US Department of Health and Human Services.[46]

COMMUNITY RESILIENCE

Resilience as defined by the United Nations is "the ability of a system, community or society exposed to hazards to resist, absorb, accommodate, adapt to, transform and recover from the effects of a hazard in a timely and efficient manner, including through the preservation and restoration of its essential basic structures and functions through risk management."[47] Resilience is a key attribute for children and families and the community to promote recovery from disasters. Protective factors among and within families, such as support for mental health and interconnectedness, support recovery.[48–52] Childcare and schools are vital stakeholders in communities that support recovery. They allow caregivers to maintain employment or respond to disasters and for children to return to routines and support their recovery. There remain many gaps in childcare/school disaster preparedness and expectations, which have been highlighted in studies, including the recent COVID-19 pandemic within school feeding programs, noting that the flexibility and planning for alternative routes for food distribution is critical to supporting the vulnerable children that rely upon these federally supported programs.[53–58] The provision of support to help families thrive is also a component of resilience for communities as demonstrated by one state during the COVID pandemic, which conducted virtual visits for non-custodial parents, and it was well received by participants and should be considered in planning by institutions that provide services to children and families.[57]

Another foundation for community resilience is family preparedness, though it is uneven and is often better among higher socioeconomic households whereas families that are in vulnerable groups (for a variety of factors, economic, cultural etc) may be less prepared. The inclusion of vulnerable community representatives can improve family and community preparedness and support resilience.[57,58]

SUMMARY

In an era where disasters are growing in frequency and impact, it is imperative that our local, state, and federal governments continue working to address the needs of children and identify ways to mitigate and eliminate gaps in their treatment before, during, and after disasters. Climate change is having the effect of increasing the severity and frequency of disasters around the world, creating an urgency to close the gaps for children. With continued work, positive differences can be made for children and families so whole communities may recover and everyone may thrive and live in a fulfilling manner.

CLINICS CARE POINTS

- Children are particularly vulnerable in a disaster not only due to their physical and psychological differences based on their age, but socioeconomic challenges can be magnified when disasters occur.

- The United States Government has regulations and processes in place to address disasters, and since Hurricane Katrina in 2005, more concerted efforts to focus on children have occurred.

- The creation of federally funded programs, disaster centers of excellence and networks will have a positive impact on addressing the needs of children and families in disasters by identifying best practices, disseminating information, identifying, and eliminating gaps in practice and information.

- Disaster science is an important means to close the information or evidence gaps for children in the disaster cycle. Data that include ethnicity, culture, and diversity needs to be explored in the disaster cycle to improve the engagement in planning for disasters in all communities.

- There remain numerous gaps in the current understanding of disasters and their effects on children. Understanding the disaster cycle, how to apply the current resources and where to close the gaps is critical to the future and advancement of disaster medicine.

DISCLOSURE

The authors have nothing to disclose.

REFERENCES

1. FEMA. State and local guide (SLG) 101 guide for all-hazard emergency operations planning. 1996. Available at: https://www.fema.gov/pdf/plan/slg101.pdf. [Accessed 7 September 2023].
2. American Academy of Pediatrics, Council on Children and Disasters, COMMITTEE ON PEDIATRIC EMERGENCY MEDICINE. Ensuring the health of children in disasters. Pediatrics 2015;136(5):e1407–17.
3. FEMA. National Preparedness Goal | FEMA.gov. www.fema.gov. Published July 20. 2020. Available at: https://www.fema.gov/emergency-managers/national-preparedness/goal. [Accessed 1 January 2024].
4. Morgan O, Ahern M, Cairncross S. Revisiting the Tsunami: Health Consequences of Flooding. PLoS Med 2005;2(6):e184.
5. Watson JT, Gayer M, Connolly MA. Epidemics after Natural Disasters. Emerg Infect Dis 2007;13(1):1–5.
6. Abdullah M, Qamar K, Umer Usman M, et al. Cholera spike following monsoon floods in Pakistan: Challenges, efforts and recommendations (short communication). International Journal of Surgery Open 2023;57:100652.
7. Patterson GE, McIntyre KM, Clough HE, et al. Societal impacts of pandemics: comparing COVID-19 with history to focus our response. Front Public Health 2021;9(9). https://doi.org/10.3389/fpubh.2021.630449.
8. Morens DM, Taubenberger JK, Fauci AS. A centenary tale of two pandemics: the 1918 influenza pandemic and COVID-19, Part I. Am J Public Health 2021;111(6): 1086–94.
9. Tayyib NM. An action plan to address the mental health impact of COVID-19 on communities: five effective strategies. Psychol Serv 2021. https://doi.org/10.1037/ser0000575.
10. Hartnett KP, Kite-Powell A, DeVies J, et al, National Syndromic Surveillance Program Community of Practice. Impact of the COVID-19 pandemic on emergency department visits — United States, January 1, 2019–May 30, 2020. MMWR Morbidity and Mortality Weekly Report 2020;69(23):699–704.
11. Snapiri O, Rosenberg Danziger C, Krause I, et al. Delayed diagnosis of paediatric appendicitis during the COVID-19 pandemic. Acta Paediatr 2020;109(8): 1672–6.
12. Cherubini V, Gohil A, Addala A, et al. Unintended consequences of coronavirus disease-2019: remember general pediatrics. J Pediatr 2020;223:197–8.
13. Markham JL, Richardson T, DePorre A, et al. Inpatient use and outcomes at children's hospitals during the early COVID-19 pandemic. Pediatrics 2021;147(6). e2020044735.
14. Ahmad FB, Cisewski JA, Anderson RN. Provisional Mortality Data — United States, 2021. MMWR Morbidity and Mortality Weekly Report 2022;71. https://doi.org/10.15585/mmwr.mm7117e1.
15. Laventhal N, Basak R, Dell ML, et al. The ethics of creating a resource allocation strategy during the COVID-19 pandemic. Pediatrics 2020;146(1). https://doi.org/10.1542/peds.2020-1243.
16. Margus C, Sarin RR, Molloy M, et al. Crisis standards of care implementation at the state level in the United States. Prehosp Disaster Me 2020;35(6):599–603.
17. Minnesota Department of Health. Health care considerations - crisis standards of care. Available at: https://www.health.state.mn.us/communities/ep/surge/crisis/hospital.html. [Accessed 23 September 2023].

18. Romney D, Fox H, Carlson S, et al. Allocation of scarce resources in a pandemic: a systematic review of US state crisis standards of care documents. Disaster Med Public Health Prep 2020;14(5):677–83.

19. Stough LM, Ducy EM, Kang D. Addressing the needs of children with disabilities experiencing disaster or terrorism. Curr Psychiatry Rep 2017;19(4). https://doi.org/10.1007/s11920-017-0776-8.

20. Driansky A, Pilapil M, Mastrogiannis A. Updating the healthcare maintenance visit for children with medical complexity. Curr Opin Pediatr 2022. https://doi.org/10.1097/mop.0000000000001116. Publish Ahead of Print.

21. American Academy of Pediatrics Committee on Pediatric Emergency Medicine and Council on Information Technology, American College of Emergency Physicians Pediatric Emergency Medicine Committee, Committee on Pediatric Emergency Medicine and Council on Clinical Information Technology, American College of Emergency Physicians. Emergency information forms and emergency preparedness for children with special health care needs. Pediatrics 2010;125(4): 829–37.

22. Health Alert Network (HAN). HAN Archive - 00479. . emergency.cdc.gov. 2022. Available at: https://emergency.cdc.gov/han/2022/han00479.asp. [Accessed 21 September 2023].

23. Centers for Disease Control and Prevention. RSV-NET Interactive Dashboard. www.cdc.gov. 2022. Available at: https://www.cdc.gov/rsv/research/rsv-net/dashboard.html. [Accessed 21 September 2023].

24. Mandavilli A. A "tripledemic"? Flu and other infections return as COVID cases rise. Available at: N Y Times 2022; https://www.nytimes.com/2022/10/23/health/flu-covid-risk.html. [Accessed 23 September 2023].

25. Weixel N. "Tripledemic" infected nearly 40 percent of households, survey finds. The Hill; 2023. Available at: https://thehill.com/policy/healthcare/3846161-tripledemic-infected-nearly-40-percent-of-households-survey-finds/. [Accessed 27 September 2023].

26. Center for Drug Evaluation and Research. Drug shortages. US food and drug administration. 2023. Available at: https://www.fda.gov/drugs/drug-safety-and-availability/drug-shortages. [Accessed 23 September 2023].

27. Administration for Strategic Preparedness and Response. HHS Increases access to tamiflu through the Strategic National Stockpile. HHS.gov 2022. Available at: https://www.hhs.gov/about/news/2022/12/21/hhs-increases-access-to-tamiflu-through-the-strategic-national-stockpile.html. [Accessed 27 September 2023].

28. Kojima N, Peterson L, Hawkins R, et al. Influenza antiviral shortages reported by state and territorial public health officials, 2022-2023. JAMA 2023;330(18):1793.

29. Cushing AM, Bucholz EM, Chien AT, et al. Availability of pediatric inpatient services in the United States. Pediatrics 2021;148(1). https://doi.org/10.1542/peds.2020-041723.

30. Potts AL, Thomas A, Bork SJD, et al. Safely caring for adult patients in a pediatric hospital during the COVID-19 pandemic: a focus on the medication-use process. Am J Health Syst Pharm 2021;78(12):1128–33.

31. Gist RE, Pinto R, Kissoon N, et al. Repurposing a PICU for adult care in a state mandated COVID-19 only hospital: outcome comparison to the MICU cohort to determine safety and effectiveness. Front Pediatr 2021;9:665350.

32. Cone DC, Brice JH, Delbridge TR, et al. Emergency Medical Services. Medical Oversight of EMS 2021;2:98. Wiley-Blackwell; Chapter.

33. Administration for Strategic Preparedness and Response. Pandemic and All hazards preparedness act. aspr.hhs.gov. Available at: https://aspr.hhs.gov/legal/pahpa/Pages/default.aspx. [Accessed 11 September 2023].

34. National Association of Emergency Medical Technicians. Emergency medical services (EMS): a valuable resource for community vaccination campaigns. NAEMT.ORG. Available at: https://naemt.org/docs/default-source/covid-19/vaccine-toolkit-07-08-2022-v2.pdf?sfvrsn=41cef693_2. [Accessed 23 September 2023].

35. Fothergill A, Peek LA. Children of Katrina. Austin, TX: University Of Texas Press; 2015.

36. National Commission on Children and Disasters. National commission on children and disasters 2010 report to the president and congress. 2010. Available at: https://www.acf.hhs.gov/sites/default/files/documents/ohsepr/nccdreport.pd. [Accessed 21 September 2023].

37. National advisory committee on children and disasters. committee recommendations. aspr.hhs.gov. Available at: https://aspr.hhs.gov/AboutASPR/Workingwith ASPR/BoardsandCommittees/Pages/NACCD/Recommendations.aspx. [Accessed 6 February 2024].

38. National Advisory Committee on Children and Disasters, Near-term strategies to improve pediatric surge capacity during infectious disease outbreaks: a report off the NACCD Surge Capacity Work Group, 2015, ASPR NACCD, Washington, DC, Available at: https://aspr.hhs.gov/_catalogs/masterpage/ASPR/Documents/Boards%20and%20Committees%20Docs/naccd-surge-capacity-rpt042815.pdf (Accessed 6 February 2024).

39. National Advisory Committee on Children and Disasters, Healthcare preparedness for children in disasters: a report of the NACCD Healthcare Preparedness Working Group, 2015, ASPR NACCD, Washington, DC, Available at: https://aspr.hhs.gov/_catalogs/masterpage/ASPR/Documents/Boards%20and%20Committees%20Docs/healthcare-prep-wg-20151311.pdf (Accessed 1 February 2024).

40. Digital S. Still at risk: U.S. children 10 years after Hurricane Katrina. Save the Children Resource Centre. Available at: https://resourcecentre.savethechildren.net/document/still-risk-us-children-10-years-after-hurricane-katrina/. [Accessed 1 February 2024].

41. National advisory committee on children and disasters. committee recommendations. aspr.hhs.gov. Available at: https://aspr.hhs.gov/AboutASPR/Workingwith ASPR/BoardsandCommittees/Pages/NACCD/Recommendations.aspx. [Accessed 1 February 2024].

42. Emergency Medical Services for Children Innovation and Improvement Center. Pediatric disaster care centers of excellence (ASPR). EMSC EIIC. Available at: https://emscimprovement.center/domains/preparedness/asprcoe/. [Accessed 6 February 2024].

43. Administration for strategic preparedness and response. homepage. aspr.hhs.gov. Available at: https://aspr.hhs.gov/Pages/Home.aspx. [Accessed 6 February 2024].

44. Emergency medical services for children innovation and improvement center (EIIC). history of EMSC. EMSC EIIC. Available at: https://emscimprovement.center/about/history-emsc/. [Accessed 6 February 2024].

45. Emergency medical services for children innovation and improvement center (EIIC). national pediatric readiness project. Available at: https://emscimprovement.center/domains/pediatric-readiness-project. [Accessed 21 September 2023].

46. Pediatric Pandemic Network. All children deserve access to high quality care. pedspandemic.org. Available at: https://pedspandemicnetwork.org. [Accessed 23 September 2023].

47. United nations office for disaster risk reduction. resilience. www.undrr.org. Available at: http://undrr.org/terminology/resilience. [Accessed 6 February 2024].

48. Sprang G, Silman M. Using professional organizations to prepare the behavioral health workforce to respond to the needs of pediatric populations impacted by health-related disasters: guiding principles and challenges. Disaster Med Public Health Prep 2015;9(6):642–9.

49. Masten AS. Resilience of children in disasters: a multisystem perspective. Int J Psychol 2021;56(1):1–11.

50. Osofsky JD, Osofsky HJ. Challenges in building child and family resilience after disasters. J Fam Soc Work 2018;21(2):115–28.

51. Lai B, Garcia A. Understanding the Impacts of natural disasters on children. Soc Res Child Devel 2020;4:10–1. Available at: www.srcd.org/policy-media/child-evidence-briefs.

52. United nations office for disaster risk reduction. sendai framework for disaster risk reduction 2015 - 2030. 2015. Available at: https://www.undrr.org/publication/sendai-framework-disaster-risk-reduction-2015-2030. [Accessed 6 February 2024].

53. Rebmann T, Elliott MB, Artman D, et al. Missouri K-12 school disaster and biological event preparedness and seasonal influenza vaccination among school nurses. Am J Infect Control 2015;43(10):1028–34.

54. Fung ICH, Gambhir M, Glasser JW, et al. Modeling the effect of school closures in a pandemic scenario: exploring two different contact matrices. Clin Infect Dis 2015;60(suppl_1):S58–63.

55. Patten EV, Spruance L, Vaterlaus JM, et al. Disaster management and school nutrition: a qualitative study of emergency feeding during the COVID-19 pandemic. J Acad Nutr Diet 2021;121(8):1441–53.

56. Kenney EL, Dunn CG, Mozaffarian RS, et al. Feeding children and maintaining food service operations during COVID-19: a mixed methods investigation of implementation and financial challenges. Nutrients 2021;13(8):2691.

57. Oehme K, O'Rourke KS, Bradley L. Online virtual supervised visitation during the COVID -19 pandemic: one state's experience. Fam Court Rev 2021;59(1):131–43.

58. Schnall AH, Kieszak S, Heiman HJ, et al. Characterizing household emergency preparedness levels for natural disasters during the COVID-19 pandemic: United States, 2020-2021. J Emerg Manage 2023;21(7):51–69.

Overcoming Vulnerabilities in Our Emergency Care System Through Pediatric Readiness

Sanyukta Desai, MD, MSc, Katherine E. Remick, MD*

KEYWORDS

- Pediatric readiness • Pediatric emergency care • Pediatric disaster preparedness
- Child vulnerability • Emergency care systems • Quality improvement

KEY POINTS

- Despite advances in emergency and trauma systems nationwide, outcomes for children lag behind those of adults.
- Pediatric readiness provides a roadmap for safe and equitable care delivery for children in all emergency department settings.
- High pediatric readiness is associated with survival benefits for critically ill and injured children.
- Until pediatric readiness becomes policy, investment in pediatric emergency care coordinators and continuous quality improvement is crucial to transform our emergency care system.

INTRODUCTION

Over 18% of the US gross domestic product is directed toward the health care system.[1] Access to high-quality emergency care—whether 9-1-1 services or a nearby emergency department (ED)—is often taken for granted. Yet, even though children account for 20% to 25% of all ED visits in the United States, emergency care systems were not designed with children in mind.[2,3]

Over the last 50 years, outcomes from trauma, stroke, and heart disease have improved significantly due to the creation of well-defined systems that include specific treatment modalities, standardized protocols, staffing models, and continuous oversight to ensure adherence to best practices.[4–10] Yet, despite significant advancements in these systems of care, the outcome benefits for children seeking emergency care have lagged behind those of adults and, alarmingly, have shown a recent uptick in mortality.[11]

Department of Pediatrics, Dell Medical School, University of Texas at Austin, Austin, TX 78723, USA
* Corresponding author. 1400 Barbara Jordan Boulevard, Suite 1.114C, Austin, TX 78723.
E-mail address: kate.remick@austin.utexas.edu

Pediatr Clin N Am 71 (2024) 371–381
https://doi.org/10.1016/j.pcl.2024.01.011
0031-3955/24/© 2024 Elsevier Inc. All rights reserved.
pediatric.theclinics.com

One in 5 children seeks emergency care every year accounting for 35 million (>20%) annual ED visits in the United States.[2,3] Nearly 90% of these visits occur in general EDs that see fewer than 10 children per day, and 25% occur in rural areas.[12,13] For an individual ED, the rate of exposure to critically ill and injured children remains exceedingly low. In the absence of universal standards or regulatory requirements for pediatric emergency care, serious adverse events and/or sentinel events remain the primary driver of system improvements. While, following such events, efforts to improve pediatric readiness are deliberate and rapid, the lack of system integration results in unsustainable gains that in turn leads to more lives lost.

Among the 35 million children who seek emergency care every year in the United States, less than 5% result in hospitalization.[3,14] Respiratory diseases remain the number one cause of hospitalizations in children under 10 years of age, while mental illness has recently become the number one cause of hospitalization in children over 10 years of age. Both have unique characteristics, nuances, and treatments in the pediatric population that challenge our emergency care systems to deliver high quality care. Furthermore, injury remains the leading cause of death in children.[15] While 45% of US hospitals are designated trauma centers, benefits in functional outcomes and mortality for most common pediatric injuries have been largely demonstrated for children presenting to pediatric-specific trauma centers.[16–22] Only 57% of children live within 30 miles of a pediatric-specific trauma center, highlighting lack of access to high-quality pediatric emergency care as a vulnerability for children with both short- and long-term consequences.[23,24]

The variability that exists in pediatric emergency care stems from a basic "unevenness" in our emergency care system's design. The Institute of Medicine, now the National Academies of Medicine (NAM), first highlighted the unique needs of children in 1993.[25,26] Subsequently, NAM issued a 3-part report "The Future of Emergency Care" that called for deep system-level changes in order to meet the emergency care needs of children.[26] Specifically, it highlighted the need for a "regionalized, coordinated, and accountable system" designed to accommodate the needs of children in all communities, where resources are easily navigated by families and health care providers and where measurable performance is linked to improved outcomes.[26]

HISTORY: THE NATIONAL PEDIATRIC READINESS PROJECT

In 1984, the Emergency Medical Services for Children (EMSC) program was first authorized by Congress to integrate the needs of children into the emergency care system and decrease pediatric morbidity and mortality due to severe illness and injury. Housed within the Health Resources and Services Administration, the EMSC is the single federal program dedicated solely to pediatric emergency care.[27] Over the last 40 years, the EMSC program has worked to develop evidence-based practice guidelines, provide educational tools and resources for health care providers, and increase awareness of the unique needs of children. The National Pediatric Readiness Project (NPRP) born out of the EMSC program to ensure high-quality emergency care for all children serves as the Program's landmark initiative (alongside the Prehospital Pediatric Readiness Project).[28]

The NPRP emerged from collaboration between the national professional societies: the American Academy of Pediatrics, the American College of Emergency Physicians, and the Emergency Nurses Association to define standards for pediatric emergency care at a system level. These standards, first published in 2001 and periodically revised, define the components of "Pediatric Readiness in the Emergency Department."[29] The NPRP initiative was strategically designed to drive improvements in pediatric readiness of EDs through 5 key interventions.

1. *NPRP Assessment*: This comprehensive assessment serves as the primary tool used to measure the pediatric capabilities of our emergency care system and identify critical and/or common deficiencies in system infrastructure.[30] It highlights 6 core domains as outlined in the joint policy statement: (1) administration and coordination, (2) pediatric competencies of health care providers, (3) pediatric quality improvement (QI), (4) pediatric patient safety, (5) pediatric protocols and policies, and (6) pediatric equipment and supplies (**Box 1**).
2. *NPRP Checklist and Toolkit*: This collection of online resources is designed to help ED-based health care teams to identify, adopt, and adapt pediatric-specific interventions to improve pediatric readiness.[31]
3. *National QI Collaboratives*: The EMSC program organizes free, informal networks of health care providers who are guided, supported, and work collaboratively to implement local system improvements.[32]
4. *National Pediatric Readiness* Quality Initiative Dashboard: This web-based, free, open access dashboard is designed to help the ED-based care teams measure and benchmark their performance on key quality metrics and engage in pediatric QI efforts.[33]
5. *Pediatric Readiness Recognition Programs*: The EMSC program highlights state and territory-based programs that verify and recognize EDs that meet pediatric readiness criteria and provides guidance for launch and maintenance of such programs.[34]

The array of activities within the NPRP umbrella is further supported through research, the validation of evidence-based practice guidelines, workforce development, and communications.

PEDIATRIC READINESS AND ITS SIGNIFICANCE

The weighted pediatric readiness score (wPRS) is derived from the NPRP assessment and is based on a 100-point scale. Individual EDs complete the self-assessment to compare their current state to similar cohorts of EDs and the national median (www.pedsready.org/).[30] Nationally, the median wPRS was 69.5 in 2021. Key findings from the 2021 assessment are outlined in **Table 1**.[13]

Box 1
Domains of pediatric readiness

Administration and Coordination: measures the presence of a dedicated physician and nurse pediatric emergency care coordinator

Pediatric Competencies of Healthcare Personnel: measures the presence of competency evaluations and maintenance of board certification for physicians and nurses

Pediatric Quality Improvement: measures the presence of patient care review processes, identification of quality indicators, collection/analysis of pediatric data, development of a pediatric QI plan, and reevaluation of performance using outcome-based measures.

Pediatric Patient Safety: measures the presence of pediatric-specific patient safety measures (eg, weight in kilograms alone, pain assessment, mental status assessment)

Pediatric Policies and Procedures: measures the presence of pediatric-specific policies for standard and disaster scenarios (eg, family-centered care, death of a child, reduced radiation dosing for imaging, disaster drills including pediatric scenarios)

Pediatric Equipment and Supplies: measures the presence of equipment (eg, pediatric blood pressure cuffs, endotracheal tubes) and appropriate staff training on location and use.

Table 1 Key findings from the 2021 National Pediatric Readiness Project assessment	
Presence of Pediatric Policies, Procedures, and Equipment	N (%) EDs N = 3557
Child maltreatment	3230 (90.8%)
Patient assessment/reassessment	2800 (78.7%)
Reduced dose radiation protocol	2701 (75.9%)
Weight in kilograms only	2651 (74.5%)
Mental health care	2599 (73.1%)
Pediatric interfacility transfer guidelines	2550 (71.7%)
Death in ED	2524 (71%)
Social services	2389 (67.2%)
Behavioral health transfer	2364 (66.5%)
Family-centered care plans	2224(62.5%)
Pediatric triage	2218 (62.4%)
100% of recommended equipment carried	2105 (59.2%)
QI process	1777 (50%)
Disaster planning	1691 (47.5%)
Immunization assessment/management	1626 (45.7%)

Several national studies have demonstrated the association between high pediatric readiness and improved outcomes for critically ill and injured children. Among children who presented to 426 EDs across 5 states, Ames and colleagues demonstrated that high pediatric readiness (wPRS >88) is associated with a 75% reduction in mortality risk for critically ill children.[35] In an evaluation of 832 trauma centers, Newgard and colleagues similarly demonstrated a 50% reduction in mortality risk among injured children seen at high pediatric-ready (wPRS >93) trauma centers.[36] Subsequently, in a cohort of 983 EDs across 11 states, Newgard and colleagues further demonstrated short- and long-term reductions in mortality among ill (76%) and injured (60%) children who presented to EDs in the highest quartile of pediatric readiness (wPRS >88).[37] This was further validated by Melhado and colleagues using data from 630 trauma centers that submit to the National Trauma Databank (wPRS ≥93).[38] Importantly, while the abovementioned studies have found a survival benefit specifically in EDs with high pediatric readiness, only 20% of EDs in the United States achieved a wPRS greater than 88 in 2021.[13]

Also of critical importance, Newgard and colleagues showed that the median time to death for children with in-hospital death was 3 hours, highlighting the importance of immediate stabilization and access to high-quality pediatric emergency care.[37] One of the primary goals behind pediatric readiness is to decrease variability in care processes with the goal of standardizing pediatric emergency care for common presentations regardless of patient demographics. Indeed, Jenkins and colleagues recently showed that high pediatric readiness is associated with a 3-fold reduction in disparities for pediatric mortality among medically ill children, most notably among the black population.[39]

The median wPRS for the United States was 55 in 2011, 68.5 in 2013, and 69.5 in 2021.[12,13] Although this overall improvement appears slow, EDs nationally demonstrated improvements in almost all key domains of pediatric readiness (ie, pediatric competencies, pediatric QI, pediatric patient safety, pediatric protocols and policies, and pediatric equipment and supplies). The overall scores reflect the strain of the

COVID-19 pandemic on the health care workforce, specifically the significant turnover and overall decrease in the presence of designated pediatric emergency care coordinators (PECCs), who are the primary drivers of pediatric readiness.[13]

PEDIATRIC EMERGENCY CARE COORDINATORS: A CRITICAL PILLAR OF PEDIATRIC READINESS

In 2006, the Institute of Medicine, now the Academy of Medicine, called for the appointment of PECCs in every ED.[26] A PECC is defined as a nurse and/or physician who serves as a pediatric champion in an administrative role to ensure that policies and procedures specific to children are in place, to coordinate QI and education, and to serve as a liaison between EDs or hospitals within a health care system to improve pediatric readiness.[29] Similar in concept to trauma stroke and ST-elevation myocardial infarction center coordinators, PECCs are charged with enacting administrative and system-level processes to ensure that their ED is ready to manage any pediatric emergency regardless of time of day or provider.

An analysis of the NPRP assessments has consistently shown that the presence of a PECC is associated with an improvement in all domains of pediatric readiness, with the most impact within the QI domain. The appointment of both a physician and a nurse PECC imparts a 16-point overall adjusted increase in pediatric readiness.[13] However, universal appointment of PECCs has been slow and impacted by large-scale stressors on the health care workforce, specifically the COVID pandemic. In 2013, 42% of EDs reported the presence of physician-nurse PECC dyads.[12] In 2021, that number decreased to 28.5%.[13] A national survey of PECCs found that 84% of PECCs have no support (eg, shift reduction, compensation) for their role, and the median time spent in the PECC role was 1 year.[40]

The continued growth and sustainability of pediatric readiness depends, in large part, on the degree to which EDs invest in PECCs. As such, there is an urgent need for a model that creates sustainability for the PECC role. Key motivators could include the provision of protected time or financial compensation and organizational commitment as demonstrated by integration of this role into the organizational chart. A job description that includes measures of impact can help attribute value to the role. Furthermore, the development of standardized training and certification and creation of collaborative shared learning networks at the regional or state level may aid in sustainability of this role. In the absence of PECCs, pediatric readiness is likely to dwindle.

QUALITY IMPROVEMENT: A KEY DRIVER OF PEDIATRIC READINESS

Perhaps one reason that pediatric readiness is not universal is lack of awareness of the quality of care provided to the pediatric population. With the majority of EDs seeing fewer than 10 pediatric patients per day, quality measures associated with high-risk, low-frequency diagnoses, such as sepsis, seem unattainable. The absence of a standardized mechanism to assess the provision of evidence-based pediatric emergency care is a critical barrier to implementing effective continuous QI in general EDs.[41–43] Although state and national registries capture global outcomes, there are no existing data repository that captures granular clinical performance metrics for children. Furthermore, low-volume EDs often lack key infrastructure including trained personnel, medical record linkage for data pulls, and automated mechanisms to visualize and track performance.[12,40] An important step toward addressing this gap is the development of nationally vetted consensus-based measures for pediatric emergency care delivery, specifically designed for low-volume EDs. Furthermore, the development of user-friendly, open access tools that allow low-resource EDs to evaluate and benchmark their performance on these metrics is a promising approach to sustain QI efforts in all ED settings.

The presence of a QI plan has been identified as one of the top 3 barriers to pediatric readiness. The 2021 NPRP assessment results demonstrate that only 50% of EDs report the presence of a QI plan and only 60% of those track pediatric-specific indicators.[13] Yet, the presence of a pediatric QI plan is one of the greatest drivers of overall pediatric readiness, imparting an average adjusted 26-point increase in the wPRS.[13] Oversight of pediatric QI efforts is one of the primary roles of a PECC. With limited pediatric quality measures and lack of resources and/or technologies to capture performance across common pediatric presentations, most emergency care provided to children remains largely unaccounted.

The National Pediatric Readiness Quality Initiative (NPRQI), funded by the Health Resources and Services Administration–EMSC Program, is an open access web-based platform that provides a mechanism for EDs to engage in pediatric Qi efforts.[33] With a real-time performance dashboard, participating EDs are able to track performance on any of 28 nationally vetted pediatric-specific quality measures focused on the most common pediatric presentations, prioritized for lower volume EDs.[44] The NPRQI provides the first window into how pediatric emergency care is provided. With integrated real-time benchmarking, it provides an opportunity to establish national standards for pediatric emergency care.

PEDIATRIC READINESS AND DISASTER PREPAREDNESS

Over the past decade, 20% of general hospitals in the United States have closed their pediatric units.[45] As a result, fewer hospitals are able to provide definitive care for common pediatric conditions, resulting in an increasing number of children being transferred to tertiary children's hospitals for definitive care.[46–48] This pattern of reliance on children's hospitals for basic pediatric care has rendered us vulnerable to critical shortages of pediatric capacity, workforce, and resources during surge events such as the "Triple-demic" of respiratory viral infections in 2022.[49,50] In the context of this inadequate national pediatric infrastructure, it is imperative that sites develop strategies to safely care for children in surge or disaster scenarios.

The NPRP recommends that all EDs develop an all-hazards disaster preparedness plan which addresses the pediatric issues detailed in **Box 2**. However, only 47.5% of US EDs have written disaster policies that specifically addressed children.[13] Surge or disaster events are also likely to worsen disparities associated with access to pediatric-ready EDs. To ensure the available resources are used judiciously to provide the greatest good for the greatest number of children, the standardized interfacility transfer guidelines should be developed and adopted regionally.

PEDIATRIC READINESS AND REGULATIONS

One of the national EMSC program performance measures is the development of statewide, territorial, or regional programs to formally recognize hospitals that can stabilize and/or manage pediatric emergencies. Currently, 18 states have developed a system for voluntary pediatric readiness recognition that includes site verification. Hospitals that have received pediatric readiness recognition have on average a 22-point higher wPRS compared to those without recognition.[51] States that have recognition programs also had a 10-point higher wPRS compared to states without such programs.[51] However, verification programs are currently voluntary and have limited reach. Only 8% of all EDs in the United States are verified as pediatric ready.[51] For the long-term sustainability of pediatric readiness initiatives, it is crucial that

---

Box 2
Essential pediatric components of disaster preparedness plans

Availability of medications, vaccines, equipment, supplies, appropriately trained providers for children in disasters

Pediatric surge capacity for injured and noninjured children

Decontamination, isolation, and quarantine of families and children of all ages

Minimization of parent–child separation and improved methods for reuniting separated children and their families

Access to specific medical and behavioral health therapies and social services for children

All disaster drills include pediatric patients; Drills that include a pediatric mass casualty incident at least once every 2 years

Care of children with special health care needs including developmental disabilities

---

verification is built into statewide or national infrastructure as a required competency for all hospitals.

Promisingly, in 2021, the American College of Surgeons (ACS) released new verification standards that require the pediatric readiness assessment to be completed by all ACS-verified trauma centers.[52] Many state trauma system verification programs are also following in situ. The implications of these new standards are potentially broad, given that 45% of all hospitals are trauma centers.

PEDIATRIC READINESS ACROSS THE CONTINUUM OF CARE

While the importance of pediatric readiness in EDs cannot be overstated, the ED is but one step along the continuum of care. For approximately 4 million children annually, the journey begins with a 9-1-1 call to emergency medical dispatch followed by an emergency medical services (EMSs) response and transport. Yet, dispatch systems and EMS agencies often experience even greater demands and resource constraints than exist in the ED setting with many agencies dependent on grants to provide continual funding.[53] The impact of prehospital care on pediatric outcomes is not well described in the medical literature, however, there is evidence of significant variability in pediatric prehospital care and outcomes compared to adults as well as limited evidence-based guidelines to support standardized clinical practice.[54–59]

Moreover, the treatment of emergencies does not end in the ED. Over 5 million children are hospitalized every year with over 80% bypassing the ED altogether. Over the last decade, over 20% of hospitals have closed their pediatric inpatient units.[45] Given the limited inpatient capacity for children, some 1737 (49%) hospitals admit children to adult inpatient units highlighting the importance of pediatric readiness beyond the ED setting.[13]

SUMMARY

Pediatric readiness is a system issue, not a workforce issue. The readiness of our emergency care system to meet the needs of children remains uneven. Yet, pediatric readiness saves lives. Pediatric readiness is achievable for all EDs but there must be a commitment to sustainability of these efforts through the identification and support of PECCs. The degree to which we elevate the PECC workforce and implement regulations that formally require compliance with pediatric readiness is the degree to which we will transform our emergency care system. Until then, families and pediatricians play a critical role in advocating for pediatric readiness in their local EDs and demanding greater transparency to help navigate our complex health care system.

As a nation, our emergency care system cannot claim high-quality, best-in-class pediatric emergency care without data to provide measurable proof. Furthermore, as "tripledemics," pandemics, floods, and man-made disasters continue to threaten our children's health and well-being, the ability to coordinate emergency care services depends on our understanding of regional capacity and capabilities. Continuous QI is the key to an accountable emergency care system. Future efforts will no doubt show that the impact of pediatric readiness on disparities in outcomes is likely far greater and less costly than imagined.

CLINICS CARE POINTS

- Pediatric readiness of emergency departments is associated with increased survival among critically ill and injured children.
- The appointment of a Pediatric Emergency Care Coordinator (PECC) in the single most important factor in driving and maintaining pediatric readiness.
- In the absence of continuous pediatric quality improvement efforts, our emergency care system cannot ensure high quality care for children.
- Pediatric readiness is a roadmap to overcoming disparities and increasing the resiliency of our emergency care system.

DISCLOSURE

The Authors have nothing to disclose.

FUNDING

The EMSC Innovation and Improvement Center (U07MC37471) is supported by the Health Resources and Services Administration (HRSA) of the U.S. Department of Health and Human Services (HHS). The contents are those of the author(s) and do not necessarily represent the official views of, nor an endorsement by, HRSA, HHS or the U.S. government.

REFERENCES

1. Martin AB, Hartman M, Benson J, et al. National Health Expenditure Accounts Team. National health care spending in 2021: decline in federal spending outweighs greater use of health care. Health Aff 2023;42(1):6–17.
2. Whitfill T, Auerbach M, Scherzer DJ, et al. Emergency care for children in the United States: epidemiology and trends over time. J Emerg Med 2018;55(3):423–34.
3. McDermott KW, Stocks C, Freeman WJ. Overview of pediatric emergency department visits, 2015. Healthcare Cost and Utilization Project (HCUP) Statistical Briefs. Agency for Healthcare Research and Quality (US). 2006. Available at: https://www.ncbi.nlm.nih.gov/books/NBK526418/. [Accessed 7 December 2023].
4. Zive DM, Schmicker R, Daya M, et al. Survival and variability over time from out of hospital cardiac arrest across large geographically diverse communities participating in the Resuscitation Outcomes Consortium. Resuscitation 2018;131:74–82.
5. Kanzaria HK, Probst MA, Hsia RY. Emergency department death rates dropped by nearly 50 percent, 1997-2011. Health Aff 2016;35(7):1303–8.

6. MacKenzie EJ, Rivara FP, Jurkovich GJ, et al. A national evaluation of the effect of trauma-center care on mortality. N Engl J Med 2006;354(4):366–78.

7. Celso B, Tepas J, Langland-Orban B, et al. A systematic review and meta-analysis comparing outcome of severely injured patients treated in trauma centers following the establishment of trauma systems. J Trauma 2006;60(2):371–8 [discussion 378].

8. Nirula R, Brasel K. Do trauma centers improve functional outcomes: a national trauma databank analysis? J Trauma 2006;61(2):268–71.

9. Heidenreich PA, Zhao X, Hernandez AF, et al. Impact of an expanded hospital recognition program for stroke quality of care. J Am Heart Assoc 2017;6(1). https://doi.org/10.1161/jaha.116.004278.

10. Friese CR, Xia R, Ghaferi A, et al. Hospitals In 'magnet' program show better patient outcomes on mortality measures compared to non-'magnet' hospitals. Health Aff (Millwood) 2015;34(6):986–92.

11. Woolf SH, Wolf ER, Rivara FP. The new crisis of increasing all-cause mortality in US children and adolescents. JAMA 2023;329(12):975–6.

12. Gausche-Hill M, Ely M, Schmuhl P, et al. A national assessment of pediatric readiness of emergency departments. JAMA Pediatr 2015;169(6):527–34.

13. Remick KE, Hewes HA, Ely M, et al. National assessment of pediatric readiness of US emergency departments during the COVID-19 pandemic. JAMA Netw Open 2023;6(7):e2321707.

14. Weiss AJ, Liang L, Martin K. Overview of hospital stays among children and adolescents, 2019. HCUP Statistical Brief #299. 2022. Agency for Healthcare Research and Quality, Rockville, MD. Available at: www.hcup-us.ahrq.gov/reports/statbriefs/sb299-Hospital-Stays-Children-2019.pdf. [Accessed 7 December 2023].

15. Goldstick JE, Cunningham RM, Carter PM. Current causes of death in children and adolescents in the United States. N Engl J Med 2022;386(20):1955–6. https://doi.org/10.1056/NEJMc2201761.

16. Notrica DM, Weiss J, Garcia-Filion P, et al. Pediatric trauma centers: correlation of ACS-verified trauma centers with CDC statewide pediatric mortality rates. J Trauma Acute Care Surg 2012;73(3):566–70 [discussion: 570-2].

17. Potoka DA, Schall LC, Gardner MJ, et al. Impact of pediatric trauma centers on mortality in a statewide system. J Trauma 2000;49(2):237–45.

18. Potoka DA, Schall LC, Ford HR. Improved functional outcome for severely injured children treated at pediatric trauma centers. J Trauma 2001;51(5):824–32 [discussion 832-4].

19. Hall JR, Reyes HM, Meller JL, et al. The outcome for children with blunt trauma is best at a pediatric trauma center. J Pediatr Surg 1996;31(1):72–6 [discussion 76-7].

20. Dreyfus J, Flood A, Cutler G, et al. Comparison of pediatric motor vehicle collision injury outcomes at Level I trauma centers. J Pediatr Surg 2016;51(10):1693–9.

21. Webman RB, Carter EA, Mittal S, et al. Association between trauma center type and mortality among injured adolescent patients. JAMA Pediatr 2016;170(8):780–6.

22. Sathya C, Alali AS, Wales PW, et al. Mortality among injured children treated at different trauma center types. JAMA Surg 2015;150(9):874–81.

23. Ray KN, Olson LM, Edgerton EA, et al. Access to high pediatric-readiness emergency care in the United States. J Pediatr 2018;194:225-32.e1.

24. United States Government Accountability Office. Report to Congressional Requesters. Pediatric Trauma Centers: Availability, Outcomes, and Federal Support

Related to Pediatric Trauma Care. 2017. Available at: https://www.gao.gov/products/gao-17-334. [Accessed 7 December 2023].

25. Weinberg JA, Medearis DN. Emergency medical services for children: the report from the Institute of Medicine. Pediatrics 1994;93(5):821–3.

26. Institute of Medicine. Emergency care for children: growing pains. Washington, DC: National Academies Press; 2007. https://doi.org/10.17226/11655.

27. Health Resources and Services Administration: Maternal and Child Health Bureau. Emergency Medical Services For Children (EMSC). Available at: https://mchb.hrsa.gov/programs-impact/emergency-medical-services-children-emsc. [Accessed 7 December 2023].

28. EMSC Innovation and Improvement Center. National Pediatric Readiness Project. Available at: https://emscimprovement.center/domains/pediatric-readiness-project/. Accessed August 16, 2023.

29. Remick K, Gausche-Hill M, Joseph MM, et al. Pediatric readiness in the emergency department. Pediatrics 2018;142(5). https://doi.org/10.1542/peds.2018-2459.

30. National Pediatric Readiness Project. The National Pediatric Readiness Project: 2021 assessment. University of Utah. Available at: https://www.pedsready.org/. [Accessed 15 June 2023].

31. Innovation EMSC, Improvement Center. Pediatric Readiness Checklist and Toolkit. Available at: https://emscimprovement.center/domains/pediatric-readiness-project/readiness-toolkit/. [Accessed 7 December 2023].

32. Innovation EMSC, Improvement Center. Quality Improvement Collaboratives. Available at: https://emscimprovement.center/collaboratives/. [Accessed 7 December 2023].

33. National Pediatric Readiness Quality Initiative. The National Pediatric Readiness Quality Initiative. University of Texas at Austin. Available at: https://sites.utexas.edu/nprqi/. [Accessed 15 August 2023].

34. EMSC Innovation and Improvement Center. Pediatric Readiness Recognition Programs. Available at: https://emscimprovement.center/domains/recognition-programs. [Accessed 7 December 2023].

35. Ames SG, Davis BS, Marin JR, et al. Emergency department pediatric readiness and mortality in critically ill children. Pediatrics 2019;144(3). https://doi.org/10.1542/peds.2019-0568.

36. Newgard CD, Lin A, Olson LM, et al. Evaluation of emergency department pediatric readiness and outcomes among US trauma centers. JAMA Pediatr 2021;175(9):947–56.

37. Newgard CD, Lin A, Malveau S, et al. Emergency department pediatric readiness and short-term and long-term mortality among children receiving emergency care. JAMA Netw Open 2023;6(1):e2250941.

38. Melhado C, Remick K, Miskovic A, et al. The association between pediatric readiness and mortality for injured children treated at US trauma centers. Ann Surg 2023. https://doi.org/10.1097/sla.0000000000006126.

39. Jenkins PC, Lin A, Ames SG, et al. Emergency department pediatric readiness and disparities in mortality based on race and ethnicity. JAMA Netw Open 2023;6(9):e2332160.

40. Foster AA, Li J, Wilkinson MH, et al. Pediatric emergency care coordinator workforce: a survey study. J Am Coll Emerg Physicians Open 2023;4(4):e13006.

41. Marin JR, Weaver MD, Barnato AE, et al. Variation in emergency department head computed tomography use for pediatric head trauma. Acad Emerg Med 2014;21(9):987–95.

42. Puffenbarger MS, Ahmad FA, Argent M, et al. Reduction of computed tomography use for pediatric closed head injury evaluation at a nonpediatric community emergency department. Acad Emerg Med 2019;26(7):784–95.
43. Sheehan B, Nigrovic LE, Dayan PS, et al. Informing the design of clinical decision support services for evaluation of children with minor blunt head trauma in the emergency department: a sociotechnical analysis. J Biomed Inform 2013;46(5): 905–13.
44. Remick KE, Bartley KA, Gonzales L, et al. Consensus-driven model to establish paediatric emergency care measures for low-volume emergency departments. BMJ Open Qual 2022;11(3).
45. Cushing AM, Bucholz EM, Chien AT, et al. Availability of pediatric inpatient services in the United States. Pediatrics 2021;148(1).
46. Hamline MY, Rosenthal JL. Interfacility transfers: a process ridden with improvement opportunities. Hosp Pediatr 2020;10(2):195–7.
47. França UL, McManus ML. Availability of definitive hospital care for children. JAMA Pediatr 2017;171(9):e171096.
48. França UL, McManus ML. Trends in regionalization of hospital care for common pediatric conditions. Pediatrics 2018;141(1).
49. Innovation EMSC, Improvement Center. The Pediatric Surge Crisis Response. Available at: https://emscimprovement.center/domains/preparedness/active/surge/. [Accessed 3 March 2023].
50. Wells K. A surge in sick children exposed a need for major changes to U.S. hospitals. National Public Radio. npr.org 2023.
51. Whitfill TM, Remick KE, Olson LM, et al. Statewide pediatric facility recognition programs and their association with pediatric readiness in emergency departments in the United States. J Pediatr 2020;218:210–6.e2.
52. American College of Surgeons Committee on Trauma. Resources for optimal care of the injured patient (2022 standards). American College of Surgeons, Chicago, IL 60611-3295. Available at: https://www.facs.org/quality-programs/trauma/quality/verification-review-and-consultation-program/standards/. [Accessed 7 December 2023].
53. National Highway Traffic Safety Agency. Federal 911 Funding. Available at: https://www.911.gov/projects/federal-funding/. [Accessed 7 December 2023].
54. Brandler ES, Sharma M, Sinert RH, et al. Prehospital stroke scales in urban environments: a systematic review. Neurology 2014;82(24):2241–9.
55. Brooks SC, Schmicker RH, Cheskes S, et al. Variability in the initiation of resuscitation attempts by emergency medical services personnel during out-of-hospital cardiac arrest. Resuscitation 2017;117:102–8.
56. Dimitrov N, Koenig W, Bosson N, et al. Variability in criteria for emergency medical services routing of acute stroke patients to designated stroke center hospitals. West J Emerg Med 2015;16(5):743–6.
57. Govindarajan P, Lin L, Landman A, et al. Practice variability among the EMS systems participating in Cardiac Arrest Registry to Enhance Survival (CARES). Resuscitation 2012;83(1):76–80.
58. Rostykus P, Kennel J, Adair K, et al. Variability in the treatment of prehospital hypoglycemia: a structured review of EMS protocols in the United States. Prehosp Emerg Care 2016;20(4):524–30.
59. Hewes HA, Dai M, Mann NC, et al. Prehospital pain management: disparity by age and race. Prehosp Emerg Care 2018;22(2):189–97.

The Role of Clinic Preparedness to Support Patients and Strengthen the Medical System During and After a Pandemic

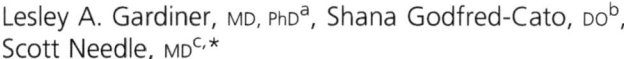

Lesley A. Gardiner, MD, PhD[a], Shana Godfred-Cato, DO[b],
Scott Needle, MD[c],*

KEYWORDS

- Pediatric pandemic preparedness • Clinic preparedness
- Pediatric disaster response

KEY POINTS

- Improving pediatric preparedness in clinics before a pandemic will improve the health of children during and after a pandemic.
- Pediatric clinics can provide much needed general pediatric care in a public health crisis to relieve the influx of patients to hospitals.
- Families of children and youth with special health care needs can benefit from specific attention before and during pandemics.
- Pediatric practices, public health, and other health care institutions can establish trusted relationships to best promote the health of children in a pandemic or disaster.

INTRODUCTION

Pediatric medical practice preparedness is necessary for all clinics. Pediatric clinics provide the bulk of health care for children across the nation and when that care is disrupted a large number of children may go without access to medical care. An essential service that pediatricians and pediatric practices can provide during a pandemic to lessen the strain on hospitals and critical care facilities is to continue to provide patient

[a] Department of Primary Care & Clinical Medicine, Sam Houston State University - College of Osteopathic Medicine, 925 City Central Avenue, Conroe, TX 77304, USA; [b] Division of Pediatric Emergency Medicine, Department of Pediatrics, Spencer Fox Eccles School of Medicine at the University of Utah, 50 North Medical Drive, Salt Lake City, UT 84132, USA; [c] Woodland Clinic Medical Group, 1207 Fairchild Court, Woodland, CA 95695, USA
* Corresponding author.
E-mail address: scott.needle@commonspirit.org

Pediatr Clin N Am 71 (2024) 383–394
https://doi.org/10.1016/j.pcl.2024.01.012
0031-3955/24/© 2024 Elsevier Inc. All rights reserved.

care. Pediatric practices will likely need to temporarily adjust their practice structure in order to best care for patients. Pediatric medical practices must not only be ready for natural disasters and man-made events but also infectious disease pandemics. Burkle and colleagues note that during a pandemic, not only will "practice as usual...temporarily cease", but "providers must look beyond their normal practice settings and become integrated within the community"; continuing to care for patients with thoughtful adjustments to practice and coordinating with community entities can decrease disease transmission and the burden on hospitals.[1]

Pediatric community practices can provide a vital role of caring for less severe patients, managing chronic conditions, and supporting and educating family members on how to care for noncritical patients at home. Prior public health events have shown that a large number of noncritical patients will pursue medical care predominately with the help of nearby family and friends; capable caregivers in the home are ideal for noncritical patient care, especially with the guidance of their primary care physician, as this prevents spread of disease and reduces unnecessarily taxing hospitals.[2]

Families of children and youth with special health care needs (CYSHCN) should be particularly prepared for disasters, including pandemics, to ensure they maintain their health during crisis. Pediatricians can assist with preparedness by helping families have all of their child's medical information in one place for easy access. If families need to access care at a new location, having their children's information on hand can be invaluable. Pediatricians can help families have extra medications and supplies on hand whenever possible, therefore decreasing their need to access care in a hospital setting which could increase their risk of exposure to infectious agents.

To fully care for children in the community, medical practices must be prepared to ensure operations can continue during or after a disaster. The lack of office preparedness can lead to operational disruption, financial loss, clinician and staff stress, patient distress, decrease in health, and increased burden on other health care settings. Prior research has shown that a large number of practices are suboptimally prepared for disasters and pandemic events.[3] The lack of time, limited financial resources, competing priorities, and lack of urgency have been suggested as some reasons for inadequate preparedness.[4] Fortunately for clinicians, resources have been developed to guide office preparedness.[5] Most resources address all-hazard preparedness, though there are some planning considerations unique to pandemics.[6,7]

MEDICAL OFFICE PREPAREDNESS

Clinics need to be prepared with a plan for disasters to improve continuity of operations during and after a disaster. A single definitive planning guide for disasters and pandemics does not exist, yet many resources share commonalities, such as the need for a written response plan, staff involvement and training, emergency supplies and equipment, and relationships with public health and other health care entities.[5,8] Continuity of operations planning involves anticipating and minimizing interruptions and disruptions of normal clinical operations and business sustainability. Planning considerations of particular importance to pediatrics include vaccine preservation, providing medical care for children with chronic conditions, communication of anticipatory guidance with families, coordination with schools and child care facilities, and addressing behavioral health concerns.

Pandemic planning generally emphasizes anticipating a surge of sick and concerned families. Visits of lower acuity, which are not time-sensitive, such as well-child visits that do not include vaccination, may be deferred. Determining which visits to safely defer can be challenging, especially when the duration or magnitude of surge cannot be anticipated. Postponement of well visits for infants in response to COVID-19, for instance, led to a decline in immunization rates, placing young children at increased risk for infectious disease.[9] Ensuring patients with chronic medical conditions are able to receive medications and other treatments in a timely manner can reduce the risk of an influx of patients to the hospital.[10] During a pandemic, infection control may further affect prioritization of visits, as well as how certain visits are conducted.

The technological, regulatory, and payment changes for telehealth and virtual visits during the COVID-19 pandemic led to an unprecedented expansion in utilization of this modality, enabling the ability to provide care without requiring an in-office visit.[11] Telehealth, however, is not a panacea for addressing clinical surge. Certain clinical conditions remain better evaluated in-person, due to telehealth's inherent limitations in physical examination and point-of-care testing. Inequitable access to broadband connectivity or private areas to conduct visits may be a barrier for some families, especially in rural or underserved communities. As the COVID-19 pandemic evolved, utilization of telehealth decreased, likely from relaxation of strict isolation precautions, improved infection control capacity in the office setting, family preference, and changes in reimbursement and state policies.[12] Telehealth should be seen as a useful measure to help address surge in a pandemic and provide infection control. Its optimal role has yet to be determined and will likely vary depending on the disaster or infectious disease outbreak, patient population, specific patient illness, technological advancements, contemporaneous regulatory framework, and local broadband infrastructure and connectivity. Other potential tools for reducing surge include telephone triage, telephone care, and Internet or smart phone-based triage applications.

Medical Office Preparedness: Infectious Disease

During an outbreak, families that need to be seen in the office may be able to utilize alternative visit accommodations to decrease the risk of infectious disease spread to and from staff as well as other patients. Consideration should be given to segregating acutely ill patients from those receiving well care or treatment for a noninfectious condition, whether by different areas within an office, different office locations, or designated appointment times through the day. One consideration for a practice with a team of providers would be to rotate who is seeing infectious patients in blocks. For example, providers could divide the care of infectious patients versus noninfectious patients over a 2 to 4 week span. This might lessen the likelihood that multiple physicians would be unable to practice due to illness or the need to isolate after exposure to illness. During the severe acute respiratory syndrome (SARS) outbreaks in Canada, in a period of days, approximately half of Toronto's emergency medical services (EMS) were exposed to the disease, resulting in the need to quarantine, and hindering the effectiveness of the EMS.[13] To mitigate this negative impact, Bielajs and colleagues suggested a model with a dedicated pandemic crew with a dedicated EMS "flu vehicle" for patients with a possible pandemic illness or exposure (vs an ordinary crew and normal EMS vehicle).[13]

For patients seen in the office, disinfection procedures should already be established for everyday infectious exposures, delineated by mode of transmission (eg, droplet vs airborne). Similarly, practices should already have small stores of personal protective equipment (PPE), including masks and respirators, gloves, eye and face protection, and gowns. Limited storage space and reluctance to commit capital to inventory of limited utility outside of a pandemic may preclude maintenance of larger stockpiles. In the early weeks of the COVID-19 pandemic, practices and hospitals alike quickly exhausted their PPE supplies, and vendors were overwhelmed and unable to ensure restocking.[14] State and federal stockpiles became vital for procuring new PPE. Clinicians with preexisting connections to local public health and health care coalitions benefited from familiarity with key coordinators and ordering systems.

Pediatricians in primary care are a trusted voice to patients and families and their guidance can help educate not only their patients but the general public on appropriate infection prevention and control measures during a pandemic. Disease containment strategies that are communicated timely, accurately, consistently, and frequently can potentially reduce transmission of the disease.[15]

Medical Office Preparedness: Vaccines

Just as pediatric primary care is where most of the children receive health care, pediatric offices provide the majority of vaccines for children. Pediatric practices should expect to be at the forefront of efforts to immunize children against any novel pathogen. Families trust their pediatricians for accurate information and the ability to comfortably and competently serve children. Not only does this trust yield parental comfort in having children receive vaccines in the pediatric office but it also has been associated with increased confidence in receiving vaccines in general.[16]

The medical home is well-versed in the logistics of immunization, particularly for children. Pediatric offices already should be thoroughly familiar with the best practices as outlined in the Centers for Disease Control and Prevention's Vaccine Storage and Handling Toolkit.[17] Most pediatric practices participate in the Vaccines for Children program, which provides a natural framework and connection for primary care pediatric practices to engage in community-wide immunization. The logistics regarding distribution of COVID-19 vaccines illustrate the importance of robust, trusted relationships between pediatric primary care practices and public health. During the COVID-19 pandemic, preexisting relationships between public health and pediatric practices aided with offices' initial ordering and procurement of COVID-19 vaccines and improved community-wide planning of vaccine distribution.[18]

Medical Office Preparedness: Communication

Pediatric practices should have established methods of communication with patients and staff and notify them of their communication plan before a disaster. It is important to discuss with families how they should expect to receive information in the event of a disaster, as stress and anxiety in a crisis can result in worried well persons seeking care at hospitals, overburdening the hospital system and resulting in unnecessary exposure to those who are infectious.[19] In addition, patients unnecessarily seeking care at emergency departments due to poor communication result in ineffective use of precious and scarce resources. Therefore, as soon as possible after a disaster or pandemic onset, clinics should update patients on changes in practice operations, including hours of operation and location. Practices can also relay health advice and anticipatory guidance to families.[20] Practice Web sites, social media, text message campaigns, automated phone calls, or secured emails are some ways families can receive updates. In addition, creation of a dedicated call center or triage line to field questions from concerned patients and families may prevent potential unnecessary visits, exposures, and transmission. The pediatric practice could establish partnerships with other groups as a way to pool resources and provide the service of a pediatric call center in the event of a medical emergency. During the SARS outbreak, a toll-free telephone helpline in Ontario, Canada, gave families valuable information and relieved the burden on hospitals by triaging concerns.[21] Not only is the opportunity to educate the public through such a system key in preventing transmission and unnecessary health care visits but also data from calls could also be used to help with surveillance efforts.[22]

The communication capacity of pediatricians and pediatric practices should be established long before the pandemic or public health emergency. The ability of pediatricians and pediatric practices to lay the framework of respect, trust, communication, and education with patients and their families, as well as community players can help decrease the burden on limited personnel and medical resources during the actual public health emergency event. Incorporating and emphasizing education regarding ways of preventing the spread of illness as part of routine visits, hand hygiene, respiratory etiquette, and appropriate time durations for quarantine or isolation can create the groundwork education required to reduce the spread of illness during a pandemic.[20] Children play a key role in the spread of illnesses such as influenza; focusing educational and risk communications early in the course of the pandemic on nonexposed but susceptible populations can decrease transmission, leading to the control of infectious spread.[15,23] Efforts to reduce the transmission of disease protect limited critical care resources that are already near capacity in non-pandemic times, increasing the likelihood that children who are truly in need of critical care will be able to access it.[1]

A key to optimizing communication is acknowledging the diverse sources that patients and families will interface with during a public health emergency and then building relationships between trusted community players and pediatricians before the event to allow for unified and consistent messaging, as well as increasing the presence of community pediatricians as a resource.[24] Patients and families interact with schools, daycare centers, colleges, universities, community, and faith-based organizations on a daily basis. Therefore, pediatricians should work to build relationships with these entities before a public health emergency to allow for established lines of communication during an event. This helps to ensure that accurate and timely information is being communicated to the public.[25,26] According to Burkle and colleagues, "pediatric professionals must be focused on both population-based and individual care when a pandemic occurs and serve a vital role as subject-matter experts and advocates."[1] Community health care preparedness coalitions are an ideal entry point for pediatric engagement with public health and broader community preparedness efforts. Health care coalitions are "partnerships among public health agencies, hospitals, EMS, emergency management agencies, and other entities to prepare for and respond to emergencies in their jurisdiction."[27] The goal of these coalitions is to ensure that all members have what is required to appropriately address emergencies, which requires coordination and planning. Participation of pediatric practices in health care coalitions can add depth and strength to pediatric disaster care efforts that have traditionally focused on hospitals.[27]

For pediatricians, these relationships can enable receipt of timely information, resources, and potential advocacy for the needs of both children and medical practices. Public health and health care coalitions in turn gain access to trusted messengers of information to families, front-line deliverers of health care, and subject matter experts in the well-being of children. Relationships can be initiated by either pediatric practices or public health; what matters is not who makes first contact, but rather that trust and mutual appreciation are established in advance of a crisis.

FAMILY PREPAREDNESS

A way that clinics and office practices can help prepare for disasters, including pandemics, is helping families understand how to be prepared. At the beginning of pandemics, movement may be limited by mandates or fear of infection, so families are often reliant on the supplies currently in their home. Ensuring that families are prepared with food, water, and medication for a few days can be immensely helpful in keeping families safe at home. Families can start by building an emergency kit, including food, water, medication, first aid supplies, blankets, and other items to keep families hydrated, warm, and fed while awaiting the crisis to subside.[28]

Children who have chronic medical conditions may require additional planning, to ensure that they can maintain their health during and after a pandemic. The CYSHCN may be cared for at home if adequate supplies, resources, and trained caregivers are available during a pandemic. Reliance on the emergency department should be discouraged for care that can be provided elsewhere in order to reduce the risk of exposure to infectious agents. Pediatricians should encourage these families to pre-stock supplies and medications in case of disaster or shortages while being cognizant that insurance and policies may limit the ability for "extra" stockpiling above regular use. If families lack an adequate supply of medication, formula, and other medical supplies, the pediatric clinics should be prepared to help them obtain supplies or know where to refer them. For example, establishing relationships with local food banks, formula companies, pharmaceutical companies, and shelters can facilitate patients and families getting needed, valuable resources during a pandemic. Families with CYSHCN should also be encouraged to have a completed emergency information form (EIF) that contains important medical history, a complete medication list, names of specialists, baseline imaging results, vaccinations, and other important information.[29] It is helpful to have a printed copy of the form in the home and at school for times when electronic access is not available.

Much of a child's life is spent in school or childcare, and therefore, ensuring preparedness for the child includes planning for these settings. Primary care clinicians are encouraged to be aware of school or childcare response plans and should encourage families to be aware of these plans as well. CYSHCN should have individualized care plans created by a care team, including medical professionals, schools, therapists, and the family.[30] Pediatricians can also provide general anticipatory guidance to schools and childcare facilities as subject matter experts in the health and well-being of children. Schools and pediatricians can partner to effectively plan for infection control, anticipatory guidance for families, and meeting children's educational and other needs if the school environment is disrupted.

MENTAL HEALTH CARE

A pandemic will likely create widespread stress, disruption, suffering, and loss. Families may require brief counseling, more in-depth evaluation, management of exacerbated preexisting conditions, and potentially referrals to additional community resources. Pediatric practices can build on their familiarity with addressing developmental, behavioral, and mental health concerns of children on an everyday basis. In addition to providing care in response to patient concerns, practices should consider how to proactively give anticipatory guidance on behavioral health best practices while universally monitoring and screening families for increased levels of distress.[31] Pediatricians may also consider special monitoring or outreach for children already being treated for mental health conditions such as depression, anxiety, or attention-deficit hyperactivity disorder.

Disruptions in the daily schedule and interruption of in-person instruction for children and adolescents can be extremely upsetting, especially for those with preexisting medical or behavioral health conditions. Teenagers thrive on interactions with peers and losing that interaction can cause significant mental health issues, which may lead to inappropriate coping mechanisms if healthy ones are not previously established, such as excessive time on electronics or use of drugs and alcohol. Rates of mental health illness and use of mental health care increased during the COVID-19 pandemic.[32] Screening children and adolescents for depression, substance use, and other behavioral concerns should be completed at every well-child visit; however, during major community stressors, including pandemics and other disasters, additional screenings and monitoring should be considered.

Pediatric practices can consider collaborating with schools or childcare centers to focus on children's mental health. Jointly developed messaging and promotion of health habits can increase the trust and consistency of community efforts. Pediatricians and schools can also develop streamlined communication and referral procedures, using each other's expertise and touchpoints with children.

ADDITIONAL OPERATIONAL CONSIDERATIONS

During a pandemic, staff themselves are likely to become acutely ill, need to care for ill family members, or fall under isolation or quarantine. For various reasons that will not be detailed here, the COVID-19 pandemic also led to broader and longer term staffing shortages. As a result, practices should plan for disruptions in usual staffing levels. Staff should be cross-trained, when possible, in order to adapt to different or multiple roles. Modifications and flexibility in duties, hours, or requirements to work in-person may help retain staff. Practices should have contingency plans for times when there is simply not enough staff for usual operations.

Communication is just as important with staff as with patients: staff need to efficiently inform the practice if they will be unable to work, whereas practices need the ability to quickly inform staff of any changes in assignments or operating procedures. Practice email, messenger or chat apps, text messages, centralized Web sites, and phone trees are some options for reaching staff.

Pediatric practices should anticipate staff experiencing the same challenges as the general public such as becoming ill, caring for family members and watching others around them suffer while additionally needing to attend to their roles as health care professionals. Clinicians should consider how to humanely promote staff resilience while remembering not to neglect their own self-care. Ideally, practices can proactively support their staff by offering flexibility, adequate time off, supportive social interactions with colleagues, access to mental health professionals, and encouragement of healthy coping strategies.

Disasters will likely create financial challenges and losses for pediatric practices; the COVID-19 pandemic proved to be no exception, starting with increased labor costs. Supply chain disruptions and shortages increased the cost of supplies. A decrease in patient encounters, whether due to public health mandates, practice-initiated changes to operations, or patient fears of infection, contributed to loss of revenue. Although the federal government authorized COVID-19-related funding to offset some losses, such measures cannot necessarily be anticipated or relied on in future pandemics. Practices need to consider options for financial stability, such as patient outreach campaigns and introducing or promoting services that do not require an in-office visit and provide convenience to families; for example, telehealth and remote patient monitoring. In addition, a surge in families seeking care may represent an opportunity for prepared practices that are able to maximize their capacity to meet the demand.

FUTURE DIRECTIONS

There are many ways that clinicians, health care systems, and policymakers can improve pandemic planning and response. Pediatric clinics affiliated with a children's hospital or large health system may have robust resources available to them, such as an increased budget, and access to alternative sites of care if their facility is not operable. Smaller community practices that care for children may not have the resources that larger practices or systems do. Improving collaboration between independent practices, larger health care entities, health care coalitions, and public health before a pandemic can improve the community response for children and families by improving coordination of care.

COVID-19 laid bare the role of health inequity, particularly in minority and underserved populations, leading to disparate morbidity and mortality. Challenges of access, such as from underinsurance or lack of insurance, transportation, or housing, require special attention and outreach. Telehealth has the potential to improve access to health care for underserved populations, yet challenges in broadband connectivity and computer or smartphone availability can also lead to worsening of disparities compared with families of higher socioeconomic status. Minority populations may require special outreach and prioritization to mitigate preexisting inequities, including linguistically and culturally appropriate communication, targeted education campaigns, and enhanced access to services, medications, or vaccines. Direct engagement with marginalized communities is essential to understand needs, appreciate cultural impacts on care, and establish trust. The reduction of disparities through improved everyday management of chronic conditions, such as asthma or diabetes, has the potential to improve both individual and community outcomes during an infectious disease outbreak.[33]

Technology has already changed the delivery of health care in a pandemic, yet its potential is still nascent. Internet-connected "smart" monitors could enhance remote care of children with special health care needs, including monitoring of vital signs or other physiologic or biochemical indicators. "Hospital at home" is now a consideration for patients who might previously have required admission to an inpatient facility. Bluetooth devices, smartphone apps or attachments, or smart watches could drastically enhance the utility of telehealth visits through collection of data or observations currently limited to in-person visits. Artificial intelligence could improve triage algorithms, including allowing patients to access care applications directly, reducing the telephone burden on clinic staff.

The implementation of electronic health records (EHRs) has improved access to health care records from off-site locations. Information sharing between EHRs, such as through interconnected platforms or Health Information Exchanges, has allowed for an even wider accessibility of medical records. The completion of the EIF can be automated through EHRs.[29] Continuing to improve technologic access to medical records as children and families move during disasters would improve care, including bidirectional communication through patient portals. Improved automation of clinical reporting and data mining can improve public health surveillance, reporting, investigation, and intervention.

State, federal, and private payor policies should address challenges with effectively preparing for pandemics and other disasters. Medicaid and private payors should ensure that families have easy access to medication refills and increased amounts of chronic medications and supplies on hand before and during pandemics and other disasters, when access to health care may be challenged. Community, state, and federal stockpiles should be stocked, maintained, and funded accordingly and should include supplies and formulations that meet pediatric needs. Supply chain disruptions need to be addressed from the national level, particularly for medications and supplies of life-saving importance and from a single source. Preparedness that explicitly addresses the unique needs of children must continue to be emphasized and required at community, state, and federal levels.[34]

Finally, though the evidence supporting and assisting clinics in developing an all-hazards plan is increasing, there is a paucity of evidence-based data on ways that pediatric practices can be most effectively prepared for pandemics or other disasters. Research linking community health outcomes to clinic preparedness efforts and specific components of preparedness planning would improve practices' ability to prudently invest and prioritize precious time, money, and other resources.

SUMMARY

Much of the literature has focused on ways for hospitals to manage surge independently; however, one powerful resource that can help mitigate surge is that of the pediatrician in primary practice. Burkle and colleagues warns, "if primary care suffers, the consequences will be immediately felt at critical care levels."[1] Community pediatric practices should be considered essential care sites during a pandemic. This requires pediatricians and primary care practices to take a vital role in planning before the event and a leadership role in coordination with the community. In a letter to members of the American Academy of Pediatrics (AAP) in September 2009, regarding the H1N1 influenza pandemic, the AAP President David T. Tayloe, Jr recommended, "at the local level, pediatricians must become leaders in the effort to convene task forces to evaluate and augment community resources for immunizing target groups, to provide access to treatment for sick people in the ambulatory setting, to develop strategies for hospitalizing seriously ill patients and to plan intensive education initiatives for the general public."[35]

Providing comprehensive care by providers that are familiar with the patient's chronic medical conditions improves the care delivered, decreases the cost, and greatly reduces the burden on local hospitals during times of high census. Families of CYSHCN can be better prepared for pandemics and other disasters by developing disaster plans in collaboration with their providers, schools, and communities.

Building relationships through coordinated efforts and communication of pediatricians and primary care practices with patient families, staff, hospitals, public health resources, and local community entities can ensure the best health outcomes for patients, limit the spread of disease, and decrease the burden of the pandemic. Pediatric clinics can be hub sites connecting patients with community resources and relaying vital information. Often community partners would like to help children and adolescents in times of need, but they do not know how to help or how to get needed supplies to the right people; having partnerships in place before a disaster allows for better coordination of resources.

Pediatricians and pediatric care practices have an important role in supporting the health of patients before and after the pandemic. Envisioning the different entities of the health care system and greater community (schools, faith-based organizations, and so forth) as part of one large team instead of siloed components of the system allows for greater coordination, better use of limited resources, and better health benefits for patients. It is essential that every member of the team, including the clinic, the hospital, and individual family members, is well-prepared, resulting in the best outcomes for patients. Pediatricians can take a leadership role in these efforts as they are natural advocates for children. Collaborations take time and require planning and preparation before the pandemic in order to lay the groundwork for effective and trusting relationships. Pediatricians and pediatric practices are essential for the optimal health of children everyday in the United States; therefore, they must be ready to provide care during a pandemic, preserve access to the health care system, and ensure the best outcomes for children.

CLINICS CARE POINTS

- All pediatric practices should undertake preparedness for disasters and pandemics, which includes having a written response plan, staff involvement, and training and emergency supplies.
- Pediatricians and pediatric practices should utilize their role as trusted sources of information to communicate with patients and their families during a pandemic and provide anticipatory guidance.
- Children and youth with special health care needs require special preparation to reduce the risk of morbidity and complications during a pandemic.

DISCLOSURE

S. Godfred-Cato received funding from the Pediatric Pandemic Network for research related to pediatric disaster preparedness and response.

REFERENCES

1. Burkle FM, Williams A, Kissoon N, et al. Pediatric emergency mass critical care: the role of community preparedness in conserving critical care resources. Pediatr Crit Care Med 2011;12(6 Suppl):S141–51.
2. Durodié B, Wessely S. Resilience or panic? The public and terrorist attack. Lancet 2002;360(9349):1901–2.
3. Needle S, Rucks AC, Wallace LA, et al. Pediatric practice readiness for disaster response. Disaster Med Public Health Prep 2021;15(3):277–81.
4. Flores G, Weinstock DJ. The preparedness of pediatricians for emergencies in the office. What is broken, should we care, and how can we fix it? Arch Pediatr Adolesc Med 1996;150(3):249–56.
5. Available at:Preparedness checklist for pediatric practices. American Academy of Pediatrics; 2013 https://downloads.aap.org/AAP/PDF/PedPreparednessCheck list1b.pdf. [Accessed 30 November 2023].
6. Available at:COVID-19: a physician guide to keeping your practice open. American Medical Association; 2022 https://www.ama-assn.org/system/files/physican-guide-keep-practice-open-covid-19.pdf. [Accessed 30 November 2023].
7. Available at:Integrating primary care providers into community pandemic influenza planning. Abbreviated pandemic influenza plan template for primary care provider offices: guidance from stakeholders. Centers for Disease Control and Prevention; 2010 https://www.cdc.gov/h1n1flu/guidance/pdf/abb_pandemic_influenza_plan.pdf. [Accessed 30 November 2023].
8. Available at:Including pediatric care providers in state-level disaster planning. American Academy of Pediatrics; 2023 https://www.aap.org/en/patient-care/disasters-and-children/professional-resources-for-disaster-preparedness/pediatric-preparedness-resource-kit/including-pediatric-care-providers-in-state-level-disaster-planning/. [Accessed 30 November 2023].
9. Ackerson BK, Sy LS, Glenn SC, et al. Pediatric vaccination during the COVID-19 pandemic. Pediatrics 2021;48(1). https://doi.org/10.1542/peds.2020-047092. e2020047092.
10. Tamariz L, Cely C, Palacio A. The forgotten need of disaster relief. Disaster Med Public Health Prep 2018;12(3):284–6.

11. Friedman AB, Gervasi S, Song H, et al. Telemedicine catches on: changes in the utilization of telemedicine services during the COVID-19 pandemic. Am J Manag Care 2022;28(1):e1–6.
12. Trends shaping the health economy value for money. Available at: Trilliant Health 2023; https://www.trillianthealth.com/reports/2023-health-economy-trends. [Accessed 30 November 2023].
13. Bielajs I, Burkle FM Jr, Archer FL, et al. Development of prehospital, population-based triage-management protocols for pandemics. Prehospital Disaster Med Sep-Oct 2008;23(5):420–30.
14. Cohen J, Rodgers YVM. Contributing factors to personal protective equipment shortages during the COVID-19 pandemic. Prev Med 2020;141:106263.
15. Burkle FM Jr. Population-based triage management in response to surge-capacity requirements during a large-scale bioevent disaster. Acad Emerg Med 2006;13(11):1118–29.
16. Nowak SA, Gidengil CA, Parker AM, et al. Association among trust in health care providers, friends, and family, and vaccine hesitancy. Vaccine 2021;39(40):5737–40.
17. Centers for Disease Control and Prevention. Available at:, Vaccine storage and handling Toolkit https://www.cdc.gov/vaccines/hcp/admin/storage/toolkit/index.html. [Accessed 30 November 2023].
18. Michaud J, Kates J. Distributing a COVID-19 vaccine across the US: a look at key issues. Available at:. Kaiser Family Foundation; 2020 https://www.kff.org/report-section/distributing-a-covid-19-vaccine-across-the-u-s-a-look-at-key-issues-issue-brief/. [Accessed 30 November 2023].
19. Kirschenbaum A. Reducing patient surge: community based social networks as first responders. Nat Hazards 2021;108(1):163–75.
20. Communications and messaging during a public health emergency. American Academy of Pediatrics. 2023. Available at: https://www.aap.org/en/patient-care/disasters-and-children/professional-resources-for-disaster-preparedness/pediatric-preparedness-resource-kit/communications-and-messaging-during-a-public-health-emergency/. [Accessed 30 November 2023].
21. Bracha HS, Burkle FM Jr. Utility of fear severity and individual resilience scoring as a surge capacity, triage management tool during large-scale, bio-event disasters. Prehospital Disaster Med 2006;21(5):290–6, discussion 297-8.
22. van-Dijk A, Aramini J, Edge G, et al. Real-time surveillance for respiratory disease outbreaks, Ontario, Canada. Emerg Infect Dis 2009;15(5):799–801.
23. MacIntyre CR, Ridda I, Seale H, et al. Respiratory viruses transmission from children to adults within a household. Vaccine 2012;30(19):3009–14.
24. Cruz AT, Tittle KO, Smith ER, et al. Increasing out-of-hospital regional surge capacity for H1N1 2009 influenza A through existing community pediatrician offices: a qualitative description of quality improvement strategies. Disaster Med Public Health Prep 2012;6(2):113–6.
25. American Academy of Pediatrics. Disaster and emergency preparedness in schools 2022.
26. Office of Public Health Preparedness and Response Division of State and Local Readiness. Public health preparedness capabilities; national standards for state and local planning March. Available at: Centers for Disease Control and Prevention 2011; https://stacks.cdc.gov/view/cdc/5902. [Accessed 30 November 2023].
27. Barnett DJ, Knieser L, Errett NA, et al. Reexamining Health-Care Coalitions in Light of COVID-19. Disaster Med Public Health Prep 2022;16(3):859–63.

28. American Academy of Pediatrics. Available at:, How to build a disaster emergency kit for your family https://www.healthychildren.org/English/safety-prevention/at-home/Pages/Family-Disaster-Supplies-List.aspx.

29. American Academy of Pediatrics, Committee on Pediatric Emergency Medicine and Council on Clinical Information Technology, American College of Emergency Physicians. Policy statement–emergency information forms and emergency preparedness for children with special health care needs. Pediatrics 2010;125(4): 829–37.

30. Available at:Disaster preparedness for children and youth with special health care needs. American Academy of Pediatrics; 2023 https://www.aap.org/en/patient-care/disasters-and-children/professional-resources-for-disaster-preparedness/preparedness-for-children-and-youth-with-special-health-care-needs/. [Accessed 30 November 2023].

31. Gold JI, Montano Z, Shields S, et al. Pediatric disaster preparedness in the medical setting: integrating mental health. Am J Disaster Med 2009;4(3):137–46.

32. Radhakrishnan L, Leeb RT, Bitsko RH, et al. Pediatric emergency department visits associated with mental health conditions before and during the COVID-19 pandemic — United States, January 2019–January 2022. MMWR Morb Mortal Wkly Rep 2022;71(8):319–24.

33. Strengthening the frontline: How primary health care helps health systems adapt during the COVID 19 pandemic. Available at: Organisation for Economic Co-operation and Development 2021; https://www.oecd.org/coronavirus/policy-responses/strengthening-the-frontline-how-primary-health-care-helps-health-systems-adapt-during-the-covid-19-pandemic-9a5ae6da/. [Accessed 30 November 2023].

34. American Academy of Pediatrics Disaster Preparedness Advisory Council, Committee on Pediatric Emergency Medicine, COMMITTEE ON PEDIATRIC EMERGENCY MEDICINE. Ensuring the health of children in disasters. Pediatrics 2015;136(5):e1407–17. https://doi.org/10.1542/peds.2015-3112.

35. Tayloe DT Jr. Pediatric leadership vital during H1N1 influenza pandemic. Letter from the president. AAP News 2009;30(9):6.

Understanding Pediatric Surge in the United States

Anna Lin, MD[a,b,*], Sarita Chung, MD[c,d]

KEYWORDS

- Pediatric surge • Crisis care standards • Surge capacity • Surge capabilities
- Contingency • Disaster

KEY POINTS

- Pediatric surge creates an imbalance of pediatric patient needs with available resources. This prompts a shift in the care paradigm away from individualized health care delivery to optimize population outcomes.
- Pediatric bed and unit closures contribute to decreased pediatric surge capacity and response capability in the United States.
- Pediatric readiness and telemedicine can improve pediatric surge capacity and response capability.
- Addressing pediatric surge will require interfacility and interagency collaboration between pediatric and community health care facilities, including real-time visibility and transparency of staffed bed availability and interfacility transfer.
- Engagement of primary care providers and the medical home in emergency planning can improve the care of children including youth with medical complexity during disaster and decrease pediatric surge burden.

INTRODUCTION

The concepts of pediatric surge in the United States continue to evolve from a theoretic framework to practical implementation. In 2006, initial definitions of surge, surge capacity, and surge response capabilities were described, including dividing surge into components of the 4 S's (staff, space, stuff, and systems).[1] These concepts were further refined by the Task Force for Mass Critical Care with specific hospital surge strategies for emergency departments (EDs), inpatient/intensive care units, and operating rooms.[2] In 2011, the Pediatric Emergency Mass Critical Care Task Force developed consensus-driven guidelines to ensure pediatric implications were

[a] Pediatric Hospital Medicine, Stanford Medicine Children's Health; [b] Department of Pediatrics, Stanford School of Medicine; [c] Disaster Preparedness, Division of Emergency Medicine, Boston Children's Hospital; [d] Pediatric and Emergency Medicine, Harvard Medical School
* Corresponding author. Division of Pediatric Hospital Medicine, 453 Quarry Road, MC 5776, Palo Alto, CA 94305.
E-mail address: alin1@stanford.edu

integrated into public health surge planning.[3] The recent coronavirus disease 2019 (COVID-19) pandemic and the subsequent 2022 to 2023 tripledemic (COVID-19/influenza/respiratory syncytial virus [RSV]) pediatric respiratory surge stressed and forced health care system transformation to meet the surge demands.[4–8] While some aspects of surge strategies were easier to implement such as alternate care sites, there were several challenges noted including an inability to increase bed capacity due to limited pediatric staffing. Novel strategies such as pediatric telehealth guidance to families and peer professionals were trialed at the local and state level.[9] There is also an increased awareness that while traditional surge science focuses on hospital surge responses, a catastrophic surge affects all aspects of the health care system. Unique surge strategies in areas such as primary care, other ambulatory clinics, and emergency medical services will be required. As the number of disasters (environmental and mass casualty events) continues to increase, pediatric implementation strategies utilized from these surge events need to be incorporated into planning at the local, state, and federal levels.

Daily, over 80% of children seek emergency care in community hospitals.[10] During a disaster, children will present with or without their families to local hospitals for emergency care.[11] Therefore, having EDs "pediatric ready" (ie, ready to care for 1 sick child) is the foundational building block for pediatric disaster surge plans. Studies have consistently shown decreased pediatric mortality in EDs with higher pediatric readiness scores.[12,13] While pediatric readiness continues to improve despite the recent COVID-19 pandemic, results from the 2021 National Pediatric Readiness Project (NPRP) revealed that less than one-half of the 3647 hospitals in the study reported the inclusion of pediatric components in their hospital disaster plans, a level of readiness which is unchanged from the previous 2013 survey.[10]

In addition, there is increasing recognition of existing health disparities for the pediatric populations seeking medical care.[14–19] Pediatric inpatient capacity in the United States continues to diminish with pediatric inpatient units and beds closing, and children are traveling greater distances to reach hospitals with pediatric capabilities, especially pediatric intensive care.[20] Pediatric care has also become more concentrated in urban settings with decreased access to pediatric subspecialties in rural settings.[21–26]

While surges due to respiratory viruses generally have seasonal predictability which can be incorporated into pediatric capacity planning, no notice events such as pediatric-based mass casualty incidents where the demand for pediatric health care capacity and resources outweigh their availability have become increasingly more prevalent. Since 2018, there has been an exponential increase in the number of K-12 school shootings.[27,28] Disturbingly, nearly 20% of these shootings occurred at elementary schools, which has implications for planning including size-appropriate medical equipment, family reunification, and mental health screening and management. Both mass casualty incidents and infectious disease outbreaks highlight the importance of pediatric surge and our ability to care for children in extenuating circumstances.

CRISIS STANDARDS OF CARE

When a surge of patients threatens to overwhelm a health care system, health care leaders may deem it necessary to shift from individualized care to population health outcomes with a basis in utilitarian ethics—"the greatest good for the greatest number."[29] With this paradigm shift, resource utilization will need to be prioritized. The Institute of Medicine issued its crisis standards of care framework in 2012,[30] outlining

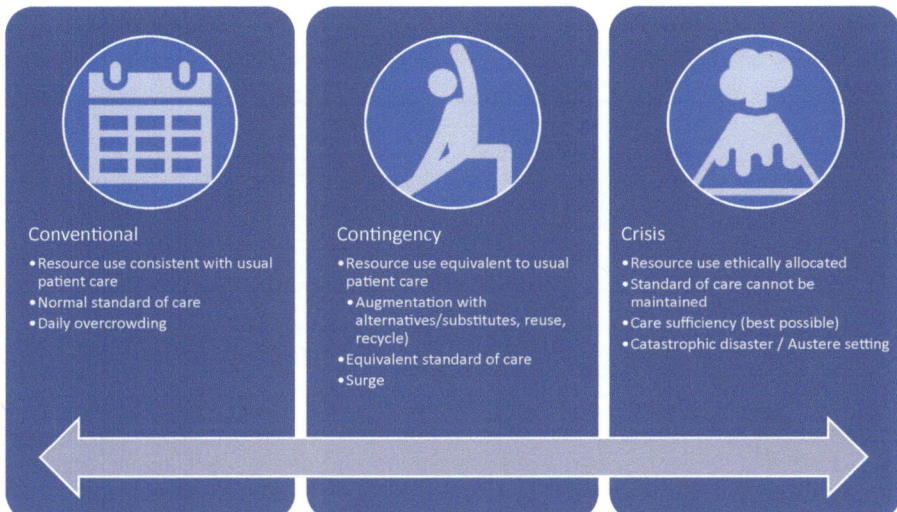

Fig. 1. Continuum of care from contingency to crisis. *Adapted from* Institute of Medicine. 2009. Guidance for Establishing Crisis Standards of Care for Use in Disaster Situations: A Letter Report. Washington, DC: The National Academies Press. https://doi.org/10.17226/12749.

a continuum of care reflected in **Fig. 1**. The 2020 COVID-19 pandemic and the subsequent 2022 to 2023 pediatric respiratory tripledemic exemplify events where health care needs of a population exceeded available resources and staff. Health care systems needed to pivot from conventional care where the "spaces, staff, and supplies used are consistent with daily practices" to contingency practices "spaces, stuff, and supplies used are not consistent with daily practice but provide care that is functionally equivalent to usual patient care."[31] In surge strategies, we shift from conventional care into contingency care. The goal of contingency and surge planning is to prevent crisis care where "adaptive spaces, staff, and supplies are not consistent with usual standards of care but provide sufficiency of care in the context of a catastrophic disaster."[29–31] There is a potential for a substantial rise in the risk of morbidity and mortality as health care systems progress along this continuum from contingency to crisis care as normal standards of care become unattainable.[30] Broader discussions incorporating local values with community members, health care providers, and public health officials must occur and should consider an ethical framework for scarce resource allocation that includes equity, justice, and transparency.

DEFINING SURGE AND ITS COMPONENTS

In 2006, a "The Science of Surge" conference funded by the Agency for Healthcare Research and Quality convened to define consensus-driven surge concepts. **Table 1** lists the definitions for surge, surge capacity, and surge response capability.

Pediatric Surge

Factors that affect surge include the type of event, its duration, and its impact on health care needs. For example, no-notice events such as a mass casualty incident require immediate health care resource availability to manage a surge but overall may be of short duration, whereas an event such as a pandemic or hurricane may

Table 1 Definitions of surge, surge capacity, and surge response capability	
Term	**Definition**
Surge	A sizable increase in demand for resources compared with a baseline demand
Surge capacity	The maximum potential delivery of required resources, either through augmentation or the modification of resource management and allocation.
Surge response capability	The ability of surge capacity (ie, the resources that can be made available) to accommodate the surge (demand for resources).

Adapted from Kelen GD, McCarthy ML. The science of surge. Acad Emerg Med. 2006; 13(11):1089-94. Doi: 10.1197/j.aem.2006.07.016.

allow additional time for resource pre-positioning and deployment, affect more children, and last for a prolonged period. In any event, we must expect that a proportion of disaster victims will be children and that disasters, in general, may disproportionately affect children due to differences in cognition and physiology,[32] and these children will require size-appropriate equipment and pediatric-specific resources. Depending on the nature of this surge, unaccompanied minors may require reunification services.[33] This emphasizes the need for pediatric readiness at all hospitals, especially community hospitals as many children live in closer proximity to community hospitals compared to pediatric tertiary hospitals. In many of these centers, a pediatric surge may only involve a handful of pediatric patients as they may lack the supplies, expertise, and systems of care to accommodate multiple acutely ill or injured children simultaneously. A pediatric medical surge will likely also be accompanied by a mental health surge. The impact of disasters on children has profound mental health consequences; therefore, early mental health intervention will be required to minimize longer sequelae.[34–36]

Pediatric Surge Capacity

Surge capacity is defined as "the ability to evaluate and care for a markedly increased volume of patients—one that challenges or exceeds normal operating capacity. The surge requirements may extend beyond direct patient care to include such tasks as extensive laboratory studies or epidemiologic investigations." Surge capacity accounts for the resources required to manage an influx of patients. Resources have historically been categorized into space, supplies, staff, and structure/systems (the 4 S's). The nature of pediatric care complicates surge capacity as described in the following sections.

Space

Depending on the nature of the surge event, the provision of pediatric care could be optimized by employing a separate space for that care. Pediatric spaces used should be inspected to ensure that they are child friendly and devoid of potential hazards (open electrical outlets, dangling cords, stairs). Cohorting pediatric patients can simplify access to pediatric expertise and supplies. Additional space considerations include the care of unaccompanied pediatric patients who may or may not require medical attention and the need for secure ingress and egress from patient care areas supporting this function. Planning must include provisions for such an area, known as a pediatric-safe area.[33]

Supplies

As children rapidly develop and grow over the course of infancy, childhood, and adolescence, the management of a large influx of pediatric patients requires age-based and weight-based supply caches. These include medical supplies such as airway and respiratory equipment, feeding tubes, and intravenous and urinary catheters.[3] Additional considerations include supplies for the nonmedical care of infants and children such as formula, age-appropriate food, diapers, portable cribs/playpens, and toys/activities. Pharmaceutical caches may require separate formulations such as liquid or chewable tablets for pediatric administration or compounding instructions to alter formulations for pediatric administration. The Strategic National Stockpile which hosts countermeasures to chemical, biological, radiological, and nuclear events must include pediatric considerations. For example, standard medication doses vary by age, body surface area, or weight as opposed to standard adult dosing. While current drug and medical supply shortages threaten any surge response, supply chain failures increase the vulnerability of pediatric medication and supplies, weakening surge capacity.

Staffing

Recently, as the health care workforce declined, staffing has challenged daily operational capacity thus constraining staffing expansion for surge capacity. Specifically, shortages in nursing, respiratory care therapy, child life specialists, and other ancillary staff create barriers in optimal care delivery. Given that pediatric-trained health care professionals typically represent only a portion of the overall health care workforce, any decrease in their number could significantly worsen the health care system's capacity to handle a surge in pediatric cases. Additional pediatric-trained, deployable assets for a more prolonged response are limited. A focus on workforce resiliency and wellness, discussed within this volume, is paramount and should be considered an organizational priority from a daily operations standpoint with likely positive impacts for surge capacity from a staffing perspective.

While all EDs should be able to stabilize any pediatric patient under normal operating conditions, many community EDs will quickly refer and transfer patients to pediatric centers.[37] Medical consultation with pediatric subspecialists including emergency medicine or critical care for concurrent or ongoing care can be lifesaving, especially if primary or secondary transfer is not feasible. Since the COVID-19 pandemic, the use of telemedicine has burgeoned.[9] This ability to provide synchronous but geographically distant care revolutionizes access to pediatric expertise, provided that regulatory and robust systems of care support this practice.

Structures/systems

Telemedicine capability is an example of a system where barriers such as multiple state licensures and credentialing of pediatric subspecialists limit its effectiveness. The catchment area of many pediatric hospitals cross state borders, so obtaining specific state licensures can be time consuming and problematic. Regulatory waivers[38] may improve flexibility for the provision of pediatric care in a disaster setting. All hospitals should have a mechanism for rapid credentialing of health care workers during disasters.[39] Pre-existing memoranda of understanding or other contractual agreements can facilitate disaster-related telemedicine but require forethought and planning prior to a crisis or event.

During any crisis, hospitals activate their hospital incident command system (HICS) which is a flexible, objective-based response system facilitating command and control, resource acquisition and allocation, and health care system communications.

Pediatric subject matter experts should serve as medical/technical specialists and recommend pediatric-specific responses after undergoing institutional HICS training. Additional training on the incident command system (ICS) can be found at the Federal Emergency Management Agency Emergency Management Institute's ICS Resource Center.[40] This team of pediatric experts could also participate in emergency management planning to ensure response guides include pediatric considerations for decontamination, triage, surge, evacuation, and family reunification. Additional information on HICS can be found at the California Emergency Medical Services Authority.[41]

Most hospitals participate in health care coalitions which partner with state preparedness and response agencies. Other stakeholders include ambulatory clinics, subacute facilities, professional societies, and community organizations. Key responsibilities include disaster readiness, response coordination, continuity of health care service delivery, and medical surge. Health care coalitions create and coordinate plans for local response to disasters, including information exchange, resource management and sharing, and delivery of medical care.[42] In 2019, the Office of Administration for Strategic Preparedness and Response (ASPR) required all health care coalitions to develop a pediatric surge annex to their mass casualty plans.[43] In addition, federal grants have funded pediatric disaster centers of excellence across the nation through the ASPR[44] as well as the Pediatric Pandemic Network through the Health Resources and Services Administration,[45] Both networks focus efforts on pediatric emergency preparedness and response.

Pediatric Surge Capability

While "The Science of Surge" article[1] looks at surge capability as the ability for resources (surge capacity) to respond to a surge, another definition for surge capability focuses on the ability to manage patients who require unusual or specialized evaluation and care.[46] As pediatric health care resources have concentrated into pediatric centers, the ability of community health care systems to provide general pediatric care wanes.[47–49] Most pediatric subspecialty care, including pediatric surgery, is now regionalized which can limit local availability and accessibility.[21–26] Even with telemedicine capabilities, pediatric expertise may not be readily available, especially if technological solutions are compromised during an event.

Because of community hospital pediatric bed closures,[20] pediatric experience and expertise may be shrinking. The maintenance of pediatric foundational knowledge can support daily pediatric readiness and augment pediatric surge capacity. Active, team-based simulation can reinforce recognition and management of pediatric emergencies in addition to fostering retention of pediatric knowledge.[50] Just-in-time pediatric education[51] and the use of pediatric treatment protocols can supplement basic medical knowledge. The Emergency Medical Services for Children's Innovation and Improvement Center (EIIC) has and continues to launch quality improvement collaboratives to improve national pediatric readiness.

PEDIATRIC SURGE PLANNING

Pediatric surge planning consists of improving pediatric surge capacity and capability. Pre-identification of alternatives and substitutes for at-risk resources allows more flexibility for augmentation. The development of processes to reuse or recycle resources as well as changes to how resources are utilized prior to crisis increases familiarity between key stakeholders and builds pre-existing relationships which foster resiliency during disaster. Building connections with other facilities, individual clinics, response agencies or organizations, and health care coalitions buffers existing structures for continuity of care during crisis. Data from the NPRP show that hospital EDs with a pediatric emergency care coordinator, a designated individual responsible for coordinating pediatric specific activities, have increased readiness and quality improvement, including pediatric patient safety and caches of pediatric-specific equipment, supplies, and medications.[10] To that end, each health care system or response agency should identify a team of pediatric disaster champions who can work within existing emergency management structures to plan for the needs of children. This team could discuss ensuring the availability of pediatric supplies and staff/expertise. Interfacility and interagency discussions around pediatric transport and transfer also require preplanning. Community hospitals can pivot from primarily adult care to serve an increased number of younger patients such as post-pubertal pediatric patients or lower acuity children. Pediatric tertiary care centers can perform regular outreach to support pediatric care in these settings. **Table 2** highlights examples of pediatric considerations in surge planning and contingency care.

LESSONS LEARNED FROM RECENT SURGES

The federal public health emergency declaration relaxed regulations related to privacy, documentation, and reimbursement during the COVID-19 pandemic which allowed state waivers and flexibility to promote the delivery of care to patients. The morbidity and mortality of the COVID-19 pandemic was largely concentrated in the adult population, so many pediatric intensive care units alleviated some of the patient burden by accepting and caring for adult patients.[52,53] Surgical case cancellation or rescheduling was another strategy that allowed for increased capacity for medical patients requiring hospitalization. This brought into question the prioritization of medical versus surgical patients. While previously available, the use of telemedicine capability skyrocketed during the pandemic.[9] Waivers during the pandemic allowed for payment for some of these services. Public health measures in response to the pandemic, including school closure, social distancing, masking, and hand hygiene, contributed to a significant decrease in the admission of acutely and critically ill children due to respiratory illness early in the pandemic.[54,55] Health care utilization in EDs as well as in outpatient pediatric clinics also decreased.[56,57] The strategy utilized by many primary care practices early in the pandemic to postpone preventative medicine visits and scheduled vaccinations, as a means of infection control and surge management, inadvertently caused substantial delay and reduction in vaccination rates.[58] Other consequences included delays in surgical care. In pediatrics, there are very few elective surgeries, and prioritization regarding the urgency of the procedure should be considered. Threat of significant complications, morbidity, or mortality with delays in surgical care[59] must weigh into the prioritization schema for admissions when limitations in pediatric capacity exist.

The recent COVID-19/influenza/RSV tripledemic respiratory viral surge of 2022 to 2023 highlighted shortages in pediatric health care capacity,[60] garnering national media attention.[61–65] The general pattern of respiratory viral illness changed unexpectedly with an early peak of illness due to RSV in addition to influenza and ongoing COVID-19 infections.[66–68] Most pediatric centers encountered issues with all aspects of pediatric surge capacity[69] — space, supplies, staff, and structures/systems (**Fig. 2**). Of all these aspects, pediatric staffing, specifically nursing and respiratory care therapists, remained the major obstacle for the expansion of services for multiple health care centers. In some regions, pediatric medical operations coordination centers (P-MOCC) were activated to manage the large surge of pediatric patients.[8,70] Multiple health care systems collaborated to support the pediatric surge and level load patients

Table 2
Example considerations for pediatric surge planning and contingency care

	Ambulatory/Pre-hospital	Hospital	State	Regional
Space	Division of spaces for sick/well visits	Repurpose existing clinical spaces to accommodate pediatric surge Open nonclinical spaces for patients or custodial care (pediatric-safe area)	Identify pediatric capacity and capability within the state	Identify pediatric capacity and capability within a region
Supplies	Work with affiliated health care systems, health care coalitions, and/or private sector to obtain supplies	Identify equivalent alternatives and substitutes for pharmaceuticals/supplies Examples: • Use of intravenous formulations intranasally or orally • Compounding instructions for the conversion of tablet or capsule formulations into palatable, liquid formulations • Use skin-to-skin care instead of incubators or warmers for neonates Create processes for extending, recycling, or reusing supplies Examples: • Reserving the use of cardiorespiratory and continuous pulse oximetry monitoring for only critically ill children • Rapid sterile processing of surgical and airway equipment	Identify critical medications and supplies specific to pediatric care Ensure processes to quickly obtain pediatric-specific supplies Request pediatric-specific supplies and pharmaceuticals from local caches or the Strategic National Stockpile Identify resources required to increase pediatric-specific supplies and pharmaceuticals Example: • Create a directory of compounding pharmacies for altering existing formulations for pediatric administration	Identify critical medications and supplies specific to pediatric care, including pediatric. countermeasures Ensure processes to quickly obtain pediatric-specific supplies. Host pediatric-specific countermeasures and supplies in the Strategic National Stockpile.

Staff	Extended hours for care Provision of minimal health care maintenance (ie, vaccine-only visits)	Identify staff/providers with pediatric expertise or training Cross train adult providers for pediatric care	Identify state-deployable assets with pediatric expertise or training Example: • Medical Reserve Corps personnel with pediatric expertise or training Deploy National Guard for nonclinical hospital support functions Create a registry of pediatric specialists who may be needed in a disaster	Identify federal-deployable assets (Disaster Medical Assistance Team) with pediatric expertise or training Identify volunteers with pediatric expertise or training within Emergency System for Advance Registration of Volunteer Health Professional
Systems/Structures	Telephone/video triage of patients Communication with hospital systems Partner with other pediatric and family practice clinics for resource sharing and creative scheduling to extend hours Provide anticipatory guidance on disaster planning for children, especially those with technology dependence	Use of telemedicine to expand pediatric expertise reach Create a process for tracking of pediatric patients throughout and mechanism for reunification for pediatric patients without adult caretakers (aka unaccompanied minors) Create or refine processes to rapidly decant highly impacted areas of the hospital (emergency departments, perioperative areas, intensive care units, acute care/medical-surgical units)	Enact state waivers to repurpose spaces for pediatric care and facilitate licensure of staff with pediatric expertise or training Coordinate pediatric care for patient level loading Incorporate pediatric expertise into planning and response activities State waivers for the use of telehealth across state borders	Ensure capability for pediatric patient movement within the National Disaster Medical System Incorporate pediatric expertise into planning and response activities

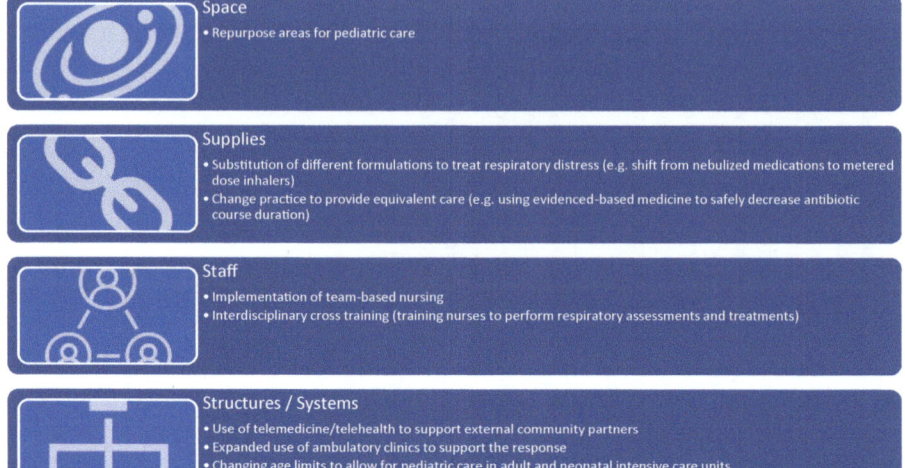

Space
• Repurpose areas for pediatric care

Supplies
• Substitution of different formulations to treat respiratory distress (e.g. shift from nebulized medications to metered dose inhalers)
• Change practice to provide equivalent care (e.g. using evidenced-based medicine to safely decrease antibiotic course duration)

Staff
• Implementation of team-based nursing
• Interdisciplinary cross training (training nurses to perform respiratory assessments and treatments)

Structures / Systems
• Use of telemedicine/telehealth to support external community partners
• Expanded use of ambulatory clinics to support the response
• Changing age limits to allow for pediatric care in adult and neonatal intensive care units
• Creation of pediatric medical operations coordination centers

Fig. 2. Strategies used to increase pediatric surge capacity during the 2022 to 2023 triple-demic surge.

requiring critical care across pediatric centers after triage through the P-MOCC. Triage decisions included level of care with decisions for admission, transfer to pediatric centers, or discharge from requesting hospitals.

CHALLENGES IN PEDIATRIC SURGE

Even with lessons learned from the COVID-19 pandemic and the 2022 to 2023 triple-demic pediatric surge, challenges in pediatric surge and surge planning continue to exist. As pediatric centers must operate near or at daily operational capacity to maintain financial viability, the ability to accommodate an additional surge of patients becomes constrained. No widely used systematic method to understand pediatric capacity exists. Regional understanding can be achieved with statewide bed tracking derived automatically from electronic health records.[8] The number of licensed pediatric beds as a proxy for pediatric capacity does not account for staff availability and may have caused an inaccurate understanding on how pediatric centers struggled during the tripledemic pediatric surge. Even in the absence of pediatric licensed beds, some hospitals may continue to care for children in nonlicensed beds.[71] The number of pediatric critical care and neonatal intensive care beds are more clearly tracked than pediatric acute care beds, yet the real-time visibility of staffed bed availability for all levels of pediatric care remains problematic. Further adding to ambiguity, no universal designation for pediatric levels of care exists to understand pediatric capabilities, with levels of care driven by local or institutional practices to some extent.[72]

Older benchmarks for general surge capacity cited the need for 500 beds per million population.[73] Using this benchmark and a pediatric population of 72.4 million, this would require over 36,000 beds. As of 2018, there were 27,496 pediatric beds,[20] and even if there was capacity and capability to surge 20%, we would be unable to achieve this benchmark. Likely there are even fewer pediatric beds if the downward trend due to pediatric unit closures over the past 5 years continues. Many existing surge plans assume the ability of health care systems to increase capacity by federally set benchmarks of 20%. A recent statewide assessment showed that pediatric capacity would only increase by about 8% during disaster in addition to a lack of access to pediatric surgical subspecialties.[74]

Pediatric pharmaceutical and supply chains remain vulnerable. While the identification of pediatric critical supplies has occurred, the maintenance of pediatric supply caches is expensive. Pediatric health care utilization remains small compared to adult utilization, and the resultant market underrepresentation underpins ongoing issues in the development and production of pediatric pharmaceuticals and supplies.[75] Recent shortages in pain medications, nebulized respiratory medications, antibiotics, and infant formula highlight the need for public policy changes.[76]

While previous projections revealed anticipated pediatric nursing shortages,[77,78] the COVID-19 pandemic and the 2022 tripledemic pediatric respiratory surge highlighted how staffing shortages severely limited pediatric surge capacity. Other staffing shortages included respiratory care therapists with pediatric expertise. As the pediatric health care workforce dwindles, a concomitant decrease in pediatric faculty puts pediatric training at risk. Systematic changes to improve resiliency and prevent burnout as well as incentives for education for the pediatric health care workforce can mitigate these shortages in the future.

From a systems and structures standpoint, challenges include the ever-increasing catchment areas with the consolidation of pediatric resources. State waivers to facilitate interstate medical care as well as flexibilities in space and staff utilization become paramount to the pediatric surge response. A full evacuation of a pediatric center will result in regional, if not national, pediatric surge.[79] Parity in reimbursement for pediatric care with respect to our adult care counterparts needs addressing as closures continue to jeopardize pediatric surge capacity and response capabilities. Additionally, investment in pediatric mental health capacity and capability can strengthen pediatric surge response, given the impact of mental health boarding within EDs and hospitals.[80] Finally, decisions made in 2023 by the Supreme Court of the United States have eroded federal regulatory powers, allowed promulgation of misinformation, and limited emergency powers as well as medication availability.[81] This has the potential to threaten future federal public health responses.

NEXT STEPS IN PEDIATRIC SURGE

While the challenges of pediatric surge loom, we can move forward in promoting pediatric surge capacity and response capability with some actionable steps.

1. Create surge exercises and drills with pediatric injects or scenarios to highlight any gaps in planning pertaining to the pediatric population. In addition, health care facilities and response agencies can then address any gaps or refine processes through after action reports.
2. Promote the concept of pediatric readiness within and beyond the ED. The EIIC is currently exploring pediatric readiness in the pre-hospital setting and readiness work could extend to both inpatient and outpatient arenas.
3. Bolster the medical home and encourage thinking around emergency management in this setting to minimize the impact of disasters on this extremely vulnerable population of children. While most of the pediatric surge literature has focused on health care facilities, the largest utilization of our intensive care units is presently by children and youth with medical complexity.
4. Explore how ambulatory settings (urgent care or pediatric/family practice clinics) can offset pediatric surge and improve capacity and response capabilities.

5. Create systematic structures for how frontline facilities and agencies can communicate needs to public health departments and other response agencies at all levels (local, state, regional, federal) as well as for general pediatric education and planning.
6. Identify triggers for a regional pediatric surge response and expand the P-MOCC model of care. Related to this, we need to promote a method for real-time visibility into staffed bed availability for pediatric acute care and intensive care.
7 Address mental health impacts in a systematic fashion to mitigate long-term sequelae.
8. Create a unified approach to pediatric crisis standards of care. This will require community forums to discuss the norms of any given locale and crisis planning which will also promulgate transparency around decisions on scarce resource allocation.

CLINICS CARE POINTS

- Addressing pediatric surge has a high level of complexity and requires collaboration at all levels.
- Pediatricians and other pediatric subject matter experts can engage with health care systems, health care coalitions, public health departments, and other response agencies to strengthen understanding of and planning for the needs of children and their families.

DISCLOSURES

Dr A. Lin received funding from Pediatric Pandemic Network and Western Regional Alliance for Pediatric Emergency Management. Dr S. Chung received funding from Pediatric Pandemic Network, Emergency Medical Services for Children Innovation and Improvement Center (EIIC), and Massachusetts Department of Public Health, United States.

REFERENCES

1. Kelen GD, McCarthy ML. The science of surge. Acad Emerg Med 2006;13(11): 1089–94.
2. Devereaux A, Christian MD, Dichter JR, et al. Summary of suggestions from the Task Force for Mass Critical Care Summit, January 26-27, 2007. Chest 2008; 133(5 SUPPL):1S–7S.
3. Kissoon N. Deliberations and recommendations of the Pediatric Emergency Mass Critical Care Task Force: Executive summary. Pediatr Crit Care Med 2011;12(6 SUPPL).
4. Mahmood T, Meda A, Trivedi S, et al. Impact of the COVID-19 pandemic on the US healthcare system. Turk J Intern Med 2023;5(3).
5. Borkan J, George P, Adashi EY. A pandemic-inspired transformation of primary care. R I Med J 2020;103(10).
6. Remy KE, Verhoef PA, Malone JR, et al. Caring for critically ill adults with coronavirus disease 2019 in a PICU: recommendations by dual trained intensivists. Pediatr Crit Care Med 2020;21(7):607–19.
7. King MA, Matos RI, Hamele MT, et al. PICU in the MICU: how adult ICUs can support pediatric care in public health emergencies. Chest 2022;161(5).

8. Mitchell SH, Merkel MJ, Eriksson CO, et al. Using two statewide medical operations coordination centers to load balance in pediatric hospitals during a severe respiratory surge in the United States. Pediatr Crit Care Med 2023;24(9):775–81.
9. Shaver J. The state of telehealth before and after the COVID-19 pandemic. Prim Care Clin Off Pract 2022;49(4):517–30.
10. Remick KE, Hewes HA, Ely M, et al. National assessment of pediatric readiness of US emergency departments during the COVID-19 pandemic. JAMA Netw Open 2023;6(7):E2321707.
11. Rebmann T, Gupta NK, Charney RL. US hospital preparedness to manage unidentified individuals and reunite unaccompanied minors with family members during disasters: results from a nationwide survey. Health Secur 2021;19(2):183–94.
12. Ames SG, Davis BS, Marin JR, et al. Emergency department pediatric readiness and mortality in critically ill children. Pediatrics 2019;144(3):e20190568.
13. Newgard CD, Lin A, Goldhaber-Fiebert JD, et al. Association of emergency department pediatric readiness with mortality to 1 year among injured children treated at trauma centers. JAMA Surg 2022;157(4):e217419.
14. Trent M, Dooley DG. Dougé J, Section on Adolescent Health, Council on Community Pediarics, Committee on Adolescent Health, et al. The impact of racism on child and adolescent health. Pediatrics 2019;144(2):e20191765.
15. Ellis C, Jacobs M, Keene KL, et al. The impact of COVID-19 on racial-ethnic health disparities in the US: now is the time to address the problem. J Natl Med Assoc 2021;113(2):195–8.
16. Phan TLT, Enlow PT, Lewis AM, et al. Persistent disparities in pediatric health care engagement during the COVID-19 pandemic. Publ Health Rep 2023;138(4):633–44.
17. Abrams AH, Badolato GM, Boyle MD, et al. Racial and ethnic disparities in pediatric mental health-related emergency department visits. Available at: Pediatr Emerg Care 2020;38(1):e214–8 http://links.lww.com/PEC/A601.
18. Wagner J, Bhatia S, Marquis BO, et al. Health disparities in pediatric epilepsy: methods and lessons learned. J Clin Psychol Med Settings 2023;30(2):251–60.
19. Arant KR, Modest JM, Gil JA, et al. What's new in pediatric orthopaedic health care disparities? J Pediatr Orthop 2022;42(9):E954–9.
20. Cushing AM, Bucholz EM, Chien AT, et al. Availability of pediatric inpatient services in the United States. Pediatrics 2021;148(1).
21. Lorch SA, Myers S, Carr B. The regionalization of pediatric health care. Pediatrics 2010;126(6):1182–90.
22. Salazar JH, Goldstein SD, Yang J, et al. Regionalization of pediatric surgery trends already underway. Ann Surg 2016;263(6):1062–6.
23. Handley SC, Lorch SA. Regionalization of neonatal care: benefits, barriers, and beyond. J Perinatol 2022;42(6):835–8.
24. Ghandour HZ, Vervoort D, Welke KF, et al. Regionalization of congenital cardiac surgical care: what it will take. Curr Opin Cardiol 2022;37(1):137–43.
25. Shay S, Shapiro NL, Bhattacharyya N. Patterns of hospital use and regionalization of inpatient pediatric adenotonsillectomy. JAMA Otolaryngol Head Neck Surg 2016;142(2):122–6.
26. Aledhaim A, Fishe JN, Hirshon JM, et al. Pediatric conditions requiring interfacility transport from emergency departments a statewide study of regionalization. Pediatr Emerg Care 2012;37(6):e319–23.
27. Riedman D. K-12 school shooting database. 2023. Available at: https://k12ssdb.org/all-shootings. [Accessed 31 October 2023].

28. Cox JW, Rich S, Chui A. Interactive school shootings database, *The Washington Post*. 2018. Available at: https://www.washingtonpost.com/education/interactive/school-shootings-database/. [Accessed 31 October 2023].

29. Institute of Medicine. Guidance for establishing crisis standards of care for use in disaster situations. National Academies Press; 2009. https://doi.org/10.17226/12749.

30. Institute of Medicine. Crisis Standards of care: a systems framework for catastrophic disaster response. National Academies Press; 2012. https://doi.org/10.17226/13351.

31. Available at:Crisis standards of care brief: principles. ASPR TRACIE; 2022 https://files.asprtracie.hhs.gov/documents/aspr-tracie-csc-principles.pdf. [Accessed 31 October 2023].

32. Peek L. Children and disasters: understanding vulnerability, developing capacities, and promoting resilience — an introduction. Child Youth Environ 2008;18(1):1–29.

33. American Academy of Pediatrics, Massachusetts General Hospital Center for Disaster Medicine. Family reunification following disasters: a planning tool for health care facilities. American Academy of Pediatrics; 2018.

34. Rousseau C, Jamil U, Bhui K, et al. Consequences of 9/11 and the war on terror on children's and young adult's mental health: a systematic review of the past 10 years. Clin Child Psychol Psychiatr 2015;20(2):173–93.

35. Jaycox LH, Cohen JA, Mannarino AP, et al. Children's mental health care following hurricane Katrina: a field trial of trauma-focused psychotherapies. J Trauma Stress 2010;23(2):223–31.

36. Zacher M, Arkin M, Rhodes J, et al. The effects of maternal disaster exposure on adolescent mental health 12 years later. Res Child Adolesc Psychopathol 2022;50(9).

37. Li J, Monuteaux MC, Bachur RG. Interfacility transfers of noncritically ill children to academic pediatric emergency departments. Pediatrics 2012;130(1):83–92.

38. US states and territories modifying requirements for telehealth in response to COVID-19 (out-of-state physicians; preexisting provider-patient relationships; audio-only requirements; etc.).Federation of State Medical Boards. 2023. Available at: https://www.fsmb.org/siteassets/advocacy/pdf/states-waiving-licensure-requirements-for-telehealth-in-response-to-covid-19.pdf. [Accessed 30 October 2023].

39. Available at:CMS releases updated emergency preparedness guidance. CMS Quality and Safety Portal; 2019 https://qsep.cms.gov/pubs/CourseMenu.aspx?cid=0CMSUIPC_ONL. [Accessed 29 November 2023].

40. ICS Resource Center. FEMA Emergency Management Institute. Available at: https://training.fema.gov/emiweb/is/icsresource/trainingmaterials/. [Accessed 29 November 2023].

41. California Emergency Medical Service Authority Hospital Incident Command System. CA EMSA. Available at: https://emsa.ca.gov/disaster-medical-services-division-hospital-incident-command-system-resources/. Accessed November 29, 2023.

42. Health care preparedness and response capabilities 2017-2022. Office of the Assistant Secretary of Preparedness and Response. Available at: https://www.phe.gov/preparedness/planning/hpp/reports/documents/2017-2022-healthcare-pr-capablities.pdf. [Accessed 30 November 2023].

43. Healthcare coalition pediatric surge annex template. ASPR TRACIE. Available at: https://files.asprtracie.hhs.gov/documents/aspr-tracie-hcc-pediatric-surge-annex-template-final-508.pdf. [Accessed 30 November 2023].

44. Available at:Pediatric disaster care centers of excellence. US Department of Health & Human Services; 2019 https://www.phe.gov/Preparedness/responders/ndms/Pages/ndpi.aspx. [Accessed 31 October 2023].

45. Available at:Regional pediatric pandemic network. Health Resources & Services Administration; 2021 https://pedspandemicnetwork.org/. [Accessed 29 November 2023].

46. Barbera J, Macintyre AG. Medical surge capacity and capability: a management system for integrating medical and health resources during large-scale emergencies. Available at:. 2nd edition. US Department of Health and Human Services; 2007 https://www.phe.gov/preparedness/planning/mscc/handbook/documents/mscc080626.pdf. [Accessed 30 November 2023].

47. Michelson KA, Hudgins JD, Lyons TW, et al. Trends in capability of hospitals to provide definitive acute care for children: 2008 to 2016. Pediatrics 2020;(1):145.

48. Cushing AM, Bucholz E, Michelson KA. Trends in regionalization of emergency care for common pediatric conditions. Pediatrics 2020;145(4).

49. França UL, Mcmanus ML. Trends in regionalization of hospital care for common pediatric conditions. Pediatrics 2018;141(1):20171940.

50. Abulebda K, Whitfill T, Montgomery EE, et al. Improving pediatric readiness in general emergency departments: a prospective interventional study. J Pediatr 2021;230:230–7.e1.

51. Watkins K, Ghasemzadeh R, Fatch S. WRAP-EM JIT - *just in time handbook: a quick pediatric reference guide for adult healthcare providers*. Available at:. WRAP-EM; 2021 http: file:///Users/steven/Downloads/WRAP-EM%20JIT%20Quick%20Pediatric%20Reference%20Guide%20for%20Adult%20Healthcare%20Providers%20(1).pdf. [Accessed 31 October 2023].

52. Wasserman E, Toal M, Nellis ME, et al. Rapid transition of a PICU space and staff to adult coronavirus disease 2019 ICU care. Pediatr Crit Care Med 2021;22(1):50–5. https://doi.org/10.1097/PCC.0000000000002597.

53. Levin AB, Bernier ML, Riggs BJ, et al. Transforming a PICU Into an adult ICU during the coronavirus disease 2019 pandemic: meeting multiple needs. Crit Care Explor 2020;2(9).

54. Wilder JL, Parsons CR, Growdon AS, et al. Pediatric hospitalizations during the COVID-19 pandemic. Pediatrics 2020;(6):146.

55. Rogerson CM, Lin A, Klein MJ, et al. School closures in the United States and severe respiratory illnesses in children: a normalized nationwide sample. Pediatr Crit Care Med 2022;23(7):535–43.

56. Yard E, Radhakrishnan L, Ballesteros MF, et al. Emergency department visits for suspected suicide attempts among persons aged 12-25 years before and during the COVID-19 Pandemic-United States. MMWR Morb Mortal Wkly Rep 2021;70(24):888–94.

57. Brown CL, Montez K, Amati JB, et al. Impact of COVID-19 on pediatric primary care visits at four academic institutions in the Carolinas. Int J Environ Res Publ Health 2021;18(11).

58. Cunniff L, Alyanak E, Fix A, et al. The impact of the COVID-19 pandemic on vaccination uptake in the United States and strategies to recover and improve vaccination rates: a review. Hum Vaccines Immunother 2023;19(2).

59. Ahluwalia R, Rocque BG, Shannon CN, et al. The impact of imposed delay in elective pediatric neurosurgery: an informed hierarchy of need in the time of mass casualty crisis. Child Nerv Sys 2020;36:1347–55.
60. Abbasi J. "This Is our COVID"—what physicians need to know about the pediatric RSV surge. JAMA 2022;328(21):2096.
61. Melhado W. Pediatric hospitals short on beds as respiratory illnesses surge among children. Available at:. The Texas Tribune; 2022 https://www.texastribune.org/2022/10/28/texas-hospitals-children-flu-covid-rsv/. [Accessed 31 October 2023].
62. Goodman B. While respiratory viruses surge, shortage of pediatric hospital beds delays care for some kids. Available at: CNN Health 2022; https://www.cnn.com/2022/10/25/health/childrens-hospital-beds-delayed-care-long-waits/index.html. [Accessed 31 October 2023].
63. Boyette C, Gumbrecht J. An "unprecedented" rise in respiratory viruses in children is overwhelming some hospitals. Available at: CNN Health 2022; https://www.cnn.com/2022/10/20/health/respiratory-viruses-hospitals/index.html. [Accessed 31 October 2023].
64. Karlamangla. RSV strains California hospitals. Available at: N Y Times 2022; https://www.nytimes.com/2022/11/29/us/rsv-california-hospitals.html. [Accessed 31 October 2023].
65. Romo V. Children's hospitals grapple with a nationwide surge in RSV infections. NPR News. October 24, 2022. Available at: https://www.npr.org/2022/10/24/1130764314/childrens-hospitals-rsv-surge. [Accessed 31 October 2023].
66. Increased respiratory virus activity, especially among children, early in the 2022-2023 fall and winter. Available at: CDC Health Alert Network 2022; https://emergency.cdc.gov/han/2022/han00479.asp. [Accessed 31 October 2023].
67. Respiratory illnesses in children-fall 2022 surge state policy actions and advocacy guidance. American Academy of Pediatrics State Advocacy. Available at: https://downloads.aap.org/doccsa/RSV_December2022.pdf. Accessed October 31, 2023.
68. Wang L, Davis PB, Berger NA, et al. Disrupted seasonality and association of COVID-19 with medically attended respiratory syncytial virus infections among young children in the US: January 2010–January 2023. medRxiv 2023. https://doi.org/10.1101/2023.05.12.23289898.
69. ASPR TRACIE roundtable. Lessons learned from the pediatric tripledemic: systems, staff, space, and supplies. ASPR TRACIE. 2023. Available at: https://asprtracie.hhs.gov/technical-resources/resource/12039/lessons-learned-from-the-pediatric-tripledemic-systems-staff-space-and-supplies-aspr-tracie-roundtable. [Accessed 30 November 2023].
70. Ruffing R, Lozon M, Bradin S, et al. Pediatric-medical operations coordinating cells (MOCC): a telehealth alternative to deployable pediatric medical assistance teams (DMATs). Pediatrics 2022;149:24, 1 Meeting Abstracts February 2022.
71. VonAchen P, Davis MM, Cartland J, et al. Closure of licensed pediatric beds in health care markets within Illinois. Acad Pediatr 2022;22(3):431–9.
72. Lin A, King MA, McCarthy DC, et al. Universal level designations for hospitalized pediatric patients in evacuation. Hosp Pediatr 2022;12(3):333–6.
73. DeLia D, Wood E. Trends - the dwindling supply of empty beds: implications for hospital surge capacity. Health Aff 2008;27(6):1688–94.
74. Li J, Baker AL, D'Ambrosi G, et al. A statewide assessment of pediatric emergency care surge capabilities. Pediatrics 2023;(4):151.

75. Hart BL, McMurtrey ME. Supply chain management: managing the supply chain in pediatric healthcare. J Strat Innovation Sustain 2018;13(3):67–74.
76. Shachar C, Gruppuso PA, Adashi EY. Pediatric drug and other shortages in the age of supply chain disruption. JAMA 2023;329(24):2127–8.
77. Lacey SR, Kilgore M, Yun H, et al. Secondary analysis of merged American Hospital Association data and US census data: beginning to understand the supply-demand chain in pediatric inpatient care. J Pediatr Nurs 2008;23(3):161–8.
78. Betz C. The call for health care reform and the pediatric nursing shortage. J Pediatr Nurs 2009;24(5):347–9.
79. Cohen RS. Regional disaster planning for neonatal intensive care. In: Arora R, Arora P, editors. Disaster management: medical preparedness, response and homeland security. 2013. https://doi.org/10.1079/9781845939298.0095.
80. McEnany FB, Ojugbele O, Doherty JR, et al. Pediatric mental health boarding. Pediatrics 2020;146(4).
81. Hodge JG, Barraza L, Piatt JL, et al. Supreme Court impacts in public health law: 2022-2023. Available at: J Law Med Ethics 2023;50(3) https://ssrn.com/abstract=4507621. [Accessed 30 November 2023].

Workforce Concerns

Professional Self Care, Personal Readiness, Impact of the Pandemic, and Other Factors that Impact the Workforce

Hilary McClafferty, MD*

KEYWORDS

- Physician burnout • COVID-19 and physician well-being
- Pediatrician burnout and wellness • Well-being centered leadership

KEY POINTS

- Pre-coronavirus disease 2019 (COVID-19) pediatricians had high burnout prevalence mirroring national trends.
- The COVID-19 pandemic took a heavy toll on physician well-being.
- Post-COVID-19 factors associated with lower burnout and increased physician well-being include a focus on organizational approaches that support physical, mental, and social well-being.

INTRODUCTION

The coronavirus disease 2019 (COVID-19) pandemic was an extraordinarily traumatic experience for individuals and organizations in healthcare. Although not necessarily the first pandemic experienced by some physicians,[1] its scope and magnitude exceeded what the majority of pediatricians in this generation have experienced. Among physicians, variables such as age, gender, educational level and stage of practice, specialty, geographic location, baseline mental health and stressors, coping skills, working conditions, workload, and levels of administrative support were some of the many demographic factors that shaped individuals' pandemic experience.

More broadly, healthcare organizations of all sizes experienced the equivalent of a stress test. Myriad pressures contributed, including staff attrition, steep financial losses, and social discord compounded by the politicization of a public health care emergency.[2] Understanding the impact of organizational stressors are important because accruing research has shown the disproportionate weight of an organization's influence

Pediatric Emergency Medicine, Tucson Medical Center, Tucson, AZ, USA
* PO Box 65865, Tucson, AZ 85728.
E-mail address: hmcclafferty@arizona.edu

Pediatr Clin N Am 71 (2024) 413–429
https://doi.org/10.1016/j.pcl.2024.03.001
0031-3955/24/© 2024 Elsevier Inc. All rights reserved.
pediatric.theclinics.com

on burnout prevalence and physician well-being. Perhaps most importantly, research has clarified that burnout is not *lack* on the part of the physician (ie, lack of resilience, stamina, empathy, compassion, and so on) but an *occupational phenomenon* resulting from a blend of organizational inertia, systems dysfunction, and ineffective leadership.[3,4] Burnout is now recognized by the World Health Organization as an occupational syndrome.[5] known to be associated with serious negative health effects.[6–9]

The COVID-19 pandemic will likely not be the last pandemic experience for many, making it critically important to analyze insights and lessons about physician well-being that will help us better prepare for the future. Although difficult to revisit, honoring the pain, trauma, and loss pediatricians experienced on both personal and professional levels is an important first step in moving forward. An overarching theme of post-pandemic analysis is the urgent need for cultural change in medicine. Identifying traits and behaviors that made us vulnerable, understanding origins, and root causes of these factors will require time, patience, and commitment.

PRE, DURING, AND POST PANDEMIC

How can we best analyze the complex trauma pediatricians experienced throughout the pandemic? For simplicity, we will consider the impact on pediatricians in a linear timeline, understanding that for many the trauma was non-linear and compounded by multiple factors.

Timeline of pediatrician's pandemic experience and impact:

- Pre-pandemic
- During pandemic
- Post-pandemic

Questions to consider at each stage:

- Where were the knowledge gaps?
- What did we learn?
- What insights should be brought forward?
- Unrepeatable mistakes?
- Unexpected benefits?
- How can these experiences help drive culture change in medicine?

Pre-Pandemic

High burnout prevalence pre-pandemic was well documented in pediatricians and pediatric trainees, mirroring that of other specialties.[10–12] One reason for this may be that character traits that initially draw trainees to the field, such as compassion and altruism, can predispose pediatricians to burnout when pushed to extremes.[13] Other factors such as caring for children who are chronically ill, maltreated, or otherwise medically vulnerable can also predispose pediatricians to compassion fatigue, vicarious traumatization, and moral distress over time, all compounders of burnout.[10] Women are also at higher risk for burnout, especially emotional exhaustion,[14–16] and now constitute a majority of pediatricians.[10,12]

Reasons for the higher burnout prevalence in women are multifactorial and under active study. Some factors may include gender bias and discrimination, especially in certain male-dominated sub-specialties, sexual harassment, and disproportionate responsibilities caring for children or elderly parents especially in mid-career physicians. Male-female salary discrepancies may also be a factor and have been documented among pediatricians. For example, a 2016 American Academy of Pediatrics survey demonstrated an earning gap of on-average 13% in early and mid-career women pediatricians compared to male colleagues after adjustment for labor force, physician-specific job, and work-family characteristics.[17] Women of color, and other underrepresented groups such as those in the physician LBGTQ community have also been shown to experience higher levels of burnout and lower levels of perceived appreciation, and control over workload, autonomy, and schedule.[18,19] Taking all into account, it is apparent that pediatricians as a group were experiencing significant levels of burnout and highly vulnerable to the forthcoming stressors of the pandemic.

During the Pandemic

During the pandemic, pediatricians like colleagues in other specialties, experienced an extraordinary array of stressors. Common themes included:

- Fear and risk of infectious exposure
- Fear of mortality
- Isolation
- Anxiety
- Depression
- Separation from family
- Potential of front-line deployment in the emergency department (ED)or intensive care unit (ICU)
- Moral distress amid ethical decisions regarding resource allocation
- Unsafe work environment, lack of protective gear
- Physical stressors such as prolonged personal protective equipment (PPE) wearing, dehydration and limited bathroom access, lack of regular meals and sleep interruption
- Loss of autonomy
- Reduction in elective procedures
- Changes to clinical schedules
- Extended or reduced work hours
- Need to continuously train new staff
- Death or illness in colleagues
- Guilt from leaving team shorthanded if one fell ill
- Workplace hostility or violence
- Extraordinary politicization of a public health emergency[2,20]

Some physicians may also have experienced triggering of the classic personality trait triad of doubt, guilt feelings, and exaggerated sense of responsibility; recognized as the compulsive triad, long recognized in normal physicians.[21]

Stressors Specific to Pediatricians

- Stressful redeployment to help manage adult patients on inpatient ward or ICU[22]
- Job security concerns due to significant drop in general pediatric patient volumes
- Drop in ED volumes, decrease in staffing hours
- Children falling behind on well-visits and immunizations
- Rebound respiratory season with pediatric respiratory illness in 2022, the "Triple-demic" of COVID/influenza/RSV.

And finally, some, primarily adult specialists in front-line care, experienced constant exposure to extreme suffering and death and the need to support patients separated from their loved ones.[2,23,24]

Women physicians in all specialties also reported compounded stress from the multiple roles they fulfilled in many households, where they often assumed primary responsibility for childcare and, during the pandemic, took a primary role in homeschooling children.[12]

Stage of Training

Stage of training was another differentiator that had a significant impact on physician experience, although a survey study from the Pediatric Resident Burnout-Resilience Consortium (PRB-RSC) failed to document significant increase in burnout among pediatric trainees during the initial stages of the pandemic compared to previous years.[25] The Accreditation Council for Graduate Medical Education (ACGME) allowed programs to selectively enforce specific requirements based on a staging system related to the severity of the pandemic at each local institution. This was in part due to a collective call for trainees to be protected both physically and emotionally from the COVID-19 pandemic.

Many trainees experienced:[26–30]

- Interruption of residency education and experiences
- Extended loss of contact to teaching faculty
- Interruption of research and lack of access to laboratories
- Increased feelings of burnout, depression, and anxiety
- Interruption in interviewing for residency and fellowship positions
- Disruption in moving into attending jobs

Post Pandemic: Insight into Action

Post pandemic an obvious need for fundamental change in health care has been highlighted based on the experiences of patients and clinicians.

What needs to change?

Identifying and understanding ingrained behavior patterns associated with higher burnout prevalence in organizations and individuals is a first step. As one example, physician, nurse, and allied health care professionals' willingness to self-sacrifice was widely publicized, and even celebrated, on media nationally and internationally during the pandemic, but at what cost? Organizations exploiting these inherent service-driven characteristics in health care workers extracted a deadly toll. A return to status quo is not sufficient.

Seeking out and normalizing attitudes and leadership behaviors associated with physician *thriving, creativity, team-building, and professional fulfillment* may be useful first steps.

In an after-action assessment of the pandemic, we have the opportunity to educate individuals and organizational leaders about how to be better prepared in the future. We can especially benefit from the research generated by the Physician Wellness Academic Consortium (PWAC)[31] and the Stanford Well MD & Well PhD Centers,[32] which have helped organize research and identify key areas, where incremental change has potential for high impact on physician health and well-being. Some of areas of active study include:

Mindset shifts

- Self-valuation
- Positive psychology
- Self-compassion

Self-care in relation to burnout prevalence

- Sleep impairment and burnout
- Nutrition in self-care and burnout

Coaching and management skills

- Physician coaching literature
- SCARF (status, certainty, autonomy, relatedness and fairness) model

Organizational well-being and leadership

- Leadership quality, self-care habits and burnout
- Organizational steps to promote sustainable well-being in individuals and teams

MINDSET SHIFTS
Self-Valuation

Self-valuation is an important emerging concept in burnout research with 2 main components:

- Appropriate prioritization of self-care rather than repeated deferment of self-care
- A growth mindset response rather than self-condemnation in response to mistakes or perceived imperfections.

Lower self-valuation may be recognizable to many readers and is associated with having lower self-compassion, treating oneself more harshly when processing mistakes, a sense of high time pressure at work, placing patient care over self-care, difficulty relaxing and reluctance to take breaks or vacations from work, difficulty allocating time for family, a feeling of excessive responsibility for things outside one's control, a sense of guilt that interferes with experiencing healthy sources of pleasure, difficulty with limit setting, and misinterpreting selfishness with healthy self-interest.[33]

Self-valuation has been shown to be significantly lower in physicians than non-physicians in national survey studies. Adjusting for self-valuation has been shown to eliminate the association between being a physician and higher risk of burnout, strongly suggesting a practice or culture of medicine influence on self-valuation.[34] Mitigating low self-valuation is a complex undertaking with high individual variability. Measuring with validated scales, raising awareness with educational initiatives, and addressing organizational practices that may consciously or unconsciously exploit physicians' low self-valuation are some potential steps forward. Physician coaching on the topic of self-valuation may be another effective way to address this issue, especially in physicians in leadership roles who have the ability to influence cultural change in institutions, or effect national policy.[34]

In addition to sense of self-valuation, which behavioral traits have been shown to be more protective and more successful in the health care setting? How can these be leveraged to effect fundamental culture change in medicine? How can individuals and organizations use this knowledge to better prepare for the next pandemic?

Positive Psychology

Another area of promising research builds on the work of Martin Seligman and Barbara Fredrickson in positive psychology.[35] At the heart of the work is the idea of cultivating positive emotion indirectly by finding positive meaning within one's current circumstances. According to Fredrickson, positive meaning can be obtained by finding benefits within adversity, by infusing ordinary events with meaning, and by effective problem solving.[35]

One example is to find benefit in an adverse situation by focusing on one's strengths and resolve rather than on the obvious negative circumstances. Meaning can help reframe ordinary events with the infusion of appreciation, love, and gratitude–even for mundane things. For example, one can find positive meaning through problem solving by supporting or initiating compassionate acts toward people in need. The initial step is positive emotion, which becomes the leverage point for finding positive meaning.

This approach helps move one away from the fear, anger, and distrust that often accompany negative emotion and allow a move into a positive "broaden and build" state of mind shown to promote creativity, more effective problem solving, discovery of novel ideas, and pro-social behavior. In turn, this promotes expansion of social bonds, enhanced social support and psychological resilience, promoting upward spirals of continued growth, and thriving. This approach can in turn positively impact your community.[36,37]

Seligman developed a shorthand name PERMA to describe the approach to enhance psychological well-being and maximize life satisfaction and creativity, which has been linked to decrease in burnout measures.[38–40]

- Positive emotion focusing on optimistic perspectives.
- Engagement, participating in enjoyable activities that stretch intellect, skills, and emotional capabilities.
- Relationships fostering meaningful social connections.
- Meaning, use of logic, religion, spirituality to gain insight into the impact of one's endeavors to lead to purposeful living.
- Accomplishments, accompaniment of goals, and recognition to create and develop sense of fulfilment.

PAUSE AND REFLECT: POSITIVE PSYCHOLOGY

- Consider how a positive psychology approach might impact your practice, department, residency program, or organization.
- Can you think of a current situation in your work life where a positive psychology approach, for example, reframing a recent event to find a positive meaning, might be helpful?

Self- Compassion

Understanding the difference between empathy (in feeling with) and compassion (concern for the suffering of others and generating a desire to help) is extremely important for health care professionals. Empathy is associated with emotional pain when witnessing another's pain or suffering, in fact, neuroimaging studies of the empathic response have shown activation of similar brain areas involved in one's own pain processing centers,[41] overall, an unsustainable approach for physicians involved in repeated exposure to suffering in day-to-day patient care.

Generating compassion for the person in pain or suffering on the other hand activates pro-social parts of the brain associated with reward, affiliation, and protection from stress as a caring perspective is adopted and a desire to help is generated.[42] Nuance here is critical; by generating compassion one is able to be aware of the other's pain without the vicarious experience of pain and suffering. Generating an excess of empathy can result in suffering, especially in repeated practice. A study by Neff[43] demonstrated that self-compassion is a skill that can be tailored and taught to health care professionals in a way that allows implementation in real-time and is associated with improvement in self-compassion scores and reduction of burnout measures and empathy fatigue.

Two large academic centers in the United States, Stanford University and Emory University, have active educational, training, and research programs in this area. The Stanford Center for Compassion and Altruism Research and Education (CCARE) investigates methods for developing compassion and promoting altruism within individuals and society through rigorous research, scientific collaborations, and academic conferences. In addition, CCARE provides compassion training programs and teacher training, as well as educational public events and programs.[44] The Emory Center for Contemplative Science and Compassion-Based Ethics offers educational programs, training, and interdisciplinary research programs.[45]

PAUSE AND REFLECT: SELF-COMPASSION

> Can you think of a recent work situation where use of self-compassion as a first response might have positively impacted your sense of self-valuation?
>
> Or may have reduced a sense of frustration or emotional exhaustion?

SELF-COMPASSION EXERCISE: ONE FOR ME, ONE FOR YOU

> - Intentionally inhale compassion for yourself.
> - Exhale compassion to the other (person, group,or situation).
> - Repeat as necessary during your workday or at home.

Self-Care Behaviors

When studied through a leadership lens, the relation of self-care behaviors and burnout prevalence is especially instructive and shows a clear association between burnout and leader's self-care behaviors.[46,47] For example, in a survey study of 1487 physicians and physician leaders at Stanford University School of Medicine, assessment of professional fulfillment, self-valuation, sleep-related impairment, and burnout showed that 9.8% of the variation in leader's aggregate leadership behavior scores was associated with their own degree of burnout. Each 1- point increase in burnout score was associated with a statistically significant drop in leadership behavior score. Interestingly, each 1-point increase in the leader's sleep-related impairment was associated with worsening sleep impairment in physicians they supervised, thought possibly related to negative role modeling of healthy sleep behavior.[46] Prioritization of personal well-being in physician leaders were also associated with lower rates of burnout and higher rating as effective leader.[47]

Evidence indicates that the leadership behaviors of physician supervisors are strongly associated with professional fulfillment and burnout among the physicians they lead. In this study, training and supporting leaders in their well-being behaviors was recommended as a particular goal of leadership development, beyond simple attention to self-care.[48] Having the confidence and organizational support to model one's own self-care behaviors in the workplace is one way to begin to effect positive culture change. This may be especially impactful for physician leaders.

Sleep

Sleep deprivation viewed as a badge of honor is embedded in the culture of medicine. It can also be considered as an occupational hazard in some regards. Sleep impairment in physicians has been well studied in relation to burnout, wellness, and clinically significant medical errors.[49]

In a study of 7700 attending physicians and house staff physicians in the Physician Wellness Academic Consortium using the well-validated Patient-Reported Outcomes Measurement Information System (PROMIS) 8-item scale that assesses tiredness, alertness, sleepiness, and functional deficits related to inadequate sleep, correlations between sleep-impairment with decreased professional fulfillment, work exhaustion, and overall burnout scores were substantial ($P < .001$) in all measures.[50] When adjusted for gender, training status, medical specialty, and burnout level and compared with low sleep-related impairment, moderate, high, and very high levels of sleep impairment in this survey study were associated with increased odds of self-reported clinically significant medical error by 53%, (odds ratio, 1.53; 95% CI, 1.12–2.09), 96% (odds ratio, 1.96; 95% CI, 1.46–2.63), and 97% (odds ratio, 1.97; 95% CI, 1.45–2.69), respectively. Additionally sleep-impairment has a high correlation with a range of negative health effects involving cardiovascular health, brain health, immune function, inflammatory response, mood, attention, and emotional processing.[51–57]

PAUSE AND REFLECT: SLEEP

- Can you bring to mind a time when you may have modeled sleep deprivation as a professional strength, especially to a trainee?
- How might you approach this differently when shaping a healthier culture in medical training?

As a foundational element of health, attention to sleep time, quality, and consistency, especially in medical training, is an area with high potential benefit as a new generation of health care professionals is trained.[50]

NUTRITION

It is widely acknowledged that physicians face significant challenges maintaining healthy nutrition in the workplace due to a variety of factors including long hours, shift work, heavy patient loads, and limited consistent access to healthy foods.[58]

In one of the relatively few studies on physician nutrition, a survey study of 245 community-based physicians evaluated associations between dietary habits and sleep related impairment.

[59] Three overarching dietary patterns were compared: plant-based, high protein, and high saturated fat and sugar. In the adjusted analysis, physicians who adhered primarily to the plant-based diet, low in saturated fats and added sugars had less sleep related impairment ($P = .027$), whereas those eating a primarily high saturated fat and added sugar had a statistically significant increase in sleep impairment measure ($P = .015$). No meaningful associations were seen in the high protein group.

Associating the nutritional component of self-care to sleep impairment builds on existing research exploring the bidirectional correlation between fatigue and cognitive performance, hormone and neurotransmitter regulation, and circadian clock disruption and inflammation.[60–62] There is a strong evidence that sleep deprivation negatively impacts dietary choices through changes in appetite related hormones that push intake of food and snacks high in sugar, sodium, fat, and saturated fat.[63–67]

PAUSE AND REFLECT: NUTRITION

Consider your nutrition during your last workday-

- Did you eat and drink fluids regularly?
- Consume healthy meals?
- Feel that you had fueled your body and brain for maximum efficiency?
- If not, what was your biggest obstacle?

There are real barriers to improving nutrition quality in physicians including lack of time, irregular schedules, heavy clinical responsibilities, lack of access to high quality food, cost, cultural factors, stigma, or embarrassment around self-care behaviors in general. However, this is an area ripe for further research, especially in medical trainees. Even incremental change will be a move in the right direction.[68]

Organizing Well-Being

There are myriad ways to organize and track individual well-being goals both independently and within a health care organization that has a 'right-mindset' toward helping physicians to improve well-bring. Menon proposes a holistic model for organizations to offer that uses 3 interrelated themes: physical wellness, wellness of mind, and social wellness, all integral to overall well-being.[69] Exploring a portfolio of options within these domains can be an important way for physicians to engage in wellness behaviors in the workplace. This may subsequently increase professional fulfillment and ultimately assist the organization maintain a healthy and engaged workforce.

Physicians can also benefit individually by following national guidelines and evidence-based health recommendations such as the American Heart Association Life's Essential 8 program.[70] The American Medical Association *STEPS forward* program also offers information about improving overall physician wellness among other topics.[71]

WELLNESS BEHAVIOR CHANGE: SIMPLY BEGIN

When considering your own well-being goals, start with a small goal that feels accessible in a domain of well-being that you are most interested in addressing. This might be as simple as committing to increasing your water intake by 10% to 15% for a week, or to taking a 5-min walk outside 3 times in a week or giving yourself a few moments of time buffer to practice self-compassion before your next clinic/surgical case/patient encounter/electronic heath record encounter. Start small and track your progress, reward yourself in a simple, healthy way as you reach your goal and move on to the next one. Build on your strengths and keep it enjoyable.

Physician Coaching

The field of physician coaching is evolving. Coaching can be used to help educate physician leaders on evidence-based practices associated with higher levels of professional fulfillment and lower burnout prevalence.[72] A 2023 systematic review by Boet, and colleagues identified 14 studies assessing the effect of coaching on physician wellness and burnout.[73] Across all studies, coaching was observed to improve several outcomes related to wellness, including work-life balance, quality of life, resilience, job satisfaction, work engagement, empowerment at work, and psychological capital. Coaching was also generally observed to decrease emotional exhaustion, distress, and burnout.

Questions remain about optimal 'dose' of coaching needed and consistency in training and preparation to effectively coach physicians. Individual physicians can independently seek out coaching in areas such as overall well-being, addressing self-valuation mindset, harnessing the power of self-compassion, mindfulness, and positive psychology to buffer from burnout and craft more enjoyable and sustainable medical careers.

One approach, especially pertinent to leadership coaching, is the SCARF model developed by David Rock, Results Coaching Systems International,[74] which builds on the work of Lieberman and Eisenberger in social neuroscience.[75,76] The SCARF model focuses on 5 domains of human social experience (status, certainty, autonomy, relatedness, and fairness). These 5 domains activate either the 'primary reward' or 'primary threat' circuitry (and associated networks) of the brain.[74]

- Status is about relative importance to others.
- Certainty concerns being able to predict the future.
- Autonomy provides a sense of control over events.
- Relatedness is a sense of safety with others, often friend rather than foe.
- Fairness is a perception of fair exchanges between people.

Familiarity with the domains teaches people, especially leaders, how to minimize unintentional threats, and activate reward responses that can help people tap into their internal reward systems. Gaining leadership skills in these areas can help increase emotional intelligence and be very useful, especially in the traditionally hierarchical academic medical setting.

PAUSE AND REFLECT: RECEIVE AND GIVE FEEDBACK

Think of a time when you received feedback from a team leader.

Could the experience have been handled more skillfully?

Now think of a time when you had to provide feedback to a team member.

Did you offer respect and acknowledgment of their importance to the team?

Provide an overview of progress and next steps?

Encourage a sense of autonomy proportional to their level of training?

Relate as a colleague invested in their success?

Give them a sense of being fairly treated?

SUMMARY

The COVID-19 pandemic acutely refocused attention on the disproportionate impact of organization culture and work environment on physician well-being. Substantial research has accrued in the field of physician burnout and well-being, which can be leveraged to shape a healthier culture of medicine. Post-pandemic, organizations have an important opportunity to move on from an outdated medical culture of unrealistic expectations and endurance.[77] When we consider the toll, is there really a choice?

Shanafelt, an internationally recognized leader in the field, has proposed a next article called 'Well-being 2.0', where the focus must shift away from the individual toward healthcare systems reform, with processes, leadership and teamwork designed to support physician well-being,[77] a philosophy endorsed by the National Academy of Medicine Action Collaborative on Clinician Well-being.[78]

In the Well-being 2.0 phase, the definition of burnout as an occupational syndrome is embraced,[5] instruments for measuring burnout have been well-validated, and clear distinctions have been made between work-driven burnout and separate mental health conditions. The focus has moved on from simply reducing burnout prevalence to deliberately cultivating organizational driven well-being. Elements of this approach include.

- Chief Wellness Officers who function at the C-suite level to address systems-based issues and infrastructure.
- Human focused information technology, engineering, and design are embraced.
- Health care professionals' needs are considered alongside patient needs.
- Self-compassion and vulnerability are accepted positive human emotions in physicians.
- Teams are cared for with professionalism, just-culture, flexibility, and support.
- Sleep and work-life integration are prioritized.
- Wellness is viewed as a core organizational strategy.
- Diversity, equity, and inclusion are foundational tenets to the organization.
- Modern training programs embrace these ideas as core competencies related to the whole health of individual physicians.

The overarching goal is to move forward in a new phase, where physicians are viewed as valued human beings who function successfully within the boundaries of normal limitations (they eat, sleep, exercise, practice routine self-care, take breaks and vacations, attend to personal and family needs and so on), without ridicule, censure, or professional penalty. Well-being is normalized, expected, and consciously cultivated on the organizational and personal levels. This will not happen spontaneously; it will take deliberate and concerted effort to make the shift.

To aid in this process, a model of Wellness Centered Leadership has been developed as an evidence-based path forward.[79] The 3 core elements of this approach include:

- Care about people always.
- Cultivate individual and team relationships.
- Professional fulfillment.

Each of these 3 components is further broken down to provide a detailed map on how to move this work forward.

- Mindset (including attitude and intention of the leader)
- Behaviors (including actions that bring out desired outcomes)
- Outcomes (interim measures of effectiveness focused on developing a culture of wellness).

CONCLUSION

Post-COVID-19, advancements in our understanding of physician well-being are encouraging, especially with respect to the impact of workplace and organizational culture. In addition to the research and programs discussed, individual physicians can take initiative to enhance to their overall well-being by exploring foundational elements of health such as sleep, nutrition, physical activity, stress management, and social connections. Positive mindset has also been shown to be a powerful protective buffer, especially in the areas of self-valuation, self-compassion, and positive psychology. Physician coaching is emerging as a potentially useful option to help support and accelerate an individual's positive behavior change.

When reflecting on one's individual experience of the COVID-19 pandemic, it may be valuable to consider on your perceived well-being pre, during, and post-pandemic. Questions to consider-

- Where were your knowledge gaps?
- What did you learn?
- What insights can you bring forward?
- Unrepeatable mistakes?
- Unexpected benefits?
- How can you use your experiences to contribute to positive culture change in medicine?

CLINICS CARE POINTS

Post-COVID-19 factors associated with lower burnout and increased physician well-being.

- Prioritization of individual and team well-being and safety, especially adequate staffing and physical resources.
- Positive well-being scores in physician leaders.
- Close alignment of values with one's physician leader.
- Perception of high psychosocial support from one's organization.
- Organizational commitment to all aspects of physician's well-being, including physical wellness, wellness of mind, and social wellness.
- Support for physician coaching to help implement wellness behaviors.
- Mindset elements such as higher self-valuation, self-compassion, and positive psychology.

DISCLOSURE

No conflicts of interest to disclose.

REFERENCES

1. Magnavita N, Chirico F, Garbarino S, et al. SARS/MERS/SARS-CoV-2 Outbreaks and burnout syndrome among healthcare workers. An umbrella systematic review. Int J Environ Res Publ Health 2021;18(8):4361.
2. Agata S, Grzegorz W, Ilona B, et al. Prevalence of burnout among healthcare professionals during the COVID-19 pandemic. Int J Occup Med Environ Health 2023;36(1):21–58.

3. Shanafelt T, Stolz S, Springer J, et al. A blueprint for organizational strategies to promote the well-being of health care professionals. NEJM Catal innov Care Deliv 2020;1(6). https://doi.org/10.1056/CAT.20.0266.

4. Shanafelt T, Larson D, Bohman B, et al. Organization-wide approaches to foster effective unit-level efforts to improve clinician well-being. Mayo Clin Proc 2023; 98(1):163–80.

5. International Classifications of Diseases. 11th revision (ICD-11). World Health Organization; 2019. Available at. https://www.Who.Int/Classifications/Icd/En/. [Accessed 30 November 2023].

6. West CP, Tan AD, Shanafelt TD. Association of resident fatigue and distress with occupational blood and body fluid exposures and motor vehicle incidents. Mayo Clin Proc 2012;87(12):1138–44.

7. Brown SD, Goske MJ, Johnson CM. Beyond substance abuse: stress, burnout, and depression as causes of physician impairment and disruptive behavior. J Am Coll Radiol 2009;6(7):479–85.

8. Shanafelt TD, Balch CM, Dyrbye L, et al. Special report: suicidal ideation among American surgeons. Arch Surg 2011;146(1):54–62.

9. van der Heijden F, Dillingh G, Bakker A, et al. Suicidal thoughts among medical residents with burnout. Arch Suicide Res 2008;12(4):344–6.

10. McClafferty H, Hubbard D, Foradori D, et al, SECTION ON INTEGRATIVE MEDICINE. AAP Section on Integrative Medicine. Physician health and wellness. Pediatrics 2022;150(5). e2022059665.

11. Kemper KJ, Schwartz A, Wilson PM, et al, PEDIATRIC RESIDENT BURNOUT-RESILIENCE STUDY CONSORTIUM. Pediatric resident burnout-resilience study consortium. Burnout in pediatric residents: three years of national survey data. Pediatrics 2020;145(1). e20191030.

12. Kumar G, Mezoff A. Physician burnout at a children's hospital: incidence, interventions, and impact. Pediatr Qual Saf 2020;5:e345.

13. Gogo A, Osta A, McClafferty H, et al. Cultivating a way of being and doing: individual strategies for physician well-being and resilience. Curr Probl Pediatr Adolesc Health Care 2019;49(12):100663.

14. McMurray JE, Linzer M, Konrad TR, et al. The work lives of women physicians: results from the Physician Work-Life Study. J Gen Intern Med 2000;15(6):372–80.

15. Dyrbye LN, Shanafelt TD, Sinsky CA, et al. Burnout among health care professionals: a call to explore and address this underrecognized threat to safe, high quality care. *NAM Perspectives.* Discussion Paper. Washington, DC: National Academy of Medicine; 2017. Available at: https://nam.edu/wp-content/uploads/2017/07/Burnout-Among-Health-Care-Professionals-A-Call-to-Explore-and-Address-This-Underrecognized-Threat.pdf. [Accessed 7 November 2023].

16. Templeton K, Bernstein CA, Sukhera J, et al. Gender-based differences in burnout: issues faced by women physicians. *NAM Perspec*tives. Discussion Paper. Washington, DC: National Academy of Medicine; 2019. Available at: https://nam.edu/wp-content/uploads/2019/05/Gender-Based-Differences-in-Burnout.pdf. [Accessed 7 November 2023].

17. Frintner MP, Sisk B, Byrne BJ, et al. Gender differences in earnings of early- and midcareer pediatricians. Pediatrics 2019;144(4):e20183955.

18. Rotenstein LS, Torre M, Ramos MA, et al. Prevalence of burnout among physicians: a systematic review. JAMA 2018;320(11):1131–50.

19. Osseo-Asare A, Balasuriya L, Huot SJ, et al. Minority resident physicians' views on the role of race/ethnicity in their training experiences in the workplace. JAMA Netw Open 2018;1(5):e182723.

20. Kiang M, Carlasare L, Israni S, et al. Excess mortality among US physicians during the COVID-19 pandemic. JAMA Intern Med 2023;183(4):374–6.
21. Gabbard G. The role of compulsiveness in the normal physician. JAMA 1985; 254(20):2926–9.
22. Belfer J, Feld L, Jan S, et al. The effect of the COVID-19 pandemic on pediatric physician wellness: a cross-sectional study. Int J Environ Res Publ Health 2022; 19(6):3745.
23. Kelker H, Yoder K, Musey P, et al. Longitudinal prospective study of emergency medicine provider wellness across ten academic and community hospitals during the initial surge of the COVID-19 pandemic. Res Square 2020;3:87786.
24. Sharafi M, Asadi-Pooya AA, Mousavi-Roknabadi RS. Burnout among healthcare providers of COVID-19; a systematic review of epidemiology and recommendations. Arch Acad Emerg Med 2020;9(1):e7.
25. Zuniga LM, Schuh A, Schwartz A, et al, Pediatric Resident Burnout and Resilience Study Consortium. Burnout during the COVID-19 pandemic: a report on pediatric residents. Acad Pediatr 2023;23(8):1620–7.
26. Accreditation Council for Graduate Medical Education. Resident/fellow education and training considerations related to coronavirus (COVID-19). ACGME; 2020. Available at: https://acgme.org/Newsroom/Newsroom-Details/ArticleID/10085/ACGME-Resident-Fellow-Education-and-Training-Considerations-related-to-Coronavirus-COVID-19. [Accessed 7 November 2023].
27. Harrington RA, Elkind MS, Benjamin IJ. Protecting medical trainees on the COVID-19 frontlines saves us all. Circulation 2020;141:e778.
28. Kadhum M, Farrell S, Hussain R, et al. Mental wellbeing and burnout in surgical trainees: implications for the post-COVID-19 era. Br J Surg 2020;107:e264.
29. Accreditation Council for Graduate Medical Education. Three stages of GME during the COVID-19 pandemic. ACGME. Available at: https://www.acgme.org/COVID-19/-Archived-Three-Stages-of-GME-During-the-COVID-19-Pandemic/. [Accessed 7 November 2023].
30. Spitzer C, Allen Sinha T, Haddad D, et al. Tips for pandemic response planning for Internal medicine training programs. MedEdPublish 2020;9:182.
31. Physician Wellness Academic Consortium (PWAC). Healthcare professional wellbeing academic consortium. Available at: https://healthcarepwac.org. [Accessed 7 November 2023].
32. Stanford W. Stanford medicine. Available at: https://wellmd.stanford.edu. [Accessed 7 November 2023].
33. Trockel M, Hamidi MS, Menon NK, et al. Self-valuation: attending to the most important instrument in the practice of medicine. Mayo Clin Proc 2019;94(10): 2022–31.
34. Trockel M, Sinsky C, West CP, et al. Self-valuation challenges in the culture and practice of medicine and physician well-being. Mayo Clin Proc 2021;96(8): 2123–32.
35. Fredrickson B. The value of positive emotions. The emerging science of positive psychology is coming to understand why it's good to feel good. Am Scientist 2003;91:330–5.
36. Fredrickson B, Joiner T. 2002. Positive emotions trigger upward spirals toward emotional well-being. Psychol Sci 2002;13:172–5.
37. Fredrickson B, Tugade M, Waugh C, et al. What good are positive emotions in crises? A prospective study of resilience and emotions following the terrorist attacks on the United States on September 11th, 2001. J Personality Soc Psychol 2003; 84:365–76.

38. Bazargan-Hejazi S, Shirazi A, Wang A, et al. Contribution of a positive psychology-based conceptual framework in reducing physician burnout and improving well-being: a systematic review. BMC Med Educ 2021;21:593.
39. Shaghaghi F, Abedian Z, Forouhar M, et al. Effect of positive psychology interventions on psychological well-being of midwives: a randomized clinical trial. J Educ Health Promot 2019;8:160.
40. Lianov L. A powerful antidote to physician burnout: intensive healthy lifestyle and positive psychology approaches. Am J Lifestyle Med 2021;15(5):563–6.
41. Klimecki O, Leiberg S, Ricard M, et al. Differential pattern of functional brain plasticity after compassion and empathy training. Soc Cognit Affect Neurosci 2014; 9(6):873–9.
42. Klimecki O, Singer T. Empathic distress fatigue rather than compassion fatigue? Integrating findings from empathy research in psychology and social neuroscience. In: Oakley B, Knafo A, Madhavan C, et al, editors. Pathological altruism. New York, NY: Oxford University Press; 2012.
43. Neff KD, Knox MC, Long P, et al. Caring for others without losing yourself: an adaptation of the mindful self-compassion program for healthcare communities. J Clin Psychol 2020;76(9):1543–62.
44. The Center for Compassion and Altruism Research and Education. Stanford University CCARE. Available at: https://ccare.stanford.edu/. [Accessed 7 November 2023].
45. Emory center for contemplative science and compassion-based ethics. Emory University. Available at: https://www.compassion.emory.edu. [Accessed 7 November 2023].
46. Shanafelt TD, Gorringe G, Menaker R, et al. Impact of organizational leadership on physician burnout and satisfaction. Mayo Clin Proc 2015;90(4):432–40.
47. Shanafelt TD, Noseworthy JH. Executive leadership and physician well-being: nine organizational strategies to promote engagement and reduce burnout. Mayo Clin Proc 2017;92(1):129–46.
48. Shanafelt T, Makowski M, Wang H, et al. Association of burnout, professional fulfillment, and self-care practices of physician leaders with their independently rated leadership effectiveness. JAMA Netw Open 2020;3(6):e207961.
49. Gates M, Wingert A, Featherstone R, et al. Impact of fatigue and insufficient sleep on physician and patient outcomes: a systematic review. BMJ Open 2018;8: e021967.
50. Trockel MT, Menon NK, Rowe SG, et al. Assessment of physician sleep and wellness, burnout, and clinically significant medical errors. JAMA Netw Open 2020; 3(12):e2028111.
51. Cedernaes J, Osorio R, Varga A, et al. Candidate mechanisms underlying the association between sleep-wake disruptions and Alzheimer's disease. Sleep Med Rev 2017;31:102–11.
52. Cappuccio F, Cooper D, D'Elia L, et al. Sleep duration predicts cardiovascular outcomes: a systematic review and meta-analysis of prospective studies. Eur Heart J 2011;32(12):1484–92.
53. Tsuno N, Besset A, Ritchie K. Sleep and depression. J Clin Psychiatry 2005; 66(10):1254–69.
54. Bernert RA, Turvey CL, Conwell Y, et al. Association of poor subjective sleep quality with risk for death by suicide during a 10-year period: a longitudinal, population-based study of late life. JAMA Psychiatr 2014;71(10):1129–37.
55. Hayley A, Williams L, Venugopa IK, et al. The relationships between insomnia, sleep apnoea and depression: findings from the American National Health and

Nutrition Examination Survey, 2005-2008. Aust N Z J Psychiatr 2015;49(2): 156–70.

56. Krause A, Simon E, Mander BA, et al. The sleep deprived human brain. Nat Rev Neurosci 2017;18(7):404–18.
57. Yoo S-S, Gujar N, Hu P, et al. The human emotional brain without sleep: a prefrontal amygdala disconnect. Curr Biol 2007;17(20):R877–8.
58. Hamidi M, Boggild M, Cheung A. Running on empty: a review of nutrition and physicians' well-being. Postgrad Med 2016;92:478–80.
59. Lemaire J, Wallace J, Dinsmore K, et al. Food for thought: an exploratory study of how physicians experience poor workplace nutrition. Nutr J 2011;10:18.
60. St-Onge M, Mikic A, Pietrolungo C. Effects of diet on sleep quality. Adv Nutr 2016; 7:938–49.
61. Parletta N, Milte C, Meyer B. Nutritional modulation of cognitive function and mental health. J Nutr Biochem 2013;24:725–43.
62. Oosterman J, Kalsbeek A, La Fleur S, et al. Impact of nutrients on circadian rhythmicity. Am J Physiol Regul Integr Comp Physiol 2015;308:R337–50.
63. Broussard J, Kilkus J, Delebecque F, et al. Elevated ghrelin predicts food intake during experimental sleep restriction. Obesity 2016;24:132–8.
64. Pardi D, Buman M, Black J, et al. Eating decisions based on alertness levels after a single night of sleep manipulation: a randomized clinical trial. Sleep 2017;40(2). https://doi.org/10.1093/sleep/zsw039.
65. St-Onge M, Wolfe S, Sy M, et al. Sleep restriction increases the neuronal response to unhealthy food in normal-weight individuals. Int J Obes (Lond). 2014;38:411–6.
66. Greer S, Goldstein A, Walker M. The impact of sleep deprivation on food desire in the human brain. Nat Commun 2013;4:2259.
67. Hanlon E, Andrzejewski M, Harder B, et al. The effect of REM sleep deprivation on motivation for food reward. Behav Brain Res 2005;163:58–69.
68. Hamidi M, Shanafelt T, Hausel A, et al. Associations between dietary patterns and sleep-related impairment in a cohort of community physicians: a cross-sectional study. Am J Lifestyle Med 2021;15(6):644–52.
69. Menon N, Trockel M, Hamidi M, et al. Developing a portfolio to support physician's efforts to promote well-being: one piece of the puzzle. Mayo Clin Proc 2019;94(11):2171–7.
70. American Heart Association Life's Essential 8 Fact Sheet. Available at: https://www.heart.org/en/healthy-living/healthy-lifestyle/lifes-essential-8/lifes-essential-8-fact-sheet. [Accessed 7 November 2023].
71. STEPS forward. American Medical Association Ed Hub. Available at: https://edhub.ama-assn.org/steps-forward. [Accessed 7 November 2023].
72. Gazelle G, Liebschutz J, Riess H. Physician coaching: a way out. J Gen Intern Med 2015;30(4):508–13.
73. Boet S, Etherington C, Dion PM, et al. Impact of coaching on physician wellness: a systematic review. PLoS One 2023;18(2):e0281406. Article e0281406.
74. Results coaching. Results Coaching Global. Available at: https://resultscoachingglobal.com. [Accessed 30 November 2023].
75. Lieberman M, Eisenberger N, Crockett M, et al. Putting feelings into words: affect labelling disrupts amygdala activity in response to affective stimuli. Psychol Sci 2007;18(5):421–8.
76. Eisenberger N, Lieberman M. Why it hurts to be left out: the neurocognitive overlap between physical and social pain. Trends Cognit Sci 2004;8:294–300.

77. Shanafelt TD. Physician well-being 2.0: where are we and where are we going? Mayo Clin Proc 2021 Oct;96(10):2682–93.
78. National Academies of Sciences, Engineering, and Medicine; Committee on Systems Approaches to Improve Patient Care by Supporting Clinician Well-being. Taking action against clinician burnout: a systems approach to professional well-being. Washington, DC: The National Academies Press; 2019.
79. Shanafelt T, Trockel M, Rodriguez A, et al. Wellness-centered leadership: equipping health care leaders to cultivate physician well-being and professional fulfillment. Acad Med 2021;96(5):641–51.

Infection Prevention and Control Implications of Special Pathogens in Children

Larry K. Kociolek, MD, MSCI[a],*, Andi L. Shane, MD, MPH, MSc[b],
Kari A. Simonsen, MD, MBA[c], Danielle M. Zerr, MD, MPH[d]

KEYWORDS

- Infection control • Infection prevention • Preparedness • Special pathogen
- High-consequence infectious diseases • Ebola • Marburg • Mpox

KEY POINTS

- Special pathogens are broadly defined as highly transmissible organisms capable of causing severe infection and disease in humans.
- Children's hospital healthcare personnel (HCP) should be prepared to screen and identify patients possibly infected with a special pathogen, isolate the patient to minimize transmission, and inform key infection prevention, clinical, and public health stakeholders.
- Special pathogen preparedness requires resources and practice with attention to education, policies and procedures, drills and training, and supplies.
- Because of the importance of family-centered and child-centered care, children's hospitals should be prepared to modify their typical care model when necessary to prevent special pathogen transmission to patient caregivers and HCP.

INTRODUCTION

Special pathogens are broadly defined as highly transmissible infectious agents capable of causing severe disease in humans. The currently practicing healthcare workforce has witnessed the emergence of several special pathogens during their careers, as well as reemergence and international spread of rarely encountered known

[a] Department of Pediatrics, Northwestern University Feinberg School of Medicine, Ann & Robert H. Lurie Children's Hospital of Chicago, 225 East Chicago Avenue, Box 20, Chicago, IL 60611, USA; [b] Department of Pediatrics, Emory University School of Medicine and Children's Healthcare of Atlanta, Emory Children's Center, 2015 Uppergate Drive Northeast, Room 504A, Atlanta, GA 30322, USA; [c] Department of Pediatrics, University of Nebraska Medical Center, 982162 Nebraska Medical Center, Omaha, NE 68198, USA; [d] Department of Pediatrics, University of Washington, Seattle Children's Hospital, Mailstop MA7.226, 4800 Sand Point Way, Seattle, WA 98105, USA
* Corresponding author.
E-mail address: Lkociolek@luriechildrens.org

Pediatr Clin N Am 71 (2024) 431–454
https://doi.org/10.1016/j.pcl.2024.01.014
0031-3955/24/© 2024 Elsevier Inc. All rights reserved.

pathogens. These include novel coronaviruses, novel influenza viruses, and ebolaviruses. Some of these reached pandemic levels and/or had profound impact on human morbidity and mortality, global economics, and healthcare delivery. Special pathogens present substantial challenges to healthcare systems for ensuring the delivery of safe and effective health care while minimizing spread of disease to healthcare personnel (HCP), patients, and families.

Hospital infection prevention and control (IPC) teams are essential for developing special pathogen policies and practices that enable HCP to *identify* patients with exposures to and/or signs and symptoms of a special pathogen as early as possible, allowing HCP to first *isolate* the patient and implement pathogen-specific and/or disease-specific mitigation measures, and then *inform* the IPC team and other stakeholders to ensure delivery of safe and high-quality care.[1] Children's hospital IPC teams and other key stakeholders have unique challenges in balancing developmentally appropriate family-centered care with keeping essential caregivers, visitors, and the community safe. In this review, we highlight the IPC implications of special pathogens in children.

CLASSIFICATION OF SPECIAL PATHOGENS

Special pathogen classification, contributing factors, available countermeasures, and risks to pediatric patients and HCP vary widely among pathogens. The following are general categories of special pathogens; some pathogens may have features of multiple categories.

High-consequence infectious diseases (HCIDs): HCIDs are special pathogens that are particularly severe and lack medical countermeasures (MCMs). HCIDs generally meet several of the following criteria[2]: (1) acute infectious disease; (2) high case-fatality rate; (3) effective prophylaxis and/or treatment are lacking; (4) difficult to recognize and detect rapidly; (5) ability to spread in the community and within healthcare settings; (6) requires an enhanced individual, population and system response to ensure it is managed effectively, efficiently, and safely. HCIDs may be novel pathogens (eg, avian influenza and novel coronaviruses) or known pathogens (eg, mpox and viral hemorrhagic fever [VHF] viruses, including ebolaviruses and Marburg virus) that reemerge and spread related to behavioral risk factors or factors associated with novel pathogen emergence and spread described in later discussion. HCIDs such as VHFs may require highly specialized biocontainment and/or other IPC practices to mitigate risk to HCP. As witnessed with coronavirus disease 2019 (COVID-19), as a pandemic evolves and MCMs are developed, knowledge of HCID treatment and prevention can increase. If the clinical consequences for individual patients decline, the pathogen may no longer be considered an HCID but it may continue to require strong hospital IPC and public health responses and management.

Novel pathogens: Many novel pathogens, including novel coronaviruses (eg, severe acute respiratory syndrome [SARS], Middle Eastern respiratory syndrome [MERS], and severe acute respiratory syndrome coronavirus 2 [SARS-CoV-2]) and avian influenza viruses, have emerged during the past 2 decades. At the time of their emergence, an understanding of pathogenesis and the clinical spectrum of disease, diagnostics, and MCMs were often lacking, leading to initial challenges in identifying the infection and mitigating disease and transmission. Novel human pathogens are often zoonotic in origin and emerge and spread when the human–animal interface is perturbed, possibly related to agricultural practices or increased infrastructure development in previously remote areas.[3] International transmission is promoted through migration and/or international travel, especially for infections that spread through the respiratory tract by those with mild or subclinical illness (eg, COVID-19). Novel pathogens can cause high incidence of disease in HCP,[4] sometimes with high mortality rates.[5]

Vaccine-preventable diseases: Factors such as vaccine hesitancy and disparities in vaccine access,[6,7] both of which were exacerbated by the COVID-19 pandemic, result in declining population vaccination rates. This has resulted in outbreaks of several vaccine-preventable diseases,[7] such as measles and poliovirus, which have hospital IPC implications.

Agents of bioterrorism: Several pathogens and/or their toxins are considered agents of bioterrorism, as defined by the US Centers for Disease Control and Prevention (CDC),[8] that vary by disease severity, ease of dissemination, and necessary level of public health preparedness efforts. The extent of person-to-person transmission varies among agents, and therefore, the risk to HCP and necessary IPC mitigation measures also varies (**Table 1**).

DISCUSSION
Identify, Isolate, and Inform

CDC guidance for optimal management of patients with special pathogens uses the construct of "Identify, Isolate, and Inform." The concept calls for healthcare institutions to determine strategies to identify patients who are at risk for a special pathogen as early as possible on entry to the organization so that they may be appropriately isolated and essential notifications can take place. These strategies should be informed by the current landscape of global, regional, and local transmission for each pathogen. For instance, a small Ebola virus disease (EVD) outbreak within the borders of one country may trigger screening of patients in neighboring countries, whereas a large EVD outbreak that has spread to involve multiple countries, may initiate more widespread screening. The CDC Health Alert Network (https://emergency.cdc.gov/han/) provides information about urgent public health incidents. These, along with local or state public health notices, can provide the trigger for active screening.

Identify

Identifying high-risk patients requires stepwise screening of exposure history and signs and symptoms of disease. The exposure history should include questions related to travel, epidemiologic risk factors, and known or potential exposures to proven cases. For example, the CDC has provided an algorithm to assist with screening for EVD.[9] The first step of the algorithm calls for screening for travel to a country with ongoing Ebola transmission or contact with an individual with confirmed EVD within the previous 21 days. If the patient answers "yes" to either of these prompts, then they are screened for fever, headache, weakness, muscle pain, vomiting, diarrhea, abdominal pain, or hemorrhage. Although this algorithm was developed for EVD, a similar approach can be implemented for any pathogen. For example, if a large measles outbreak has spread beyond an isolated region, screening can include travel to the affected region or known exposure to a case and symptoms and signs of measles. With measles and other vaccine-preventable pathogens, it is also important to collect vaccination history to better understand the likelihood of infection. Washington State Department of Health[10] developed an assessment tool[11] to help clinicians assess the risk of measles in patients presenting with concerning exposure history or symptoms of disease. Electronic health record systems are important tools that can be leveraged to enable travel and symptom screening.[12]

Table 1
Agents of bioterrorism[8] and patient isolation precautions after infection is confirmed

Agent	Precautions
Category A (highest priority): easily disseminated or transmitted from person to person; high-mortality rate; potential for major public health impact; may cause public panic and social disruption; and requires special action for public health preparedness	
Anthrax (Bacillus anthracis)	Contact precautions (cutaneous) and standard precautions (gastrointestinal or respiratory)
Botulism (Clostridium botulinum toxin)	Standard precautions
Plague (Yersinia pestis)	Droplet precautions
Smallpox (variola major)	Airborne-contact precautions
Tularemia (Francisella tularensis)	Standard precautions
VHFs, including Filoviruses (Ebola, Marburg)	HCID special precautions/biocontainment
Arenaviruses (Lassa, Machupo)	HCID special precautions/biocontainment
Category B: moderately easy to disseminate; moderate morbidity rate and low mortality rate; and require specific enhancements of CDC's diagnostic capacity and enhanced disease surveillance	
Brucellosis (Brucella species)	Contact precautions (if patient diapered or incontinent), otherwise standard
Epsilon toxin of Clostridium perfringens	Standard precautions
Food safety threats (Salmonella species, Escherichia coli O157:H7, Shigella)	Contact precautions
Glanders (Burkholderia mallei)	Airborne-contact precautions
Melioidosis (Burkholderia pseudomallei)	Airborne-contact precautions if pneumonia, otherwise standard precautions
Psittacosis (Chlamydia psittaci)	Standard precautions
Q fever (Coxiella burnetii)	Airborne precautions (when performing aerosol-generating procedures), otherwise contact precautions
Ricin toxin from Ricinus communis (castor beans)	Level B PPE, self-contained breathing apparatus, disposable Tyvek suite coated with Saranex or polyethylene to prevent penetration, air purifying respirator with P-100 filter, and eye and face protection such as a full-face respirator
Staphylococcal enterotoxin B	Contact precautions
Typhus (Rickettsia prowazekii)	Standard precautions
Viral encephalitis (alphaviruses, such as eastern equine encephalitis, Venezuelan equine encephalitis, and western equine encephalitis])	Standard precautions
Water safety threats (Vibrio cholerae and Cryptosporidium parvum)	Contact precautions
Category C: emerging pathogens that could be engineered for mass dissemination in the future because of availability; ease of production and dissemination; and potential for high morbidity and mortality rates and major health impact	
Nipah virus	HCID special precautions/biocontainment
Hantavirus	Standard precautions

Abbreviation: HCID, high-consequence infectious disease.

Isolate

Once a patient of concern is identified, they should be isolated immediately using optimal rooming and personal protective equipment (PPE) for the specific organism of concern (**Table 2**). Depending on the pathogen, such as for VHFs, high-level biocontainment may be needed. Few hospitals have dedicated biocontainment units but all hospitals should determine where they would care for patients with special pathogens such as VHFs. Identification of the space in advance allows for planning for traffic control, how the space will be used (locations for donning and doffing, and so forth), and simulation within the space. Healthcare organizations should document where their negative pressure and airborne infection isolation rooms (AIIRs)[13] are located and plan for how these rooms will be utilized. Notably, not all negative pressure rooms are AIIRs. AIIRs are not only negatively pressured but they also have at least 6 to 12 air changes per hour and directly exhaust the air from the room to the outside of the building (or recirculate it through a high-efficiency particulate air [HEPA] filter before returning to circulation). Depending on the size of the room, higher air exchange rates may reduce the amount of time the room needs remain vacant after a patient with an airborne infection occupies it. AIIRs are the best option for patients with suspected or confirmed airborne transmitted infectious diseases; however, their numbers are limited in many institutions. If an AIIR is not available, patients should be transferred to an institution with AIIRs as soon as is feasible. While awaiting transfer, a negative pressure room should be used. If a negative pressure room is not available, then a single occupancy room should be used with the door closed. Additional steps that may be taken to prevent transmission while awaiting transfer are to place a face mask on the patient when possible and/or utilize a portable HEPA filtered air purifier.

The transport of patients with special pathogens within the facility should be limited and routes through the facility should be mindfully planned to limit exposure to others. When a patient with a suspected or proven airborne infection is outside the AIIR, respiratory etiquette should be encouraged, including placing a face mask on the patient when possible, or for patients unable to wear a mask, placing a light blanket over their head. For diseases spread through other routes, such as through infectious skin lesions, lesions should be covered with a sheet and/or gown.

PPE varies by pathogen (see **Table 2**); however, in all cases, the importance of donning and doffing cannot be overstated. Using the recommended sequence[14] for donning PPE will enable efficient and appropriate application of the PPE to help prevent contamination events during patient care. Careful and deliberate doffing, including following the recommended sequence and noting opportunities for PPE cleaning and disinfection, will decrease the risk of self-contamination during the process. Use of a dedicated space and a trained observer for donning and doffing will help ensure that correct donning and doffing sequences are followed. These steps would ideally be followed for all special pathogens and should be considered required for patients with VHF.

Environmental cleaning and waste management recommendations vary according to the pathogen (see **Table 2**). The labels of cleaning and disinfection products should be reviewed for claims against specific pathogens, and the manufacturer's instructions and recommended disinfectant dwell times should be followed. When planning for waste management, the relevant local and federal regulations should be incorporated.

Keeping a log of all individuals entering the patient room is recommended for patients with VHF viruses or MERS-CoV. Strategies for staffing ratios will vary by pathogen and should consider the type of PPE being worn by healthcare workers (eg, Occupational Safety and Health Administration [OSHA] requirements for rest time)

Table 2
Minimum requirements for room placement and personal protective equipment per CDC guidance by pathogen

	Proven EVD[a] OR Unstable[b] PUI	Stable EVD[a] PUI without Vomiting, Diarrhea or Bleeding	Emerging Respiratory Viruses (eg, MERS-CoV, Avian Influenza)[14]	Mpox[52]	Measles[53]
Room placement	Single patient room with closed door and private bathroom or covered bedside commode *AIIR if AGPs will be performed*	Single patient room with closed door and private bathroom or covered bedside commode *AIIR if AGPs will be performed*	AIIR	Single patient room with closed door and private bathroom *AIIR if AGPs will be performed*	AIIR
PPE					
Gloves	Single-use (disposable) gloves with extended cuffs. Two pairs of gloves should be worn. At a minimum, outer gloves should have extended cuffs Frequently decontaminate gloves during care with an alcohol-based hand rub	Single-use (disposable) gloves with extended cuffs. Two pairs of gloves should be worn. At a minimum, outer gloves should have extended cuffs	Single-use (disposable) gloves	Single-use (disposable) gloves	Standard precautions
Eye protection	Single-use (disposable) full face shield	Single-use (disposable) full face shield	Single-use (disposable) eye protection or reusable eye protection, which is cleaned and disinfected prior to reuse	Single-use (disposable) eye protection or reusable eye protection, which is cleaned and disinfected prior to reuse	Standard precautions

Mask/respirator	Fit-tested N95 or a respirator with a higher level of protection, such as a PAPR	Single-use (disposable) facemask	Fit-tested N95 or a respirator with a higher level of protection	Fit-tested N95 or a respirator with a higher level of protection	Fit-tested N95 or a respirator with a higher level of protection
Gown/coveralls	Single-use (disposable) fluid-*impermeable*[54] coveralls without integrated hood OR gown that extends to at least midcalf. Single-use (disposable) apron that covers the torso to the level of the midcalf	Single-use (disposable) fluid-*resistant*[55] coveralls without integrated hood OR gown that extends to at least midcalf	Clean, disposable gown	Clean, disposable gown	Standard precautions
Shoe/boot covers	Single-use (disposable) boot covers that extend to at least midcalf	Not required	Not required	Not required	Not required
Other	Consider standardized garment under PPE: scrubs or disposable garments and dedicated washable footwear	Consider standardized garment under PPE: scrubs or disposable garments and dedicated washable footwear	N/A	N/A	Healthcare workers entering the room should have evidence of immunity to measles

Environmental infection control

(continued on next page)

Table 2
(continued)

	Proven EVD[a] OR Unstable[b] PUI	Stable EVD[a] PUI without Vomiting, Diarrhea or Bleeding	Emerging Respiratory Viruses (eg, MERS-CoV, Avian Influenza)[14]	Mpox[52]	Measles[53]
Environmental cleaning	A product recommended for use against Ebola virus[56] should be used for environmental cleaning and disinfection Immediately clean visibly contaminated equipment and surfaces Regularly clean and disinfect in the absence of visible contamination	A product recommended for use against Ebola virus[56] should be used for environmental cleaning and disinfection Immediately clean visibly contaminated equipment and surfaces Regularly clean and disinfect in the absence of visible contamination	Standard cleaning and disinfection procedures using a product with a MERS-CoV or other human coronavirus claim	Standard cleaning and disinfection procedures using a product with an emerging viral pathogen claim[57] Soiled laundry should be gently and promptly contained avoiding contact with lesion material that may be present on the laundry Wet rather than dry dusting preferred	Standard cleaning and disinfection procedures
Waste management	Manage as Category A[58,59] waste following local and federal regulations	Manage as Category A[58,59] waste following local and federal regulations	Manage as regulated medical waste following local and federal regulations	Clade II: Manage as regulated medical waste following local and federal regulations Clade I: Manage as Category A waste[59]	Manage as regulated medical waste following local and federal regulations

Abbreviations: PUI, person under investigation; VHF, viral hemorrhagic fever.
[a] Although the CDC website[54] specifies Ebola virus disease, efforts are underway to broaden to other VHF viruses, including Marburg Virus.[60]
[b] Unstable: clinically unstable PUI or PUI with vomiting, diarrhea, or bleeding.

and the need for site managers, observers, and runners. Available HCP should include nurses, respiratory therapists, and acute and critical care providers. When considering necessary HCP skillsets to add to the team, those with skills in airway management and vascular access should be represented. In general, only those HCP who are required for patient-facing care should enter the hospital room of a patient with a special pathogen, particularly for HCIDs, such as Ebola virus. This recommendation is particularly important for HCIDs, such as Ebola virus. To minimize exposures of staff to children with special pathogens, staff who provide face-to-face care should be trained to perform tasks beyond direct patient care, including environmental cleaning and restocking of patient supplies. Additional steps should be considered when caring for children with special pathogens such as confirmed EVD. Site managers should be used to oversee the implementation of precautions and protocols, and consideration should be given to activating the hospital incident command system to ensure efficient communication and decision-making regarding staffing, supplies, and communication.

Inform
As patients are identified and isolated because of concern for a special pathogen, the facility's IPC team should be contacted immediately. The IPC team will help ensure appropriate isolation and PPE has been implemented, and they will assist in navigating communications with public health. The decision to test a patient is ideally made in collaboration with public health officials, and in many settings, the public health department is the "gatekeeper" for accessing testing resources. Importantly, public health officials will manage community-level exposures and follow-up, which includes managing family and household exposures and setting guidance for quarantine or isolation of family members at home or in another setting. After these initial communications are accomplished, consideration should be given to internal and external organizational communications, oftentimes coordinated through the hospital incident command system. Establishing a framework or communication plan in advance of an event can help ensure an appropriate communication cascade when it is needed.

Occupational Health

The occupational health team in a children's hospital has important challenges, including identifying organizational occupational health leaders that bridge the skills of managing adult healthcare workforce needs and understanding the pediatric patient care environment. Physicians with training in public health and/or internal medicine and pediatric infectious diseases are among those with relevant expertise to help lead occupational health teams and provide stakeholder engagement to special pathogen preparedness activities.

Preparedness activities for the occupational health team include developing systems to identify and record HCP involvement in the care of patients with special pathogens, especially within a biocontainment unit. This includes a system for tracking potential exposures, daily monitoring of the team for any disease symptoms, and procedures for managing potentially infectious adult HCP such as transfer agreements with an adult biocontainment unit. The occupational health team can additionally support clinical operations for HCP vaccination and/or other MCMs. Preparing these dedicated policies and procedures in advance is essential.

Occupational health models in a pediatric facility
Many models exist to provide care to HCP in pediatric healthcare facilities. An in-house model where an occupational health professional provides clinical care to employees of the same healthcare system may provide benefits by having employees

receive occupational health services from a trusted colleague who is familiar with the healthcare system's operations and the provision of pediatric care. A disadvantage of an in-house model is that the employees of the occupational health system may not be able to provide wellness care or behavioral health services and may not have the expertise to provide occupational injury care. Additionally, some employees may be concerned about confidentiality issues when a colleague is providing occupational care.

Alternatively, a children's hospital may have a contractual agreement for occupational health services from an external company or partner hospital. As a contractual model often has an adult medicine-trained occupational health physician overseeing care, a pediatric physician must often be engaged to adjudicate exposures involving children. An advantage of the contractual model is that wellness, behavioral health care, and occupational injury care and prevention can be delivered to employees in the workplace. A disadvantage of contractual occupational health care in a pediatric facility is that the contractors may not be familiar with the pediatric healthcare system, may not have access to or familiarity with the electronic medical record, and may not be familiar with the unique aspects of pediatric infectious disease exposures.

The implication is that whichever model of employee and occupational health a system adopts—in-house, contractual, or a blend of the 2—the model must be able to accommodate the monitoring and surveillance required for caring for employees potentially exposed or infected with a highly transmissible pathogen and to effectively communicate potential occupational risks and risk mitigation strategies with a healthcare workforce caring for pediatric patients.

Caring for healthcare personnel of children with known or suspected special pathogen infections

Although caring for employees with exposures to vaccine-preventable and/or special pathogens may be straightforward among healthy and highly immunized HCP, exceptional circumstances exist; unimmunized and/or seronegative HCP and/or HCP with underlying medical conditions may be delivering care to children with a known or suspected pathogen. These situations illustrate the need for excellent communication between the employee/occupational health, clinical team, and hospital epidemiology teams. We learned a tremendous amount about monitoring HCP during the COVID-19 pandemic[15] that translates well into the surveillance and monitoring needed to care for HCP caring for children with known or suspected special pathogens. Automated applications and self-reporting strategies with temperature monitoring utilizing smartphone applications (apps) that communicated with a hospital occupational health database became an accepted form of surveillance. Despite challenges with several commercial devices and reports that temperature screening was ineffective in preventing ill HCP with SARS-CoV-2 infections from entering the healthcare environment,[16] temperature elevation may be an initial presentation of several non-SARS-CoV-2 infections. Furthermore, due to diurnal variation in body temperatures, twice daily temperature assessments, as practiced by several facilities who cared for adults with VHFs, may be required to optimally detect body temperature excursions. In combination with symptom reporting, temperature monitoring could provide an early indication of illness onset in HCP caring for a child with a special pathogen.[17] Apps and electronic entry facilitated data collection and review but also resulted in data entry fatigue. Attestation statements may have encouraged more honest responses but many factors contribute to accurate symptom reporting.[18]

Suggested strategies to optimize HCP surveillance include identifying those with direct patient contact through electronic proximity linkage of HCP ID badges and the patient identification band. A similar strategy can be used between HCP ID badges and labeled waste/body fluids to identify those HCP that did not have direct contact with the patient but who had contact with infectious materials. Surveillance of HCP who do not have direct contact with a child with a known or suspected special pathogen but rather with their bodily fluids or waste may benefit from being included in occupational health symptom surveillance.

To optimize reporting and to minimize presenteeism (ie, the act of providing clinical care while ill), policies that support HCP self-exclusion from the healthcare environment when ill are essential. Public health involvement may be necessary if quarantining of HCP is indicated or when a report of a symptomatic employee is made.

In addition to physical health maintenance of HCP, a focus on their psychological and mental health is essential. The care of children with known or suspected special pathogens can be isolating. Healthcare workers may be shunned by their families, colleagues, and communities.[19] It is therefore critical to have counselors and/or an occupational health assistance program to debrief and discuss challenges and their emotions with employees in a nonjudgmental and supportive venue. Whether delivering care in a high-resource or limited-resource setting, HCP encountered many of the same mental health challenges during earlier Ebola virus outbreaks. The stigma often extended beyond direct-care HCP to any individual associated with an institution where care was being provided.[20] Incorporating the hospital chief communication or public relations officer to assist with constructing thoughtful internal and external messaging about the care of children with special pathogens can assist with reducing stigma.

Respiratory protection programs and specialized personal protective equipment training

To ensure that employees are optimally prepared to care for children with a known or suspected special pathogen, respiratory protection and additional PPE may be required. For enhanced respiratory protection from pathogens with airborne transmission, N95 respirator fit testing should be prioritized for clinical and nonclinical HCP who may have prolonged face-to-face contact with patients or prolonged presence in individual patient rooms. Under OSHA standard 1910.134,[21] fit testing must be performed initially (before the employee is required to wear the respirator in the workplace) and must be repeated at least annually. Fit testing must also be conducted whenever respirator design or facial changes occur that could affect the proper fit of the respirator. Fit testing may also need to be repeated whenever a new type of respirator is acquired by an institution, which may be needed during a pandemic when supply chain constraints for previously fit-tested respirators may occur. During the COVID-19 pandemic, annual fit testing was deferred to preserve supplies of N95 respirators. Developing a prioritization program to dedicate resources to those who will benefit optimally may be required as part of resource preservation. Respiratory protection programs should also include a respiratory health questionnaire, clinician review with recommended respiratory clearance, employee education and training, hands-on training of respirator use and maintenance, and education on donning and doffing respiratory protection apparatus. When annual fit testing cannot be performed, education and training along with questionnaire administration may be substituted to prioritize fit testing for direct clinical care. For those unable to safely wear N95 respirators, hospitals should have alternative respiratory protection devices, such as powered air-purifying respirators (PAPRs) or controlled air-purifying respirators. Care for children with certain special pathogens, such as ebolaviruses and Marburg virus, requires policies for and training with additional high-level PPE, as detailed by the CDC[22] and the National Emerging Pathogen Education and Training Center (NETEC)[23] and described in **Table 2**.

Vaccination programs

Programs and policies should be implemented that support HCP to be fully vaccinated per the HCP-advised adult immunization schedule. This may include establishing receipt of certain vaccines as a condition of employment for those without a documented and verified medical exemption; accommodating philosophic exemptions may be required per local laws or regulations.[24,25] Vaccine access can be optimized by offering immunizations in HCP-friendly venues and locations, such as between-shift clinics, evening-staffed clinics, and rolling vaccination carts. Caregivers of high-risk (eg, premature neonates, immunocompromised, and critically ill) pediatric patients, who may be unable to leave the hospital to receive a vaccine, could benefit from receiving vaccinations at the children's hospital; this increases vaccine uptake and decreases risk of caregivers infecting HCP. In certain situations, such as the emergence of a novel pathogen, prioritization of vaccines and other countermeasures may be indicated.[26] A risk-stratification program by heath condition, age, or patient care location may be time-intensive and could result in perceptions of bias. When local conditions require prioritization of MCMs or vaccines because of limited supply, organizational responses may include equitably designating a subset of HCP for vaccination and expanding eligibility criteria as vaccine supply allows.

Drills and Training

One of the essential elements of developing and maintaining a program for providing care to children with a special pathogen, including care within a dedicated biocontainment unit, is the preparation of the personnel who will manage future patients. The necessary training will provide both knowledge of the epidemiology, diagnosis, and treatment of specific potential pathogens, as well as skills to help build confidence and safe patient care practices within the unit. Team members must be educated on policies and procedures, including infection control practices, environmental cleaning and safety, PPE, and any unit-based clinical care pathways.[27] Team composition must ensure that all potential patient care can be safely conducted both within a dedicated biocontainment unit as well as dedicated space for special pathogen care within general patient care areas. If there are specific patient care activities that cannot safely be coordinated because of risk of transmission to HCP, contingencies must be arranged to address these potential deviations from usual practice. Examples from the 2014 to 2015 EVD epidemic included modification of laboratory studies to point-of-care testing[28] and recommendations to not offer highly specialized interventions to support multiorgan failure such as extracorporeal membrane oxygenation.[29]

Typical patient care teams will include multiple physician specialties, nurses, laboratory technicians, and critical care personnel. Biocontainment units preparing to care for children will need to ensure that an appropriate complement of pediatric staff are available and well trained.[30] Clinical care teams require initial substantial training to develop the knowledge and skills to provide safe care to children with special pathogens and ongoing continuing education and drilling to maintain a constant state of readiness and high-level competency. IPC teams are essential to this preparedness education for frontline clinical staff.

Another important element of ongoing team-based training is building trust, camaraderie, and support among the team members. This baseline trust is critical to high functioning teams once activation occurs and stress levels increase. Trust in one's colleagues is critical when caring for a child with a special pathogen and is a critical requirement for safe care. For example, HCP must work as a team and monitor for breeches in PPE and inadvertent exposures. Teams with high levels of trust are also more likely to effectively sustain the required "flattening" of typical institutional hierarchies that is needed for all team members to effectively raise concerns, call out potential safety risks, and ask questions that drive the safest possible care for patients and team members. Establishing an environment without hierarchy, where in-room cleaning or bagging of waste, for example, are done by any person in the room, regardless of their usual scope of practice. These effective and trusting relationships are built and maintained with drills and exercises.

Teams responsible for caring for children with special pathogens should routinely practice donning and doffing PPE that is utilized within their unit, including working with partners to check and validate practices and to monitor for errors that could lead to self-contamination. Drills should also incorporate clinical scenario testing within the patient care space, using high-fidelity simulation mannequins or patient actors when possible, to identify and resolve challenges in the care environment related to the biocontainment conditions. Potential challenges include safe examination practices such as practicing auscultation with safer stethoscopes, managing sharps through practicing IV placement and phlebotomy procedural skills, and medication handling within the unit. Clinical care team members should be trained to perform enhanced environmental cleaning, including safely managing spills contaminated with patient bodily fluids. Doing so will limit the need for environmental services personnel to enter the patient room and prevent special pathogen exposure to these HCP. For example, training in endotracheal intubation, resuscitation, and managing safe handling and transportation of deceased patients should occur. Safe patient transport is another area that teams require scenario planning and practice to execute effectively. For HCP within the biocontainment unit, training could include admission procedures for the unit, such as handoffs from the EMS team who may be transporting the patient from the community directly into the biocontainment unit. Specialized transport equipment, such as isopods, should also be incorporated into these drills so that unit care teams are familiar with their use.[31]

Drills are also important opportunities to practice unexpected scenarios for the care team. Unexpected scenarios can be incorporated into training exercises to identify potential system-level and/or HCP-level gaps in preparedness. Examples include managing a patient who acutely decompensates or codes within the biocontainment setting, managing a laboring patient through newborn delivery, a frightened and uncooperative child, and safely responding to a needed facility repair or HCP medical emergency within the biocontainment area. Environmental scenarios to consider include blood and body fluid spills within the patient space or cleaning/bathing a patient who has extensive bodily fluid contamination, including managing bedding and environmental surface cleaning. Training activities and support for many of the above scenarios are available through NETEC.[23]

Access to Medical Countermeasures

MCMs[32] for special pathogens include drugs (eg, antimicrobial medications), biologics (eg, vaccines, blood products, and antibodies), and devices (eg, PPE, diagnostic tests, and ventilators). MCMs are regulated by the US Food and Drug Administration (FDA). The availability of MCMs varies widely depending on the pathogen and its public health impact. The stage of clinical development and clinical experience of MCMs also vary among pathogens, and this is particularly problematic in pediatrics where clinical investigation and/or clinical experience in children may be limited or nonexistent.

Children's hospitals' emergency management and supply chain teams should work closely to ensure both a sufficient pipeline of necessary MCMs for day-to-day use and also for potential periods of increased need. This is not only necessary to maintain clinical operations during anticipated seasonal surges in viral respiratory illness but also as an emergency stockpile to support unpredictable events related to emergence of a novel pathogen that leads to epidemic levels of pediatric illness. Staff training exercises, especially for special pathogen preparedness, also necessitates an inventory of additional supplies.

Pandemic conditions can affect supply manufacturing, and the global supply chain can experience delays. For these reasons, MCM procurement during pandemics may become exceedingly difficult because demand significantly exceeds supply. Freestanding children's hospitals and small health systems may lack leverage in the marketplace to secure adequate MCM inventory. Several preparatory and contingency strategies are needed to address this. First, supply chain teams can maintain multiple MCM options at baseline to provide more options in the case of an emergency. Notably, children's hospitals should anticipate additional operational and educational needs if a new supply alternative is attained. For example, changing to a different type of N95 respirator will require fit testing to the new mask; a different diagnostic assay or reagent (eg, viral transport media) will require laboratory validation; a different brand of vaccine may have different dosing and administration instructions. These needs should be anticipated to maintain staff and patient safety. During a public health emergency when MCMs may be limited, children's hospitals have adopted several contingency measures to maintain clinical operations. For example, early in the COVID-19 pandemic, some laboratories developed in-house diagnostic assays for SARS-CoV-2 and/or created their own viral transport media; some hospitals 3D printed nasal swabs. One children's hospital managed limited N95 respirator inventory by developing a multidisciplinary team to serve as stewards for ensuring appropriate use of N95 respirators and real-time PPE education; this was well received by frontline staff.[33]

To ensure equitable availability to pediatric populations, generally, and to children in underserved areas, several additional measures need to be taken. Children are often the last group to participate in clinical trials for new MCMs. Therefore, children's hospitals may need to work with their clinical investigation and pharmacy teams to ensure access to potentially life-saving MCMs under an FDA-approved individual patient investigational new drug application[34] or expanded access (ie, compassionate use)[35] mechanism directly. Caregivers may have concerns about products that have received FDA Emergency Use Authorization[36] or new products that have received full FDA approval. For new vaccines, for example, these concerns may be more prevalent among disadvantaged populations, such as non-Hispanic Black individuals[37–39] and individuals lower income or education levels.[38] Being proactive with education and countering misinformation may reduce misconception and improve equitable access. One children's hospital improved access of COVID-19 therapeutics to socially vulnerable children by screening for and contacting newly diagnosed patients in real-time rather than relying on physician referral.[40] Mobile health teams and community partnership can also improve access to MCMs in the community.[41,42]

Family-Centered and Child-Centered Care

During the 2014 to 2015 EVD outbreak, US pediatricians undertook the evaluation and management of a large number of children for whom there was a concern for an exposure or infection. During a 7-month period between July 2014 and January 2015, CDC provided guidance to clinicians caring for 89 children: 33 had an epidemiologic link; 15

were tested, and all were negative for EVD.[43] From this experience, delays were noted in the provision of care for other conditions and management of family members was an articulated challenge.

This report,[43] supported by observations of physician stakeholders experienced with care of children under investigation for EVD, prompted ongoing discussions about balancing the clinical and psychosocial needs of children and families. Family-centered care[44] respects each child and their family's innate strengths and cultural values and views the healthcare experience as an opportunity to build on these strengths. As pediatricians, incorporating family-centered care into clinical care is our usual practice and the foundation of our approach. Familial presence provides social and emotional support that optimizes clinical care. However, when a child is under investigation for a special pathogen, the provision of traditional family-centered care requires reevaluation.[45] As with all aspects of the care of children, a "one-size-fits-all approach" is not ideal, although there are some common themes that may be leveraged in the provision of care. In addition, a child's condition may change during their hospitalization from critically ill to needing rehabilitative services, during which the provision of both clinical and family-centered care will vary. **Table 3** illustrates some of the considerations for family-centered care for children with known or suspected special pathogens.

One of the most challenging aspects of providing care to children with a known or suspected special pathogen is balancing the provision of clinical care while respecting the psychosocial needs of pediatric patients and their caregivers and maintaining a protected environment for HCP. Although each facility will need to consider and develop a plan for various scenarios related to family visitation and engagement based on the unique needs as outlined in **Table 3**, it will be helpful to develop guidance for where and how engagement will occur. Depending on the location of presentation, the pathogen, and exposures, family members may need to be excluded from being physically present until a child is stabilized, and additional information is obtained. Physically distant options to maintain family engagement, such as telephonic and/or video technology, may fulfill some of the mutual need to view children and their family members. Communication may be additionally challenged if the patient and/or family is not proficient in the English language, which should be anticipated for many special pathogens that originate in travelers or migrants from non-English-speaking countries. Telephonic and/or video interpreter services will be needed in these situations. If a family member is exposed to or infected with the special pathogen, they may be subject to temporary isolation or quarantine with guidance from the local health department.

The engagement of hospital ethics committees, clinicians, child-life specialists, social workers, patient advocates, chaplains, and public health partners may be beneficial in developing guidance.[46] Once guidance has been developed, it is critical that guidance is communicated to all stakeholders so that a consistent message is delivered to clinicians and families. Guidance is based on the best available evidence at the time and that it may be subject to refinement as additional information is obtained. It is critical to communicate that clinicians are balancing the provision of effective and safe care with infection prevention with the goal of bringing children and family members together as expeditiously as possible.

Organizational and Systems Support for Preparedness

The 2014 West Africa Ebola outbreak prompted US health systems to substantially expand their preparedness efforts for special pathogens. As a part of that response, the Department of Health and Human Services Office of the Assistant Secretary for

Table 3
Considerations for family-centered care for children with known or suspected special pathogens

	HealthCare Staffing Issues	Family Presence Without PPE	Family Presence While Wearing PPE	Alternatives to Family Presence	Family Engagement in End-of-Life Care
Developmental Stage	Higher staff-to-patient ratios for younger or less independent children	More acceptable for younger and/or developmentally delayed children who may be frightened by PPE	More acceptable for children who are comfortable with caregiver wearing PPE	Telephonic and/or video technology: younger and/or developmentally delayed children may not understand that a parent is not present	Challenging at any developmental stage
Pathogen	Higher staff-to-patient ratios needed for novel and special pathogens such as those associated with VHFs or for those for which vaccines are unavailable or ineffective	May be reasonable if family members are vaccinated/immune	Will be dependent on availability of PPE; ability of family members to don, doff, and wear PPE without contamination; and ability of healthcare monitoring of family members after exposures (ie, *Who will monitor and how will monitoring occur? Who will be responsible if a family member becomes ill during the encounter or as a consequence of the encounter?*)	Telephonic and/or video technology may be an optimal replacement for being in the room for children with particularly virulent pathogens	Telephonic and/or video technology could provide comfort to family who are unable to be present at the end of life

Stage of illness	Higher staff-to-patient ratios for more acute stages of illness	May be reasonable if family members are vaccinated/immune	Will be dependent on availability of PPE; ability of family members to don, doff, and wear PPE without contamination; and ability of healthcare monitoring of family members after exposures (ie, *Who will monitor and how will monitoring occur? Who will be responsible if a family member becomes ill during the encounter or as a consequence of the encounter?*)	Telephonic and/or video technology may be an optimal replacement for being in the room with particularly virulent pathogens	May be disadvantageous to have a direct family presence for end-of-life care, especially with particularly virulent pathogens
Family members exposed and without evidence of disease	Staff may express concerns with caring for children whose exposed family members are in the room because family members may become ill and require care and/or be an additional source of pathogen exposure	Family members would require PPE if they were present within the incubation period of the child's illness to protect against ongoing exposure and risk of developing disease. PPE for family requires consideration of education for proper use and disposal of PPE PPE allocation to family may not be possible if supplies are limited	Will be dependent on availability of PPE; ability of family members to don, doff, and wear PPE without contamination; and ability of healthcare monitoring of family members after exposures (ie, *Who will monitor and how will monitoring occur? Who will be responsible if a family member becomes ill during the encounter or as a consequence of the encounter?*)	Telephonic and/or video technology could substitute for in-person interaction, reducing opportunities for pathogen transmission	May be less of a risk for clinical disease if the family member is infected with the same organism and at the same stage of illness. End of life is often associated with peak level of viremia, especially for VHF pathogens, increasing risk of pathogen transmission

(continued on next page)

Table 3
(continued)

	HealthCare Staffing Issues	Family Presence Without PPE	Family Presence While Wearing PPE	Alternatives to Family Presence	Family Engagement in End-of-Life Care
Family members infected with evidence of disease	Staff may express concerns with caring for children whose exposed family members are in the room because family members may be an additional source of pathogen exposure. Family members could acutely worsen and require care. Family members may be at a different stage of illness than their child	Family members would likely require PPE to prevent additional pathogen exposure	Will be dependent on availability of PPE; ability of family members to don, doff, and wear PPE without contamination; and ability of healthcare monitoring of family members after exposures (ie, *Who will monitor and how will monitoring occur? Who will be responsible if a family member becomes ill during the encounter or as a consequence of the encounter?*)	Telephonic and/or video technology could substitute for in-person interaction, reducing opportunities for pathogen transmission	May be less of a risk for disease if the family member has or has had recent clinical disease with the same organism; however, acute stages of illness may not be identical. End of life is often associated with peak level of viremia, especially for VHF pathogens, increasing risk of pathogen transmission

Preparedness and Response (since renamed the Administration for Strategic Preparedness and Response [ASPR]) developed a 3-tiered system to network hospitals into treatment, assessment, and frontline facilities with specific capabilities. In 2015, the National Ebola Training and Education Centers were established (since renamed the NETEC) with 10 dedicated regional Ebola Treatment Centers[47]; efforts by ASPR to expand the number of centers are ongoing.[48] Children's hospitals should work with their public health department and regional emergency preparedness coalition to define their specific tiering for special pathogen care and develop a business plan to support the clinical program and preparedness activities. Lessons learned following the only documented cases of Ebola transmission to HCP within the US highlight the critical needs for special pathogen preparedness.[49] In addition, the COVID-19 pandemic led to new challenges and opportunities to utilize existing preparedness frameworks to expand the scope of preparedness activities beyond special pathogens readiness.

One of the key drivers for sustainability of these special pathogen treatment centers is a dedicated effort to maintain high levels of facility and staff readiness at all times and not only during major global events that heighten visibility of these illnesses. Sustainable preparedness efforts are challenging when organizations are continuously faced with competing pressures for resource allocation of equipment and staff time and energy. A comprehensive national preparedness framework requires all hospitals to be capable of identifying and appropriately triaging patients with potential emerging and special pathogens and to safely support transfer to an appropriate site of care for treatment.

The required organizational support to maintain a state of readiness at smaller hospitals, community hospitals, and specialty hospitals, including children's hospitals, is particularly burdensome and less likely to be partially offset by extramural support under the existing national response framework. For example, one freestanding children's hospital designated as an assessment center for Ebola in 2014 to 2015 reported an estimated unbudgeted hospital capital investment of greater than US$250,000 in materials and equipment, greater than 3000 hours of staff training and planning time, estimated at more than US$100,000 in staff worked hours, for an annualized preparedness total cost of US$181,350 during the 2014 to 2015 outbreak response.[50]

The imperative remains to continuously improve preparedness at all acute care hospitals, including children's hospitals, which may serve as sites of potential initial presentation, triage, and treatment of pediatric patients with special pathogens. Initially, within the networks for national preparedness, provision of care for children received limited visibility and dedicated resource allocation. Expansion of nationally networked preparedness for children was addressed more recently with the development of the Pediatric Pandemic Network[51] (supported by the Department of Health and Human Services, Health Resources and Services Administration) during the COVID-19 response. This is an important step toward enhancing preparedness nationally to effectively incorporate management of special pathogens at the children's hospitals dedicated to caring for the most complex pediatric patients.

SUMMARY

Preparing children's hospitals and HCP for special pathogens is complex. Effective preparedness requires committed resources for ongoing planning and practice with attention to education, policies and procedures, drills and training, and supplies. Although dedicated resources are required, successfully preparing for special pathogens is an important measure toward keeping communities, HCP, and patients and their families safe in this global age that brings pathogens from across the world to our doorstep. Preparedness for special pathogens is an investment that will not only enhance safety in the event of a special pathogen but also elevate preparedness for everyday pathogens.

CLINICS CARE POINTS

- Children's hospital HCP should be prepared to identify special pathogens by being familiar with special pathogen alerts, epidemiologic risk factors, signs, and symptoms.
- After identifying a patient with a possible special pathogen, children's hospital HCP should be prepared to minimize risk of transmission to themselves and others by isolating the patient in the appropriate room type and utilizing appropriate PPE.
- After isolating a patient with a possible special pathogen, children's hospital HCP should be prepared to inform their IPC colleagues and other key clinical and public health stakeholders to ensure appropriate clinical evaluation and implementation of best practices for safe clinical care.
- Children's hospitals should develop policies, practices, and preparedness activities to equip their HCP to safely care for children with special pathogens.
- Effective preparedness requires committed resources for ongoing planning and practice with attention to education, policies and procedures, drills and training, and supplies.
- Because of the importance of family-centered and child-centered care, children's hospitals should be prepared to modify their typical care model when necessary to prevent special pathogen transmission to patient caregivers and HCP.

DISCLOSURE

L.K. Kociolek reports grant support from Merck, United States and the Department of Health and Human Services, United States, Health Resources and Services Administration, United States. A.L. Shane reports grant support from the Department of Health and Human Services, Administration for Strategic Preparedness and Response, United States (BARDA). K.A. Simonsen reports grant support from Merck, Alinta, and the Department of Health and Human Services, Administration for Strategic Preparedness and Response to support her salary. D.M. Zerr reports grant from Merck and consultancy for Allovir.

REFERENCES

1. Centers for Disease Control and Prevention. Identify, Isolate, Inform: Emergency Department Evaluation and Management for Patients Under Investigation (PUIs) for Ebola Virus Disease (EVD). Available at: https://www.cdc.gov/vhf/ebola/clinicians/emergency-services/emergency-departments.html. [Accessed 4 August 2023].
2. UK Health Security Agency. High consequence infectious diseases (HCID). Available at: https://www.gov.uk/guidance/high-consequence-infectious-diseases-hcid#definition-of-hcid%202021. [Accessed 4 August 2023].
3. Jones KE, Patel NG, Levy MA, et al. Global trends in emerging infectious diseases. Nature 2008;451(7181):990–3.
4. Elkholy AA, Grant R, Assiri A, et al. MERS-CoV infection among healthcare workers and risk factors for death: Retrospective analysis of all laboratory-

confirmed cases reported to WHO from 2012 to 2 June 2018. J Infect Public Health 2020;13(3):418–22.

5. Suwantarat N, Apisarnthanarak A. Risks to healthcare workers with emerging diseases: lessons from MERS-CoV, Ebola, SARS, and avian flu. Curr Opin Infect Dis 2015;28(4):349–61.

6. Deal A, Halliday R, Crawshaw AF, et al. Migration and outbreaks of vaccine-preventable disease in Europe: a systematic review. Lancet Infect Dis 2021; 21(12):e387–98.

7. Phadke VK, Bednarczyk RA, Salmon DA, et al. Association Between Vaccine Refusal and Vaccine-Preventable Diseases in the United States: A Review of Measles and Pertussis. JAMA 2016;315(11):1149–58.

8. Centers for Disease Control and Prevention. Bioterrorism Agents/Diseases. Available at: https://emergency.cdc.gov/agent/agentlist-category.asp. [Accessed 4 August 2023].

9. Centers for Disease Control and Prevention. Identify, Isolate, Inform: Emergency Department Evaluation and Management of Patients Under Investigation for Ebola Virus Disease. Available at: https://www.cdc.gov/vhf/ebola/pdf/ed-algorithm-management-patients-possible-ebola.pdf. [Accessed 5 August 2023].

10. Washington State Department of Health. Measles. Available at: https://doh.wa.gov/public-health-healthcare-providers/notifiable-conditions/measles. [Accessed 5 August 2023].

11. Washington State Department of Health. Measles Assessment Checklist for Providers. Available at: https://doh.wa.gov/sites/default/files/legacy/Documents/Pubs/348-490-MeaslesAssessmentQuicksheetProviders.docx?uid=64cdcbc6da59a. [Accessed 5 August 2023].

12. Burkholder TW, Dziadkowiec O, Bookman K, et al. Adherence to Universal Travel Screening in the Emergency Department During Epidemic Ebola Virus Disease. J Emerg Med 2019;56(1):7–14.

13. Centers for Disease Control and Prevention. Glossary. Guideline for isolation precautions: preventing transmission of infectious agents in healthcare settings. Available at: 2007 https://www.cdc.gov/infectioncontrol/guidelines/isolation/glossary.html.

14. Centers for Disease Control and Prevention. Interim Infection Prevention and Control Recommendations for Hospitalized Patients with Middle East Respiratory Syndrome Coronavirus (MERS-CoV). Available at: https://www.cdc.gov/coronavirus/mers/infection-prevention-control.html. [Accessed 5 August 2023].

15. Bielicki JA, Duval X, Gobat N, et al. Monitoring approaches for health-care workers during the COVID-19 pandemic. Lancet Infect Dis 2020;20(10):e261–7.

16. Maung Z, Kristensen M, Hoffman B, et al. Temperature Screening of Healthcare Personnel Is Ineffective in Controlling COVID-19. J Occup Environ Med 2022; 64(5):382–4.

17. Carter P, Megnin-Viggars O, Rubin GJ. What Factors Influence Symptom Reporting and Access to Healthcare During an Emerging Infectious Disease Outbreak? A Rapid Review of the Evidence. Health Secur 2021;19(4):353–63.

18. Lichtman A, Greenblatt E, Malenfant J, et al. Universal symptom monitoring to address presenteeism in healthcare workers. American journal of infection control 2021;49(8):1021–3.

19. Srivatsa S, Stewart KA. How Should Clinicians Integrate Mental Health Into Epidemic Responses? AMA J Ethics 2020;22(1):E10–5.

20. New York Times. Bellevue Employees Face Ebola at Work, and Stigma of It Everywhere. Available at: https://www.nytimes.com/2014/10/30/nyregion/bellevue-

workers-worn-out-from-treating-ebola-patient-face-stigma-outside-hospital.html. [Accessed 5 August 2023].

21. Occupational Safety and Health Administration. 134: Respiratory Protection. 1910. Available at: https://www.osha.gov/laws-regs/regulations/standardnumber/1910/1910.134. [Accessed 5 August 2023].

22. Centers for Disease Control and Prevention. Ebola Disease: Personal Protective Equipment. Available at: https://www.cdc.gov/vhf/ebola/healthcare-us/ppe/index.html. [Accessed 5 August 2023].

23. National Emerging Special Pathogens Training and Education Center. Available at: https://netec.org/. [Accessed 5 August 2023].

24. Weber DJ, Al-Tawfiq JA, Babcock HM, et al. Multisociety statement on coronavirus disease 2019 (COVID-19) vaccination as a condition of employment for healthcare personnel. Infection control and hospital epidemiology : the official journal of the Society of Hospital Epidemiologists of America 2022;43(1):3–11.

25. Gallagher MC, Haessler S, Babcock HM. Influenza Vaccination and Healthcare Personnel Compliance. Curr Treat Options Infect Dis 2020;12(1):71–6.

26. Hughes K, Gogineni V, Lewis C, et al. Considerations for fair prioritization of COVID-19 vaccine and its mandate among healthcare personnel. Curr Med Res Opin 2021;37(6):907–9.

27. Flinn JB, Hynes NA, Sauer LM, et al. The role of dedicated biocontainment patient care units in preparing for COVID-19 and other infectious disease outbreaks. Infection control and hospital epidemiology : the official journal of the Society of Hospital Epidemiologists of America 2021;42(2):208–11.

28. Hill CE, Burd EM, Kraft CS, et al. Laboratory test support for Ebola patients within a high-containment facility. Lab Med 2014;45(3):e109–11.

29. DiLorenzo MA, Baker CA, Herstein JJ, et al. Institutional policies and readiness in management of critical illness among patients with viral hemorrhagic fever. Infection control and hospital epidemiology : the official journal of the Society of Hospital Epidemiologists of America 2021;42(11):1307–12.

30. Herstein JJ, Le AB, McNulty LA, et al. An update on US Ebola treatment center personnel management and training. American journal of infection control 2020;48(4):375–9.

31. Centers for Disease Control and Prevention. Guidance for Developing a Plan for Interfacility Transport of Persons Under Investigation or Confirmed Patients with Ebola Virus Disease in the United States. Available at: https://www.cdc.gov/vhf/ebola/clinicians/emergency-services/interfacility-transport.html. [Accessed 5 August 2023].

32. Food and Drug Administration. What are Medical Countermeasures?. Available at: https://www.fda.gov/emergency-preparedness-and-response/about-mcmi/what-are-medical-countermeasures. [Accessed 5 August 2023].

33. Patel AB, O'Donnell A, Bonebrake A, et al. Stewardship of personal protective equipment (PPE): An important pandemic resource for PPE preservation and education. Infection control and hospital epidemiology : the official journal of the Society of Hospital Epidemiologists of America 2021;42(5):636–7.

34. Food and Drug Administration. Expanded Access Categories for Drugs (Including Biologics). Available at: https://www.fda.gov/news-events/expanded-access/expanded-access-categories-drugs-including-biologics#:~:text=Individual%20Patient%20Expanded%20Access%20IND,may%20not%20be%20under%20development. [Accessed 5 August 2023].

35. Food and Drug Administration. Expanded Access. Available at: https://www.fda. gov/news-events/public-health-focus/expanded-access. [Accessed 5 August 2023].

36. Food and Drug Administration. Emergency Use Authorization. Available at: https:// www.fda.gov/emergency-preparedness-and-response/mcm-legal-regulatory- and-policy-framework/emergency-use-authorization. [Accessed 5 August 2023].

37. Alfieri NL, Kusma JD, Heard-Garris N, et al. Parental COVID-19 vaccine hesitancy for children: vulnerability in an urban hotspot. BMC Publ Health 2021;21(1):1662.

38. Yasmin F, Najeeb H, Moeed A, et al. COVID-19 Vaccine Hesitancy in the United States: A Systematic Review. Front Public Health 2021;9:770985.

39. Kociolek LK, Elhadary J, Jhaveri R, et al. Coronavirus disease 2019 vaccine hesitancy among children's hospital staff: A single-center survey. Infection control and hospital epidemiology : the official journal of the Society of Hospital Epidemiologists of America 2021;42(6):775–7.

40. Parzen-Johnson S, Sun S, Patel AB, et al. Sociodemographic Comparison of Children With High-risk Medical Conditions Referred vs Identified Through Screening Plus Outreach for COVID-19 Therapeutics. JAMA Netw Open 2022;5(12): e2248671.

41. Jiménez J, Parra YJ, Murphy K, et al. Community-Informed Mobile COVID-19 Testing Model to Addressing Health Inequities. J Public Health Manag Pract 2022;28(Suppl 1):S101–10.

42. Alcendor DJ, Juarez PD, Matthews-Juarez P, et al. Meharry Medical College Mobile Vaccination Program: Implications for Increasing COVID-19 Vaccine Uptake among Minority Communities in Middle Tennessee. Vaccines (Basel) 2022;10(2). https://doi.org/10.3390/vaccines10020211.

43. Goodman AB, Meites E, Anstey EH, et al. Clinical Inquiries Received by CDC Regarding Suspected Ebola Virus Disease in Children–United States, July 9, 2014-January 4, 2015. MMWR Morbidity and mortality weekly report 2015; 64(36):1006–10.

44. Family-centered care and the pediatrician's role. Pediatrics 2003;112(3 Pt 1): 691–7.

45. Mehrotra P, Shane AL, Milstone AM. Family-Centered Care and High-Consequence Pathogens: Thinking Outside the Room. JAMA Pediatr 2015; 169(11):985–6.

46. Davies HD, Byington CL. Parental Presence During Treatment of Ebola or Other Highly Consequential Infection. Pediatrics 2016;138(3). https://doi.org/10.1542/ peds.2016-1891.

47. Assistant Secretary for Preparedness, Response. Regional Treatment Network for Ebola and Other Special Pathogens. Available at: https://www.phe.gov/ Preparedness/planning/hpp/reports/Documents/RETN-Ebola-Report-508.pdf. [Accessed 5 August 2023].

48. Administration for Strategic Preparedness, Response. ASPR Awards $21 Million to Health Facilities to Enhance Nation's Preparedness for Special Pathogens. Available at: https://aspr.hhs.gov/newsroom/Pages/RESPTC-Prep-Award-24Oct2022. aspx. [Accessed 5 August 2023].

49. Chevalier MS, Chung W, Smith J, et al. Ebola virus disease cluster in the United States–Dallas County, Texas, 2014. MMWR Morbidity and mortality weekly report 2014;63(46):1087–8.

50. Simonsen KA, Phipps AR, Hall M, et al. Costs Associated with Ebola Preparedness at a Freestanding Pediatric Assessment Center. Infection control and hospital epidemiology 2017;38(11):1367–9.

51. Pediatric Pandemic Network. Available at: https://pedspandemicnetwork.org/. [Accessed 10 September 2023].

52. Centers for Disease Control and Prevention. Infection Prevention and Control of Mpox in Healthcare Settings. Available at: https://www.cdc.gov/poxvirus/mpox/clinicians/infection-control-healthcare.html. [Accessed 24 August 2023].

53. Centers for Disease Control and Prevention. Interim Infection Prevention and Control Recommendations for Measles in Healthcare Settings. Available at: https://www.cdc.gov/infectioncontrol/guidelines/measles/index.html. [Accessed 24 August 2023].

54. Centers for Disease Control and Prevention. Guidance on Personal Protective Equipment (PPE) To Be Used By Healthcare Workers during Management of Patients with Confirmed Ebola or Persons under Investigation (PUIs) for Ebola who are Clinically Unstable or Have Bleeding, Vomiting, or Diarrhea in U.S. Healthcare Settings, Including Procedures for Donning and Doffing PPE. Available at: https://www.cdc.gov/vhf/ebola/healthcare-us/ppe/guidance.html. [Accessed 5 August 2023].

55. Centers for Disease Control and Prevention. For U.S. Healthcare Settings: Donning and Doffing Personal Protective Equipment (PPE) for Evaluating Persons Under Investigation (PUIs) for Ebola Who Are Clinically Stable and Do Not Have Bleeding, Vomiting, or Diarrhea. Available at: https://www.cdc.gov/vhf/ebola/healthcare-us/ppe/guidance-clinically-stable-puis.html. [Accessed 24 August 2023].

56. United States Environmental Protection Agency, List L. Disinfectants for Use Against Ebola Virus. Available at: https://www.epa.gov/pesticide-registration/list-l-disinfectants-use-against-ebola-virus. [Accessed 24 August 2023].

57. United States Environmental Protection Agency. What is an emerging viral pathogen claim?. Available at: https://www.epa.gov/coronavirus/what-emerging-viral-pathogen-claim. [Accessed 24 August 2023].

58. Centers for Disease Control and Prevention. Ebola-Associated Waste Management. Available at: https://www.cdc.gov/vhf/ebola/clinicians/cleaning/waste-management.html. [Accessed 24 August 2023].

59. United States Department of Transportation. Pipeline and Hazardous Materials Safety Administration. Available at: https://www.phmsa.dot.gov/transporting-infectious-substances/planning-guidance-handling-category-solid-waste. [Accessed 24 August 2023].

60. Centers for Disease Control and Prevention. Interim Guidance for U.S. Hospital Preparedness for Patients Under Investigation (PUIs) or with Confirmed Ebola Virus Disease (EVD): A Framework for a Tiered Approach. Available at: https://www.cdc.gov/vhf/ebola/healthcare-us/preparing/hospitals.html. [Accessed 24 August 2023].

Mental Health Impact of Pandemics and Other Public Health Emergencies in Children

David J. Schonfeld, MD[a,b,*], Thomas Demaria, PhD[b]

KEYWORDS

- Pandemic • COVID-19 • Public health emergency • Children • Mental health • Grief
- Health communication • Professional self-care

KEY POINTS

- Pediatric health care providers can provide universal support to children and families to mitigate potential risk factors to adjustment while fostering protective factors to promote resiliency in children and families and offer practical guidance to parents and other caregivers on how to talk to and support their children.
- It is important to distinguish between transient distress and sadness, which is virtually universal during a pandemic, from mental illness that requires clinical intervention.
- Public health emergencies often tax the personal resources of health care providers, underscoring the need to integrate self-care strategies in personal and professional practice routines.

Disasters become public health emergencies when the scale, timing, and/or unpredictability threatens to overwhelm the capacity of existing public health services. Public health emergencies are often defined by their potential health consequences rather than their specific causes or precipitating events.[1] Children have limited independent coping skills and fewer prior life experiences that may have promoted personal resiliency. They may lack the developmental maturity required to manage worries about the infection, disability, and death of self and others close to them. As such, the mental health of children during public health emergencies such as a pandemic may be impacted more than that of adults.

Much of what we know about the metal health impact on children of pandemics and other public health emergencies is based on the COVID-19 pandemic. The research conducted on the mental health impact on children of the pandemic is, at this point in time, limited and preliminary. Data collected during the pandemic often relied by

[a] Keck School of Medicine of the University of Southern California; [b] National Center for School Crisis and Bereavement at Children's Hospital Los Angeles
* Corresponding author. Children's Hospital Los Angeles, 4650 Sunset Boulevard, #53, Los Angeles, CA 90027.
E-mail address: schonfel@usc.edu

Pediatr Clin N Am 71 (2024) 455–468
https://doi.org/10.1016/j.pcl.2024.01.015   pediatric.theclinics.com
0031-3955/24/© 2024 Elsevier Inc. All rights reserved.

necessity due to appropriate concerns of infection especially early in the pandemic, on proxy measures (such as health care utilization and billing data), parent reports of children's symptoms (as opposed to children's self-reports or clinical interviews), and on-line surveys. For this study, extrapolations will therefore be made from learnings, as well as the authors' experience, after other disasters. Recommendations will focus on practical suggestions for pediatric practitioners.

STAGES OF THE PANDEMIC AND ASSOCIATED ADJUSTMENT CHALLENGES

The COVID-19 pandemic extended over several years and consisted of a series of waves of increasing and then waning levels of infection and death. It appears the most difficult period for children's adjustment was the initial wave; children demonstrated improvement or even normalization of mental health in subsequent waves, even prior to the availability of vaccines. Caregivers showed a more persistent pattern of distress especially for those with the primary responsibility for childcare. In the early stages of the pandemic, a higher prevalence of anxiety and depressive symptoms in children and adolescents was reported and attributed to the many changes due to the pandemic itself, social isolation, and caregiver distress.[2] Caregiver adjustment to stress and emotional difficulties, however, did show an improvement in later waves of the pandemic.[3] This pattern highlights the need for greater support of both children and caregivers at the initial stages of a public health crisis and more focus on longer-term support for caregivers with persistent adjustment difficulties.

ROLE OF COMMUNICATION IN DISASTERS ON CHILD ADJUSTMENT

Children are better able to cope with a difficult situation if they feel they understand it. They can learn more about a crisis through public or social media, as well as from explanations and discussion with caregivers, educators, pediatric health care providers, and other trusted adults.

The amount of media coverage during a public health emergency often seems inversely proportional to the amount of accurate new information. In an evolving public health crisis, media coverage often includes misinformation (characterized by unintentional mistakes), disinformation (that is intentionally fabricated or manipulated in order to cause harm), and malinformation (involving correct information that is used to harm others such as the deliberate release of private information). Complicating things further, children may have an incomplete knowledge base, limited understanding of underlying concepts, and difficulty discerning accurate from inaccurate information. They therefore have a particular need for trusted adults to help them understand and process feelings related to evolving and often conflicting information present in the media during a public health emergency. In turn, parents and caregivers will benefit from trusted pediatric health care providers providing similar assistance.

It is helpful to remember that there are 2 main purposes for public health communications during a crisis: to provide realistic reassurance or to provide practical advice that can be used to decrease risk to self or others close to the individual. Informing people of a new or potential new risk (such as a newly identified variant) without providing any practical new information on steps that can be taken to decrease risk is not helpful and may only foster fear and feelings of helplessness. Although media coverage may be continuous during an evolving crisis, children and adults alike should monitor their consumption of media, and make sure it is a healthy diet and that they do not consume too much. If the media is not providing reassurance nor offering relevant new preventive strategies, it is best to disconnect from media (television, print, radio, and social media) for the time period and connect instead with families and friends (in-person or remotely).

It is important for pediatric and public health professionals during an evolving public health emergency to prepare the public that our understanding of the situation will, appropriately, also evolve. For example, during the early stages of the COVID-19 pandemic a lot of attention was focused on sanitizing surfaces as a preventive mea-sure which led to a depletion of available cleaning supplies. Later the focus shifted to the use of masking and social distancing as a primary prevention strategy. Rather than representing an example of conflicting information that illustrates that public health advice cannot be trusted, it represented an appropriate shift to more accurate infor-mation as knowledge was gained collectively among professionals.

Concerns also relate to evolving information about the mental health impact of the pandemic especially during the period when people were isolating at home. Initial re-ports, based largely on caregiver reports of their impressions of children's adjustment, not surprisingly identified increased concerns of depressive and anxious reactions in children,[4] which were readily attributed to social isolation, activity restrictions, uncer-tainly of the future, and a fear of infection, sickness, and death. Although this research helped alert the public to potential mental health complications, it may have overesti-mated the prevalence of clinical depression or anxiety disorders and left caregivers worried that their own children may be permanently "damaged" by their pandemic experiences.

While not minimizing or pretending that adjustment reactions do not or should not be experienced by children, pediatric health care providers should help to provide uni-versal support to children and families with a goal of promoting resiliency. They can help families distinguish between transient distress and sadness (which should be ex-pected to be near universal during a pandemic) from clinical mental illness such as anxiety, post-traumatic stress disorder (PTSD) or clinical depression (which would require additional mental health treatment). Pediatric health care providers should be cautious in overuse and overreliance on screening instruments for mental health conditions that were not validated for use during a public health crisis.

The negative news reporting bias may also minimize potentially positive aspects of the recovery process such as the potential for increases in family cohesiveness because of the increased time together, or reductions in distress in some children who had experienced high levels of anxiety related to peer interactions or academic demands that predated the pandemic. The quality of the caregiver–child relationship remained as a strong predictor of resiliency in children.[5] Some children reported that they benefitted from the lockdown during the pandemic as there was a reduction in bullying and more opportunities for sleep and exercise.[6] These potentially positive im-pacts should not be exaggerated or be used to discredit the widespread and signifi-cant distress otherwise felt by virtually everyone.

Pediatric health care providers can also provide guidance to caregivers on how to talk to and support their children. Adults should not tell children (or other adults) that they should not be worried or minimize their concerns. A first step before offering reassurance is to find out the individual's personal fears or concerns. Children may have very different fears or worries than adults; fears also differ among adults them-selves. Effective reassurance is not possible until there is an awareness of what is most relevant to the individual.

It is important to help children express and cope with their uncertainty and fear. Adults should share and model effective strategies of dealing with distress, discom-fort, anxiety, and sadness. This might include reading or hobbies that promote healthy distraction. It may also include talking to others, journaling or blogging, or art and music to promote expression of feelings. In the midst of an ongoing crisis, people need to do both—at times they must face and process their distress and at other times use distraction to temporarily reduce distress. Exercise and yoga and the appropriate use of respectful humor are also useful strategies. Relaxation techniques and mindfulness, which can be taught even to very young children, and self-hypnosis and guided imagery can be learned to deal with anxiety. Cognitive behavioral strategies can help people replace negative thoughts with more positive interpretations that result in improvements in feelings and behaviors.

PANDEMIC CHANGES IN SCHOOL PROCESSES

The UNICEF estimated that 99% of the world's 2.36 billion children lived in a country that imposed at least some restrictions on social gathering, with more than half experiencing some form of lockdown.[7] This response to COVID-19 led to an estimated 1.6 billion children being out of school for an extended period[8,9] and the necessity to deliver instruction remotely despite a hasty transition. This resulted in the use of under-developed online teaching materials by school staff often unfamiliar with online platforms and with inadequate and often disproportionate access to Internet service and computers. This resulted in a dramatic change in the lives of children and families as schools serve an important role in the daily life of children. Besides offering academic instruction, schools serve as a place where children obtain meals, routine/structure, peer and adult socialization, screening for mental health and medical problems and a variety of other important services. Many families had difficulty addressing these needs and the many challenges of remote learning.

Overall academic performance was negatively affected by COVID-19 lockdowns, with lower scores in standardized tests found compared to previous years. Academic, motivational, and socioemotional factors contributed to lower performance. Educators, caregivers, and students reported disorganization, increased academic demands, and motivational and behavioral changes.[10] Indeed, the quality of instruction children received as remote learning varied dramatically—with some children only getting mailed worksheets and others getting online live lessons with their own teachers. Students appeared to benefit most from remote learning during the pandemic when educators were able to actively engage students in this new mode of learning and when families had resources to supervise the child's remote instruction and assignments.

Students who required special academic accommodations and students from low-income families with limited technological access had more difficulties.[11] Remote learning was difficult for families with multiple children and caregivers holding jobs that also required remote access if they all needed access to a shared family computer. Other transitions in normal school processes further increased the stress of children, such as the suddenness of school closing limiting access to school resources, the infection/mortality of members of the school community, and the subsequent reopening of school buildings with special modifications to prevent potential infection which still limited interactions among educators and students. Pediatricians can encourage the families they serve (and the school systems they work with) to consider proactively how to ensure continuity of learning when an individual child or the entire school must temporarily transition to remote learning.

Caregivers and educators can be reminded by pediatricians that academic expectations should be modified during a public health emergency. Even if children are able to return to class, the ongoing threats to health and numerous deaths in the community will have a significant impact on children's academic functioning, as well as the ability of teachers to continue to teach effectively. It should not be expected that students can rapidly resume their pre-emergency rate of learning; it is unrealistic to think that they can somehow "catch up" and make up for considerable lost instructional time (eg, in some cases a year in length) without making significant changes to the curriculum and educational content. Pre-existing learning challenges often become worse following prolonged stress and new learning problems may emerge. Many children will have difficulty concentrating and be more distracted thus limiting their learning and/or remembering of new facts or concepts. Pediatricians can also assist caregivers and schools to find a balance between maintaining reasonable expectations for academic growth while also providing additional support and academic accommodation. If academic expectations even temporarily exceed children's learning capacity, school may emerge as a source of additional distress for children rather than as a source of support to promote recovery.[12]

FAMILY AND CAREGIVER DISTRESS DURING THE PANDEMIC

Caregivers and families faced many challenges during the pandemic beyond those resulting from school closings and the need to supervise remote instruction (often while trying to work remotely themselves). Many caregivers experienced financial insecurity due to job loss or a reduction in working hours. The impact of financial stress was especially pronounced in families with children who had pre-existing vulnerabilities.[13,14] This has led some to worry that there may have been an increase in child maltreatment as a result of caregivers feeling overwhelmed and lacking sufficient resources that have remained undocumented, in part because of the social isolation when schools were closed and the lack of adults outside the home regularly monitoring children's well-being.[15,16]

Especially during the first year of the pandemic, caregivers had little in their control to ensure the safety of their family, especially if their occupation was considered "essential" or their financial situation did not afford an opportunity for them to remain home. The perception of loss of control was heightened by the uncertainty of information provided by previously trusted sources about the prevention of infection and clinical course of COVID-19, difficulty obtaining resources that they believed would protect their family (eg, masks, vaccines), and misinformation about potential shortages of household necessities which led to limited access to supplies and hoarding of resources (eg, toilet paper, paper towels, soap). Pediatricians can help caregivers by not only communicating information about an evolving public health emergency, but also by helping caregivers and children to accurately assess personal risk. In this way, caregivers are better positioned to distinguish between the possibility of a potential risk and the actual probability of a negative outcome occurring, thereby reducing anxiety in caregivers.

MENTAL HEALTH NEEDS DURING THE PANDEMIC

Children may demonstrate a wide range of adjustment reactions after a disaster including both internalizing and externalizing problems as well as somatic reactions,[17] but most children will return to their pre-existing emotional state after the threat is no longer present. **Table 1** lists some of the more common symptoms of adjustment reactions in children after a disaster. Many children will hide their distress in order to support adult caregivers who may be visibly distressed or because they sense that their reactions are abnormal or inappropriate. As a result, adults often underestimate the degree of distress experienced by children in the aftermath of a disaster. For this reason, supports should be offered to children when major stressors are experienced

Table 1 Common symptoms of adjustment reactions in children after a disaster[19]	
Sleep problems	Difficulty falling or staying asleep, frequent night awakenings or difficulty awakening in the morning, nightmares, or other sleep disruptions.
Eating problems	Loss of appetite or increased eating.
Sadness or depression	May result in a reluctance to engage in previously enjoyed activities or a withdrawal from peers and adults.
Anxiety, worries, or fears	Children may be concerned about a repetition of the traumatic event (eg, become afraid during storms after surviving a tornado) or show an increase in unrelated fears (eg, become more fearful of the dark even if the disaster occurred during daylight). This may present as separation anxiety or school avoidance.
Difficulties in concentration	The ability to learn and retain new information or to otherwise progress academically may be compromised.
Substance abuse	The new onset or exacerbation of alcohol, tobacco, or other substance use may be seen in children and adults after a disaster.
Risk-taking behavior	Increased sexual behavior or other reactive risk-taking can occur, especially among older children and adolescents.
Somatization	Children with adjustment difficulties may present instead with physical symptoms suggesting a physical condition.
Developmental or social regression	Children (and adults) may become less patient or tolerant of change or become irritable and disruptive.
Post-traumatic reactions and disorders	

Adapted from the Textbook of Clinical Pediatrics, 2nd ed; with permission.

(such as the death of a close family member) even in the absence of apparent distress. Psychological resilience can be enhanced in children through multilevel systems including school, family, the medical home, and community resources, working together to reduce risks during a pandemic.[18]

Screening instruments generally used in pediatric practice settings to identify early signs of mental illness may not be valid in the context of a pandemic or other public health crisis, when distress (eg, stress, sadness, worries) would be expected to be essentially universal. This may lead to overdiagnosis of PTSD, depression, or anxiety respectively.

Population-level or universal support should be a primary focus of providing psychosocial support rather than following a primary medical model of screening, identification, diagnosis, and referral to treatment of individuals with perceived mental illness—with a goal of universal support to promote resiliency as the primary goal rather than treatment of mental illness. Within the United States, there was a disproportionate burden of both COVID-19 infection and mortality, as well as related stressors (eg, financial stresses and housing instability), among individuals from marginalized minorities and/or socioeconomically disadvantaged families. The increase burden of illness and disadvantage was compounded by the pre-existing limited access to services and supports within these communities. This highlights the need to provide universal support during a public health emergency while taking added steps to ensuring equitable access to resources and supports in such disadvantaged groups.

The principles of Psychological First Aid (PFA) provide a useful framework to pediatric practices on how to support patients and families during a public health emergency. PFA includes psychoeducation—to help individuals understand common reactions coupled with practical advice on how to cope with these reactions; attention to ensuring basic needs; and supportive services to promote coping strategies and adjustment and to accelerate the natural recovery process. Research supports that PFA training significantly improves knowledge of appropriate psychosocial response and PFA skills in supporting people in acute distress.[20] All staff in pediatric health care settings should have basic skills in PFA. Given that the same strategies can used in the context of a personal or family crisis, it represents a basic skill set that health care providers can use daily.

As an ongoing public health emergency lasting for several years, the COVID-19 pandemic taxed pre-existing coping strategies of children and resources and systems of support. The many losses experienced; the prolonged fear/threat of infection, serious illness or death; the isolation, loneliness, and suppression of social needs; and the wide range of secondary stressors created additional coping challenges.[21] Risk and protective factors that can help identify those children at higher risk for mental health difficulties in the setting of a public health emergency can be found in **Box 1**.

Pediatric health care providers should work to mitigate the impact of risk factors, while fostering protective factors to increase children's resilience. They should share

---

Box 1
Risk and protective factors for mental health difficulties among children in the setting of a public health emergency

Risk Factors
- Prepandemic functioning and vulnerabilities including history of adverse experiences as well as acute or chronic medical or mental health issues.[22,23] Children with pre-existing anxiety or depression should be encouraged to continue or resume mental health services remotely as soon as possible after the beginning of the public health emergency.
- Younger school-age children may be more at risk because of the missed routines and stimulation of early childhood education.[24,25]
- Death or serious/chronic illness of caregiver.
- Impairments of caregiver functioning, with the risk being more pronounced with single caregiver families and caregivers suffering from a mental illness.[26,27]
- Caregivers at greater risk of COVID-19 exposure such as caregivers considered "essential workers" including front line health care workers during the pandemic. Essential workers dealt during the pandemic with the fear of personal infection and potentially spreading the virus to family members.
- Reduced access to peers resulting in loneliness and isolation.[28]
- When special needs of the child cannot be met through remote instruction, especially those children with neurodevelopmental, intellectual, or language disorders.[29]
- When the family and/or child's perception of risks posed by the public health emergency are increased.
- Children of marginalized minorities and/or socioeconomically disadvantaged families or others with less pre-existing resources and support.

Protective Factors
- Maintenance of routine/structure in the home.
- Effective family communication about the public health emergency.
- Positive familial relationships and improved family connections due to time together.
- Social support,[30] which has been identified as the main protective factor for children identified in nearly all disaster research studies.[31]
- Appropriate play and leisure.
- Physical exercise such as athletics which decreases sedentary behavior and overreliance on screen time.
- Access to entertainment and learning opportunities to decrease boredom and provide stimulation.

these strategies with caregivers. Family attentiveness to the emotional needs of their children during a pandemic becomes more important because of their child's isolation from peers and important adults outside the home (such as educators). Pediatricians can share tips about active listening strategies so that caregivers can be better attuned to the emotional needs of the children. Families should establish and maintain predictable routines in the home such as established times for meals and bedtime, and encourage family play and activities, and the teaching of life skills (eg, cooking, maintenance of the home).

Resiliency can be fostered by promoting problem-solving, enhancing motivation to overcome challenges, fostering a sense of purpose and hope, encouraging supportive relationships, and by providing security through the demonstration of leadership by role models.[32] Caregivers can offer age-appropriate opportunities for their children to gain a sense of control and engage in decision-making so that children can restore meaning in their lives and achieve confidence that they can master challenges they may face and contribute to their own recovery[32] and that of others. Finding ways to help others can also help people feel some sense of agency during a time when many are feeling powerless.

Caregivers should be encouraged to attend to their own needs as continued vigilance to the needs of their children during the many waves of a pandemic can otherwise lead to emotional burnout and the neglect of personal needs of adults.

COMPLICATIONS OF GRIEVING DURING THE COVID-19 PANDEMIC

Children who experienced the death of a close family member or a friend as a result of a disaster are more likely to have prolonged post-traumatic stress symptoms[33] and to develop later emotional difficulties.[17] Even outside the context of a pandemic, bereavement can have both immediate and long-lasting impacts on children's emotional adjustment, psychological functioning, academic achievement, developmental trajectory, and social and behavioral adaptation.[12]

More than one million people in the United States are estimated to have died during the pandemic; this increases the likelihood that a child knew someone who died whether in their family or community. Dying is a natural part of life; however, death is often a frightening event for children. Deaths in the midst of the COVID-19 pandemic magnified normative fears. Social distancing often separated those that were dying from family and friends, limiting the opportunity to share feelings and support during the end-of-life stage and thereby interfered with a healthy grieving process.[34] Communicating feelings to a sick family member in a restricted health care setting via a cell phone or computer limited the expression of feelings, especially if the infected family member could not actively participate because of their health status. Death due to COVID-19, or even deaths from unrelated causes that occurred during the period of strict isolation of patients due to fears of the spread of COVID-19, was often a lonely and dehumanized process for patients and families. Families often found difficulty obtaining information about the health status of their family member which resulted in their feeling powerless and unable to help or be with their loved ones.[35] Family members often made difficult decisions (eg, suspending life support) from a distance and with limited information and support. Children and their families were not permitted to participate in the funeral rituals of their culture or visit their family members before their death. When patients and families find themselves facing death and grief in unexpected ways that deviate from preconceived expectations, unresolved family issues and prolonged grief may become more common.[34]

Secondary Losses

A number of significant and profound secondary losses were also experienced by children and families during the COVID-19 pandemic beyond those losses due to death. These events and experiences may be considered by children as a significant and persistent "gap" or "hole" in their lives. Pediatricians can help children by broadening their questions related to grief to include these other losses, including

1. Loss of pleasurable experiences such as time with extended family and friends, dating, vacations, travel, participation in sports, attending theater, restaurants, concerts, and religious services.
2. Quality of life losses due to reduced family income and concern about savings.
3. Loss of milestones and one-time experiences such as graduations, special birthdays or anniversaries, prom, college visits, athletic championship games, etc.

Communicating with and Supporting Grieving Children

Pediatricians may find it stressful supporting grieving children in the midst of a public health emergency. They may not know what to say or not say, feel profoundly sad witnessing children in distress when they themselves are experiencing distress and loss, or when they find prior feelings of loss and trauma are activated in the setting of widespread death and distress. Pediatricians may feel that they should not show emotions to their patients and worry about the cost of this emotional engagement especially when they already feel overwhelmed by stress they have encountered during the pandemic.

Pediatricians may worry that simply asking children about the death of someone close to them may upset them further. In the immediate aftermath of a major loss, the loss is almost always on a child's mind. Although a question about the death may lead to an expression of sadness, it is the death itself, and not the question, that is the cause of the distress. Inviting children to express their feelings allows them to express their sadness; it does not cause it. In contrast, avoiding the subject may create more problems. Children may interpret the silence as evidence that the pediatrician is unaware of their loss, feels that their loss is trivial and unworthy of comment, is disinterested in their grief, is unwilling or unable to assist, or views the child as unable to cope even with support. Instead, **Box 2** lists steps that can be used to initiate the conversation.

Further information on how pediatricians can support grieving children and families can be found in the clinical report from the American Academy of Pediatrics.[36]

PROFESSIONAL SELF-CARE AND WELLNESS DURING A PANDEMIC

The COVID-19 pandemic pushed doctors and health care workers to the limits of their professional competence and took a considerable toll on their health and well-being.[37] Many pediatricians needed to change the way they worked with children, often relying on the self-report of caregivers and telemedicine sessions where possible to evaluate the emerging and chronic needs of their patients. Pediatricians also needed to weigh their personal risk of exposure when they resumed in-person visits with their duty to care for their patients. The vigilance about potential personal infection and spreading the infection to their families was an additional burden. In turn, the need to self-isolate if they or their family members had tested positively for COVID-19 took pediatricians away from their clinical practice. All these factors can cause guilt, tension, and moral injury—the challenge of knowing what care patients need but being unable to provide it due to constraints beyond their control.[37]

A 2021 online survey of physicians collected 1 year after the start of the pandemic found that 80% were impacted as a result of COVID-19: 49% reported

---

Box 2
Initiating the conversation with grieving children during a pandemic or public health emergency

- *Express your concern*: It is okay to be tearful or simply to let them know you feel sorry that someone they care about has died during the pandemic or about other losses they have experienced because of the pandemic.

- *Be genuine: children can tell when adults are authentic*: Do not tell the child you will miss her grandfather if you have never met him; instead, let the child know that you appreciate that he was important to her and you feel sorry that she had to experience such a loss.

- *Listen and observe; talk less*: Simply being present while the child is expressing grief and tolerating the unpleasant emotional display can be very helpful. Children often fear that the strong feelings they have will frighten others so active listening to their emotional expressions can help them find the courage to share their concerns.

- Invite discussion using open-ended questions such as "How are you doing since your mother died?", "How is your family coping with all the changes caused by the pandemic?", "What did you miss out on enjoying because of the pandemic?"

- Limit the sharing of your personal experiences or losses during the pandemic. Keep the focus on the child's loss(es) and feelings.

- Offer practical advice, such as suggestions about how to answer questions about the death that might be posed by peers or how to talk with teachers about associated learning challenges.

- Ask children what they already know about or have heard about the public health emergency. Look for misinformation, misunderstandings, and misconceptions, especially those that may cause or add to fears or concerns or contribute to feelings of guilt or shame. Children may feel shame if their family member died because of COVID-19 or guilt because they believe they could have helped their family member avoid becoming infected or helped them obtain treatment that would have prevented the death.

- *Offer appropriate reassurance*: Do not minimize children's concerns about worries they may still have about the pandemic or the future but let them know that over time you do expect that they will become better able to cope with their distress.

- Provide basic information in simple and direct terms. Avoid medical jargon and unnecessary detail.

- Communicate your availability to provide support over time. Do not require children or families to reach out to you for such support, but rather, make the effort to schedule follow-up appointments and reach out by phone or e-mail periodically.

---

a reduction in income and 32% experienced a reduction in staff. More than half of physicians (57%) had felt inappropriate feelings of anger, tearfulness, or anxiety because of COVID-19; 46% of physicians had withdrawn or isolated themselves from others; and 34% reported feeling hopeless or without a purpose. Despite the high incidence of mental health symptoms, only 14% of physicians sought professional support.[38]

Pediatricians play a vital role for children and families by demonstrating emotional regulation and availability, promoting a reasonable approach to problem-solving, and modeling coping strategies. Indeed, to help ensure that patients receive the best care possible during a public health crisis, and to prevent burnout and foster job satisfaction, pediatricians have a responsibility to take care of themselves and their colleagues—both physically and psychologically.[39] Pediatricians may wish to ignore signs of personal distress and "unpacking" of their own "emotional baggage" until the crisis period passes, but this is unrealistic during a long-term public health crisis

---

Box 3
Core elements of a comprehensive self-care plan for professional and personal wellness

Decrease levels of stress activation
- Reduce stress levels through relaxation activities
- Reduce the impact of stressors through the use of time and practice management tools

Increase the amount of pleasurable activities
- Engage in hobbies and areas of personal interest
- Participate in activities that encourage personal growth or the acquisition of new skills
- Allow time to appreciate and celebrate personal achievements

Change the way you think about problems and challenges
- Practice creativity, flexibility, and positivity
- Maintain an openness to change, feedback, learning, and growth
- Use problem-solving tools to be more decisive
- Increase acceptance of the limitations (imperfections) of self, others, and the world

Increase appreciation of emotions
- Experience all emotions freely and see them as helpful feedback
- Process emotions at a level you control

Increase body/health/wellness activities

Improve satisfaction from relationships and the satisfaction others have with you
- Increase social support from family members and colleagues
- Assert personal needs and set clear boundaries to the requests of others
- Improve the quality of social interactions
- Limit exposure to negative and pessimistic conversations

Seek balance and predictability in your life
- Strive to maintain a balance among professional, personal, and family roles
- Incorporate daily routines that provide comfort and predictability

---

such as the COVID-19 pandemic. Pediatricians may also be reluctant to focus on their own needs when patients and their own family members are struggling.

The first step in making self-care a priority is to recognize barriers which prevent you from following through with your wellness plan as well as signs that your self-care plan is not helping you manage your lifestyle. Health care providers should monitor themselves and their colleagues for warning signs including emotional overload, neglect of health and relationships, professional burnout, and compassion fatigue.

Box 3 includes suggested elements that health care providers should consider when they develop their own comprehensive self-care plan for professional and personal wellness.

CLINICS CARE POINTS

- During a pandemic or other public health emergency, pediatric health care providers should focus on providing universal support to promote resiliency in all children and families.

- It is important to distinguish between transient distress and sadness, which is virtually universal during a pandemic, from mental illness that requires clinical intervention.

- Pediatric health care providers can offer valuable practical guidance to parents and other caregivers on how to talk to and support their children during a pandemic.

- There are 2 main purposes for public health communications during a crisis: to provide realistic reassurance and to provide practical advice that can be used to decrease risk. Informing patients and their families of a new and potential risk without providing any practical information on steps to decrease risk may only foster fear and feelings of helplessness.

- Telling children that they should not be worried or minimize their concerns during a pandemic is not helpful. Discuss with children their concerns and help them learn strategies to cope with feelings of distress, fear, anxiety, or sadness.

DISCLOSURE

The authors have nothing to disclose.

REFERENCES

1. Nelson C, Lurie N, Wasserman J, et al. Conceptualizing and defining public health emergency preparedness. Am J Publ Health 2007 Apr;97(Suppl 1):S9–11.
2. Deolmi M, Pisani F. Psychological and psychiatric impact of COVID-19 pandemic among children and adolescents. Acta Biomed 2020;91(4):e2020149.
3. Feldman G, Martin S, Donovan E. Psychological flexibility as a predictor of mental health outcomes in parents of pre-school children during the COVID-19 pandemic: a two-year longitudinal study. J Contextual Behav Sci 2023;27:116–9.
4. Madigan S, Racine N, Vaillancourt T, et al. Changes in depression and anxiety among children and adolescents from before to during the COVID-19 pandemic: a systematic review and meta-analysis. JAMA Pediatr 2023;177(6):567–81.
5. Essler S, Christner N, Paulus M. Short-term and long-term effects of the COVID-19 pandemic on child psychological well-being: a four-wave longitudinal study. Eur Child Adolesc Psychiatr 2023;1–14.
6. Kaess M, Hoekstra PJ. Child and adolescent psychiatry in the post-COVID era: lessons learned and consequences for the future. Eur Child Adolesc Psychiatr 2023;32:917–9.
7. Available at:Don't let children be the hidden victims of COVID-19 pandemic. UNICEF; 2021 https://www.unicef.org/reports/hidden-victims-of-covid-19-pandemic. [Accessed 23 September 2023].
8. Alban Conto C, Akseer S, Dreesen T, et al. Florence, Italy. Available at:, . COVID-19: effects of school closures on foundational skills and promising practices for monitoring and mitigating learning loss. Innocenti Working Paper 2020-13. UNICEF Office of Research; 2020 https://www.unicef-irc.org/publications/pdf/COVID-19_Effects_of_School_Closures_on_Foundational_Skills_and_Promising_Practices_for_Monitoring_and_Mitigating_Learning_Loss.pdf. [Accessed 23 September 2023].
9. Newlove-Delgado T, Russell AE, Mathews F, et al. Annual research review: the impact of COVID-19 on psychopathology in children and young people worldwide: systematic review of studies with pre- and within-pandemic data. J Child Psychol Psychiatry 2023 Apr;64(4):611–40.
10. Cortés-Albornoz MC, Ramírez-Guerrero S, García-Guáqueta DP, et al. Effects of remote learning during COVID-19 lockdown on children's learning abilities and school performance: a systematic review. Int J Educ Dev 2023 Sep;101:102835.
11. Morgan H. Alleviating the challenges with remote learning during a pandemic. Educ Sci 2022;12(2):109. https://doi.org/10.3390/educsci12020109.
12. Schonfeld DJ, Quackenbush M. The grieving student: a guide for schools. 2nd edition. Baltimore, MD: Brookes Publishing; 2021.
13. Adegboye D, Williams F, Collishaw S, et al. Understanding why the COVID-19 pandemic-related lockdown increases mental health difficulties in vulnerable young children. JCPP Adv 2021;1:e12005.

14. Thompson SF, Shimomaeda L, Calhoun R, et al. Maternal mental health and child adjustment problems in response to the COVID-19 pandemic in families experiencing economic disadvantage. Res Child Adolesc Psychopathol 2022;50(6): 695–708.

15. Whaling KM, Der Sarkissian A, Larez N, et al. Child maltreatment prevention service cases are significantly reduced during the COVID-19 pandemic: a longitudinal investigation into unintended consequences of quarantine. Child Maltreat 2023 Feb;28(1):34–41.

16. Qu M, Yang K, Cao Y, et al. Mental health status of adolescents after family confinement during the COVID-19 outbreak in the general population: a longitudinal survey. Eur Arch Psychiatry Clin Neurosci 2023 Mar;273(2):335–45.

17. Pfefferbaum B, Shaw JA, American Academy of Child and Adolescent Psychiatry AACAP Committee on Quality Issues CQI. American Academy of Child and Adolescent Psychiatry (AACAP) Committee on Quality Issues (CQI). Practice parameter on disaster preparedness. J Am Acad Child Adolesc Psychiatry 2013 Nov;52(11):1224–38.

18. Masten AS, Motti-Stefanidi F. Multisystem resilience for children and youth in disaster: reflections in the context of COVID-19. Advers Resil Sci 2020;1(2): 95–106.

19. Schonfeld DJ, Gurwitch RH. Children in disasters. In: Elzouki AY, Stapleton FB, Whitley RJ, et al, editors. Textbook of clinical pediatrics. 2nd edition. Berlin, Germany: Springer-Verlag; 2012. p. 687–98.

20. Wang L, Norman I, Xiao T, et al. Psychological first aid training: a scoping review of its application, outcomes and implementation. Int J Environ Res Publ Health 2021 Apr 26;18(9):4594.

21. Gkatsa T. A systematic review of psychosocial resilience interventions for children and adolescents in the COVID-19 pandemic period. J School Educ Psychol 2023;3(1):34–48.

22. Stinson EA, Sullivan RM, Peteet BJ, et al. Longitudinal impact of childhood adversity on early adolescent mental health during the COVID-19 pandemic in the ABCD study cohort: does race or ethnicity moderate findings? Biol Psychiatry Glob Open Sci 2021 Dec;1(4):324–35.

23. Tso WWY, Wong RS, Tung KTS, et al. Vulnerability and resilience in children during the COVID-19 pandemic. Eur Child Adolesc Psychiatr 2022 Jan;31(1): 161–76.

24. Samji H, Wu J, Ladak A, et al. Review: Mental health impacts of the COVID-19 pandemic on children and youth - a systematic review. Child Adolesc Ment Health 2022 May;27(2):173–89.

25. Egan SM, Pope J, Moloney M, et al. Missing early education and care during the pandemic: the socio-emotional impact of the COVID-19 crisis on young children. Early Child Educ J 2021;49:925–34.

26. Babore A, Trumello C, Lombardi L, et al. Mothers' and children's mental health during the COVID-19 pandemic lockdown: the mediating role of parenting stress. Child Psychiatr Hum Dev 2023 Feb;54(1):134–46.

27. Gonzalez M, Zeidan J, Lai J, et al. Socio-demographic disparities in receipt of clinical health care services during the COVID-19 pandemic for Canadian children with disability. BMC Health Serv Res 2022;22:1434.

28. Farrell AH, Vitoroulis I, Eriksson M, et al. Loneliness and well-being in children and adolescents during the COVID-19 pandemic: a systematic review. Children 2023;10(2):279.

29. Asbury K, Toseeb U. A longitudinal study of the mental health of autistic children and adolescents and their parents during COVID-19: part 2, qualitative findings. Autism 2023 Jan;27(1):188–99.

30. Ehrler M, Hagmann CF, Stoeckli A, et al. Mental sequelae of the COVID-19 pandemic in children with and without complex medical histories and their parents: well-being prior to the outbreak and at four time-points throughout 2020 and 2021. Eur Child Adolesc Psychiatr 2023 Jun;32(6):1037–49.

31. Lai BS, Lewis R, Livings MS, et al. Posttraumatic stress symptom trajectories among children after disaster exposure: a review. J Trauma Stress 2017 Dec; 30(6):571–82.

32. Masten AS. Resilience of children in disasters: a multisystem perspective. Int J Psychol 2021 Feb;56(1):1–11.

33. King LS, Osofsky JD, Osofsky HJ, et al. Perceptions of trauma and loss among children and adolescents exposed to disasters: a mixed-methods study. Curr Psychol 2015;34:524–36.

34. LeRoy AS, Robles B, Kilpela LS, et al. Dying in the face of the COVID-19 pandemic: contextual considerations and clinical recommendations. Psychol Trauma 2020;12(S1):S98–9.

35. LeRoy AS, Knee CR, Derrick JL, et al. Implications for reward processing in differential responses to loss: impacts on attachment hierarchy reorganization. Pers Soc Psychol Rev 2019;23(4):391–405.

36. Schonfeld DJ, Demaria T, DISASTER PREPAREDNESS ADVISORY COUNCIL AND COMMITTEE ON PSYCHOSOCIAL ASPECTS OF CHILD AND FAMILY HEALTH. Providing psychosocial support to children and families in the aftermath of disasters and crises. Pediatrics 2015;136(4):e1120–30.

37. Goddard AF, Patel M. The changing face of medical professionalism and the impact of COVID-19. Lancet 2021 Mar 13;397(10278):950–2.

38. Available at:2021 Survey of America's physicians COVID-19 impact edition: a year later. The Physicians Foundation; 2021 https://www.physiciansfoundation. org/research-insights/the-physicians-foundation-2021-physician-survey/. [Accessed 23 September 2023].

39. Madrid PA, Schacher SJ. A critical concern: pediatrician self-care after disasters. Pediatrics 2006;117(5 Pt 3):S454–7.

Strengthening Pediatric and Public Health Collaboration to Protect Children's Health During a Pandemic

Zanah K. Francis, PhD[a], Elizabeth M. Dufort, MD[b],
Bernadette A. Albanese, MD, MPH[c], Wendy M. Chung, MD, MS[d],
Ellen H. Lee, MD, MPH[e], Zack Moore, MD, MPH[f],
Laurene Mascola, MD, MPH[g], Erica Pan, MD, MPH[h,i],
Caitlin Pedati, MD, MPH[j], George Turabelidze, MD, PhD[k],
Sarah Y. Park, MD[l],*

KEYWORDS

- Pandemic preparedness • Public health • School closure • Vaccination
- Science communication

KEY POINTS

- Pediatric health care providers serve a critical role in support of children and their families during a pandemic.
- Public health and pediatric providers need to maintain a strong partnership to best support children and their families through a pandemic.

Continued

[a] United States Department of Health and Human Services, 200 Independence Avenue Southwest, Washington, DC 20201, USA; [b] Albany Medical College, 43 New Scotland Avenue, Albany, NY 12237, USA; [c] Adams County Health Department, 4430 South Adams County Parkway, Brighton, CO 80601, USA; [d] Texas Medical Association, 3600 Gaston Avenue, Dallas, TX 75246, USA; [e] New York City Department of Health and Mental Hygiene, 42-09 28th Street, CN-22A, Long Island City, NY 11101, USA; [f] Division of Public Health, Epidemiology Section, Department of Health and Human Services, 225 N. McDowell Street, Raleigh, NC 27603, USA; [g] Los Angeles County Department of Public Health, 313 N. Figueroa Street, Los Angeles, CA 90012, USA; [h] Center for Infectious Diseases, California Department of Public Health, 850 Marina Bay Parkway, Richmond, CA 94804, USA; [i] Pediatric Infectious Diseases, University of California, San Francisco, CA, USA; [j] Virginia Beach Department of Public Health; 4452 Corporation Lane, Virginia Beach, VA 23462, USA; [k] Missouri Department of Health and Senior Services, 220 South Jefferson Street, St Louis, MO, 63103, USA; [l] John A. Burns School of Medicine Department of Pediatrics, Kapiolani Medical Center for Women & Children, University of Hawaii at Manoa, 1319 Punahou Street, Room 739, Honolulu, HI 96826, USA
* Corresponding author.
E-mail address: sypark@alum.mit.edu

Pediatr Clin N Am 71 (2024) 469–479
https://doi.org/10.1016/j.pcl.2024.01.016
0031-3955/24/© 2024 Elsevier Inc. All rights reserved.

pediatric.theclinics.com

Continued

- Key actions for pediatric providers include the following:
  - ○ Build connections with your state, tribal, or territorial and local public health infrastructure in advance of an emergency, and develop and maintain connections with your local pediatric organizations (eg, local AAP chapter, children's hospital) to facilitate timely communications and ready access to support during a public health emergency.
  - ○ Leverage public health and clinical professional connections to stay current regarding public health issues and provide input or feedback regarding public health recommendations and plans addressing children and their families.
  - ○ Engage in pandemic preparedness now to identify children and families in your care who would likely be at higher risk for severe illness, ensure appropriate staff support, and facilitate evidence-based care and timely communication for your patients and their families in alignment with a public health response.

INTRODUCTION

The widespread and significant impact of the coronavirus disease 2019 (COVID-19) pandemic on children and their families, characterized by its global scale, rapid transmission, and extensive mitigation measures, serves as a stark reminder that our communities remain susceptible to such events and these events may not be confined to once-in-a-century occurrences. As current or former public health pediatricians reflecting on this crisis as well as past pandemics such as the 2009 H1N1 influenza pandemic (pH1N1), it is clear our strategies for pediatric readiness for future pandemics need substantial transformation. A major objective of any pandemic is to implement mitigation measures, including non-pharmaceutical intervention measures such as testing/screening, masking, and school closures that can slow the incidence of new infections and reduce the impact of ill patients on health care systems, with the least disruptions on families' lives, until effective vaccines or treatments are widely available (**Fig. 1**).[1] However, deciding what interventions to implement and when is often complicated by multiple factors, and children may be particularly vulnerable to the effects of these interventions, both direct and indirect. COVID-19, especially, has highlighted the importance of proactive pandemic planning, response, and recovery for pediatric health care providers to ensure the health and well-being of children during a public health emergency. Future plans must effectively address the unique needs and concerns of pediatric populations. This article provides an overview of lessons learned and key components that should be considered by pediatric health care providers, practice sites, health systems, and public health for establishing pandemic preparedness focused on children and their families, including identifying and managing risks, communicating with patients and families, and implementing public health measures, in support of the overall public health response. By understanding the key components of pandemic planning, pediatric health care providers can play a critical role in protecting the health of children and their families.

APPROACH

Current and former pediatric public health physician co-authors from across the United States were convened for multiple sessions to discuss lessons learned and strategies to strengthen pediatric health care provider partnerships and pandemic preparedness. The experts were selected based on their training and broad

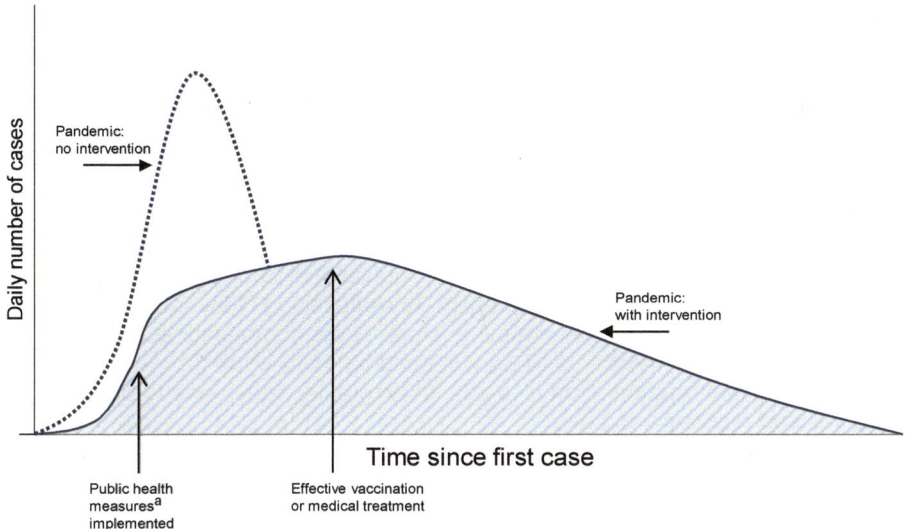

Fig. 1. Public health objectives of pandemic response. [a]Examples of public health measures include non-pharmaceutical intervention measures such as social distancing, testing/screening, masking, and school closures. Demonstrated is a simplified concept to convey basic public health objectives. Other complex factors such as the potential for no effective vaccine or medical treatment and subsequent need to reassess, modify, or reconsider intervention measures or demonstrating the impact of an overwhelmed health care capacity are important considerations but not depicted in this figure. (*Adapted from* Qualls N, Levitt A, Kanade N, et al. Community Mitigation Guidelines to Prevent Pandemic Influenza — United States, 2017. MMWR Recomm Rep 2017;66(No. RR-1):1–34. DOI: https://doi.org/10.15585/mmwr.rr6601a1.)

experience in a variety of areas, including child health, public health policy, community-based interventions, and pandemic response within local, large city or county, and state public health departments. These authors were asked to discuss the following topics surrounding lessons learned and pandemic planning: the role of the pediatric provider in a pandemic, the impact of disease severity on children, coordination and communication with local public health officials, effective communication, and issues unique to children such as school closing and reopening as well as vaccination logistics and challenges. The discussions were recorded, transcribed, and analyzed to identify common themes and recommendations. The findings from the discussion meetings were used to develop the content of this article.

LESSONS FROM PAST PANDEMICS: H1N1 INFLUENZA PANDEMIC VERSUS. CORONAVIRUS DISEASE 2019

Comparing lessons learned from public health and health care system responses to pH1N1 and COVID-19 demonstrates important differences in public perception and decision-making as they relate to risk among pediatric populations. One example of differing acceptance of mitigation measures based on relative risk to pediatric populations is that regarding school closures. Given the increased relative risk to younger populations during pH1N1, many parents and communities advocated for temporary school closures, reflecting a sense of fear and uncertainty related to the impact of the virus on children and young adults, although such closure was not always warranted given the incubation and transmission dynamics of pH1N1.[2] In contrast, although COVID-19 posed specific concerns for children (eg, multisystem inflammatory syndrome in children (MIS-C), severe acute COVID-19), COVID-19 has posed a greater risk for severe disease among older adults.[3–6] Although many schools elected to close quickly in the spring of 2020, this different dynamic plus multiple additional factors, including the disease impact and restriction measures in any given region, resulted in often mixed responses to COVID-19 mitigation measures.

These different relative and perceived risks posed unique challenges for decision-makers in balancing data-driven public health interventions against levels of community concern related to perceived impacted populations. Further, these differences underscore the need for a more comprehensive examination of the factors that shape public perception during pandemics as this can affect community acceptance and adoption of mitigation measures. By understanding these dynamics, we can better tailor future communication strategies and foster greater adherence to public health measures and recommendations.

COORDINATION AND COLLABORATION ACROSS PUBLIC HEALTH AND PEDIATRIC PROVIDERS

In a pandemic response, timing is critical. To ensure timely dissemination of vital information, communication channels between public health officials and pediatric providers should be efficient and well-established a priori. However, the existing communication landscape still includes gaps that demand immediate attention. Early in a pandemic or other public health crises, this void has hindered the timely dissemination of accurate information to parents and patients, contributing to misinformation and confusion. Establishing these channels before a crisis ensues is essential, allowing health care providers to receive real-time updates, guidance, and recommendations. This communication gap was evident during pH1N1, and similar challenges occurred during the COVID-19 response which underscores the need for further progress in addressing misinformation and confusion during pandemics.

Encouraging proactive involvement of pediatric providers in public health initiatives can bridge knowledge gaps, align strategies, and promote a unified response (**Fig. 2**). By fostering relationships, pediatric providers can contribute valuable clinical insights while public health officials can provide vital epidemiologic perspectives, emerging public health guidance and recommendations, and access to tools and resources. Collaborative efforts are essential to ensure children receive optimal care and families receive appropriate guidance during emergencies. Health communicators within public health departments can bolster this effort by crafting and sharing with pediatric providers clear, evidence-based messages that resonate with diverse audiences, thus promoting consistent and accurate information dissemination. Leveraging communications-related technology could further enhance communication between public health officials and pediatric providers through efficient and scalable means of sharing information, disseminating guidelines, and engaging in real-time discussions. Early communication structures lay the foundation for effective response and ensure public health officials and pediatric providers present a united front in the face of uncertainty.

The landscape of pediatric care is diverse, encompassing a wide array of providers, with each group possessing a unique vantage point in children's health care, thus making their involvement in pandemic response important. However, there are challenges in ensuring communication reaches the full spectrum of providers. Identifying and reaching every provider can pose an immense challenge. Tailoring messages to

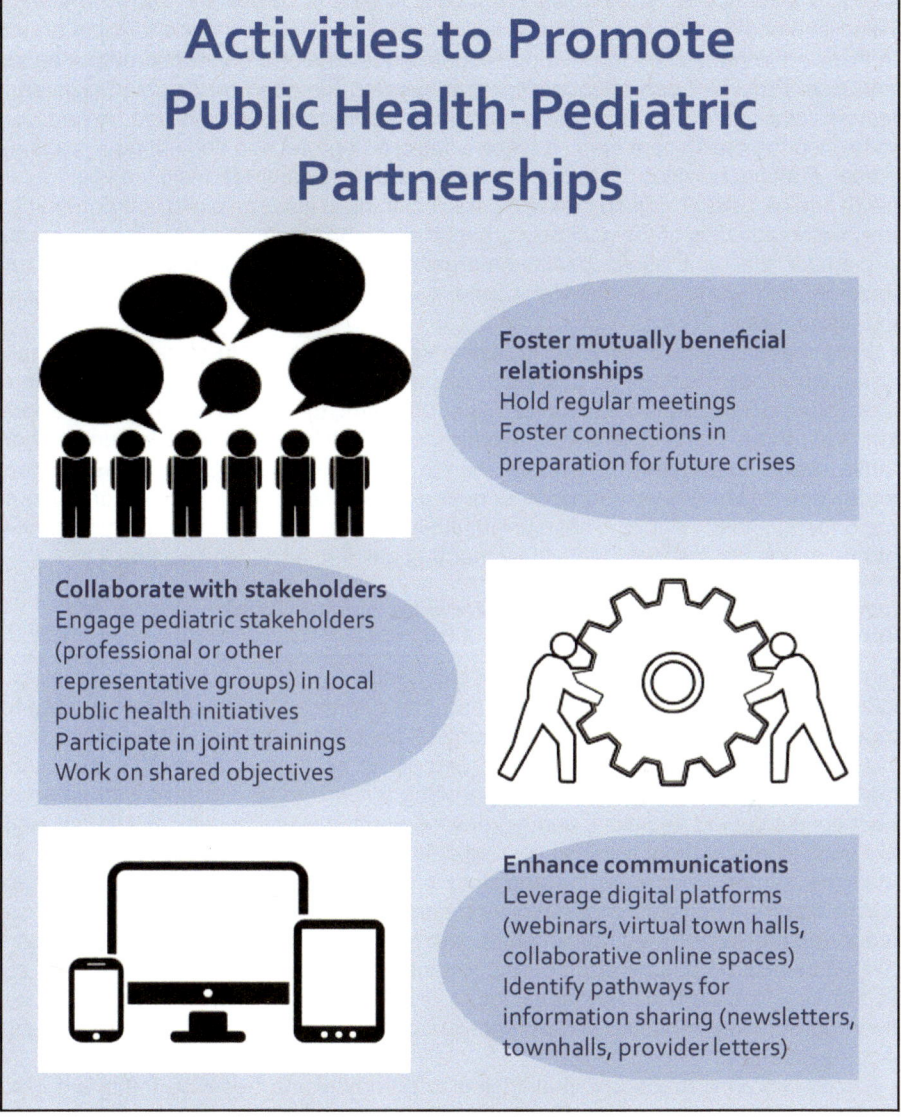

Fig. 2. Building bridges to support a unified response in a crisis.

resonate with each group's expertise, while maintaining consistency, poses a complex yet imperative task. Recognizing the nuances of these roles and targeting communication can facilitate harnessing the full potential of the pediatric care network to contribute to a community's pandemic response and eventual recovery. Identifying and rectifying these communication gaps can enhance the collective ability to deliver comprehensive and well-coordinated pediatric care during pandemics.

Local public health jurisdictions are on the front lines of pandemic response, facing legal, political, and logistical challenges in community engagement and in recommending and enforcing public health measures. Multiple challenges have the potential to undermine evidence-based public health decisions, which should be based on scientific evidence and unbiased responses. Pediatric providers and community-based stakeholders engaged in the wellbeing of children and their families should be involved in processes to develop recommendations and pandemic response approaches. Providers can advocate for emphasizing the need for decisions rooted in best available data and scientific expertise to optimize prevention and patient care while ensuring health care staff infection control and protection and mitigating against mutual staffing burnout. Establishing and funding collaborations involving public health and pediatric-focused stakeholders, including in academia and in communities, now, well in advance of the next public health emergency, could be an effective means to plan for the next public health emergency, fill the gaps in pediatric data and research, and work on pediatric-focused evaluations of public health emergencies and responses.

While preparedness activities and considerations can never fully prepare our health systems and communities for unknown risks and scenarios, it is essential to have pre-established connections and relationships, platforms for coordination and collaboration, and modes of effective communication across all levels of our communities from public health to pediatric providers, health systems, academia and researchers, community-based organizations, other government officials, emergency management responders, and the public. These pre-established platforms are necessary requisites for any pandemic response activities affecting children and their families.

Communication for Patients and Their Families: Pediatric Providers as Trusted Messengers

Primary care providers together with public health agencies can serve as important sources of information for children and their families. Clear, concise easy-to-understand communication is paramount to rapidly inform the public, build trust, and promote the adoption of recommended public health measures. Effective public health messaging strategies must juggle being timely and transparent with reflecting the rationale behind decisions and acknowledging the evolving nature of the situation and gaps in information. Meanwhile, pediatric providers, especially pediatricians, are often the trusted messengers, translating complex scientific concepts and varying risks into comprehensible information and recommendations for families.[7] Their experience and pre-established relationships with patients and families foster trust, making them influential communicators during a pandemic. Further, pediatric providers can be the key to adapting messages for their unique communities, especially those disproportionately impacted and potentially lacking trust in the larger health and public health systems.

Events like pandemics are challenging to communicate because there is a great degree of early uncertainty coupled with ongoing updates to recommendations as new information emerges. This might mean children and their families will have questions before there is sufficient information, or information may change over time, which can affect trust. Acknowledging uncertainty openly, coupled with transparent updates as knowledge unfolds, maintains credibility. This can help interrupt the flow of misinformation, which poses a significant challenge during pandemics, fueling fear, and sometimes creating apathy. In the digital age, misinformation can spread rapidly, fueling misconceptions and undermining public health efforts.[8,9]

Pediatric providers are viewed as health literacy experts, armed with accurate information and scientific understanding, and therefore essential in debunking false claims and counteracting misinformation by providing evidence-based information to families. Similar to other required continuing professional education, providers should consider training and consulting resources as needed to better equip themselves to discern credible sources and critically evaluate information, especially from social media. Given the popularity of social media as a primary source of information for many portions of the population, maintaining awareness of potential misinformation on these platforms will help identify key topics about which to educate patients and their families.[10]

Addressing common myths directly, supported by evidence, and highlighting reputable sources, contribute to building a solid foundation of accurate knowledge among families. The influx of studies and articles, coupled with the issue of increased non-peer reviewed as well as retracted papers, makes discerning reputable sources from sensationalized content a daunting task. Medical (eg, the American Academy of Pediatrics [AAP] and academic medical centers or children's hospitals) and public health (eg, the Centers for Disease Control and Prevention or state, tribal, or territorial, and local health departments) authorities can play valuable roles in disseminating accurate information to pediatric providers and the public. When evidence and understanding of a new disease or situation is evolving quickly and there may not be certainty yet about disease characteristics or how to prevent infection, consistency and alignment of messages can foster public trust.

PEDIATRIC HEALTH CARE PREPAREDNESS ALIGNING WITH PUBLIC HEALTH OBJECTIVES

The scale of a pandemic can strain health care systems and supply chains, underscoring the need for preparedness. Having systems and specifically a clinic or health care preparedness plan in place to manage patients during public health emergencies is crucial. Specifically, providers should establish plans to ensure staffing, including tracking staff vaccination status whether for vaccine-preventable or the pandemic disease, maintaining appropriate infection control procedures as well as overall operations policies, and plan options to address staff absenteeism during a pandemic. Depending on capacity, providers may opt to partner with larger practices or health systems for support. Additionally, resource strategies, telehealth approaches, and protocols and personal protective equipment for managing potentially infected patients are essential components of overall preparedness. Electronic health records can be used to facilitate tracking and analyzing critical data, including those regarding infected patients, identifying high risk patients and families, and sharing and receiving data regarding patient vaccinations.

Equitable access to care, for example, in the form of testing resources, should be addressed in all response activities. Disparities in testing availability can hinder early case identification and possible treatment, leading to potentially greater transmission and more severe illness within marginalized communities. Pediatric providers can advocate for equitable access to testing, vaccinations, and health care to ensure all children, regardless of socioeconomic status or geographic location, have access to the same standard of care. Active collaborations with local health departments and community-based or health care organizations to facilitate mobile testing units, outreach efforts, and partnerships can make health care more accessible for underserved patients.

RESPONSE MEASURES WITH UNIQUE CHALLENGES AFFECTING CHILDREN
Vaccination

In any pandemic, scarcity of vaccines is inevitable in the initial stages related to the lag in developing an effective vaccine, followed by logistical and supply chain challenges. With pH1N1, developing a vaccine seemed straightforward although frustrating given the dependence on traditional egg-based technology which automatically meant a 5–7-month delay.[11] COVID-19 posed new challenges given the lack of a previous coronavirus vaccine and limited experience beyond the 2002–3 severe acute respiratory syndrome with a novel coronavirus having serious clinical impact. However, newer or rapidly advanced technologies have emerged in the form of, for example, mRNA vaccines, a technology that had been previously developed and may change the landscape for all future vaccines.[12,13] Vaccine demand during the pH1N1 and COVID-19 pandemics were both high initially and then declined, although the decline for pH1N1 was more precipitous,[14] while the rapid emergence of new COVID-19 variants that led to breakthrough infections and the need for frequent boosters led to some vaccine fatigue. Although overall demand for COVID-19 vaccines has declined,[15] the continuous emergence of new variants and findings suggesting seasonality[16] as COVID-19 evolves have translated to a certain level of sustained need. Add to this that every day as new babies are born there will always be a new wave of susceptible, COVID-19-naïve individuals also contributing to eroding overall herd immunity. A strategic approach to prioritization is needed with special attention directed toward messaging and outreach to ensure populations with risk factors, including, for example, younger and older age groups as well as those with underlying medical conditions associated with higher risk of severe illness receive the protection they and their families need.

Navigating the logistical challenges of enrolling pediatric providers in Vaccines for Children (VFC), other vaccine distribution programs, and immunization registries can be a pressing concern. Small practices face hurdles with multi-dose vials and the intricacies of cold chain logistics. Large health systems and institutions, including children's hospitals, can assume leadership roles in managing these logistics by partnering with small practices. This collaborative approach will not only address the challenges faced by such practices but also streamline the distribution process, ensuring vaccines reach the intended recipients without delay.

School-based vaccination programs and other non-traditional community-based delivery of health services may be potentially powerful strategies for ensuring widespread vaccine coverage and maintaining capacity to conduct mass prophylaxis for other large outbreaks.[17] Administering vaccines in a familiar and accessible environment like schools can reach a broader population and increase overall vaccination rates.[17–19] Keys to success require having strong stakeholder relationships and developing plans in advance. Assuming the vaccine cold chain requirements can be managed as with pH1N1, this approach holds promise for pediatric vaccinations, as schools serve as hubs of social interaction and potential disease transmission as well as provide a unique opportunity to reach large numbers of children, including those whose families might face barriers to accessing vaccines and medical care in other settings.

Immunization information systems and registries can help facilitate the tracking of vaccinations and the seamless sharing of information between different providers. Moreover, data gleaned from these systems have been instrumental in informed planning, particularly in light of the decline in routine vaccination coverage that occurred during the COVID-19 pandemic. Such planning is critical to avert future outbreaks of vaccine-preventable diseases associated with a wane in administering routine vaccinations. Pediatric providers should be familiar with their state's immunization information system and their VFC program or public health immunization program as public health communications regarding vaccines, both pandemic and routine, are often provided through or adapted from the VFC or similar public health immunization network.

School Closures

Few challenges have been as complicated and multifaceted as the decision-making processes surrounding the closure and reopening of schools and daycares during a pandemic. The decision to close schools and for how long during an outbreak or a pandemic is complex, requiring careful consideration of pathogen characteristics and transmission including the role of children in disease transmission, asymptomatic transmission, severity of disease in children, and the primary at-risk population for a given pandemic. Other factors that may also contribute to the decision include potential public health benefits, equity concerns, and adverse consequences not only for children but also staff and parents or the community in general. Pediatric providers should maintain awareness of these factors through the scientific literature and through those established communication channels with public health partners as recommended earlier in this article, as well as an awareness of the issues at their local schools and school districts.

At the beginning of the COVID-19 pandemic, while there was an absence of a clear understanding of transmission dynamics within educational settings and no access to more tailored mitigation strategies like vaccination or treatment, authorities grappled with the question of whether children might serve as vectors of infection to others including more vulnerable elders in their communities. Several papers published before and during pH1N1 explored the challenges and issues associated with school closures including effectiveness of school closures in reducing transmission, the economic and social costs of school closures, and the ethical considerations involved in making decisions about school closure.[20,21] School closures, while disruptive, can provide invaluable time to develop protocols, comprehend the nuances of the disease, and develop vaccines and medical treatments. Closures can be most effective when implemented early and in combination with other mitigation measures, such as social distancing and mask-wearing.[22]

There can also be a number of negative consequences, such as disruption to education, school-based services for children with special needs, childcare concerns affecting work and income in the family, acute mental health challenges or exacerbation of existing mental health conditions, compromised physical well-being, and food insecurity.[23,24] Any negative impacts will disproportionately affect low-income families who may lack the resources for remote learning, other learning experiences, and childcare. Acknowledging these disparities and tailoring interventions to address them is pivotal to ensure that public health measures do not inadvertently exacerbate societal inequities.

A continual evaluation of the impacts and best evidence considerations for return to school must be considered with relevant childcare stakeholders and advocates including pediatric providers with an aim toward the least necessary disruption to the mental and physical well-being of children and their families. In general, pediatric-focused assessment and modeling studies with key stakeholder involvement are needed to inform public health decisions and ensure measures prioritize both children's health and educational equity. The ABC Science collaborative started in 2020 by the Duke School of Medicine is one example of a collaborative effort between public health, educators, schools, academic researchers, and pediatric providers to provide data to inform evidence-based decision making in schools, including those related to school closing and reopening decisions.[25]

SUMMARY

Past experience but especially the COVID-19 pandemic has highlighted the need for an integrated approach to pandemic response and impacts on children, leveraging the strengths of both public health departments and pediatric health care providers. Proactive communication channels and strong relationships between public health and pediatric providers are imperative for effective pandemic preparedness. Transparent communication, even when faced with limited information, is pivotal in building trust and increasing public acceptance of recommended measures. Combating misinformation necessitates a joint effort to educate and empower pediatric health care providers, enabling them to serve as reliable sources of accurate and consistent information for families. By devising strategies for managing patients and maintaining open lines of communication, pediatric providers serve a key role in ensuring the safety of children, young adults, and families in the face of future pandemics. Recognizing that future epidemics and pandemics will occur, public health and pediatric providers must collaborate to minimize consequences and address the unique impacts on children and their families.

CLINICS CARE POINTS

- Collaboration and communication between public health and pediatric providers facilitates exchanging current and locally relevant information and guidance, which are essential to protect children's health during public health emergencies.

- Pediatric care providers are trusted messengers and important sources of information for children and their families; acknowledging uncertainty openly, coupled with transparent updates as knowledge unfolds, maintains credibility during a pandemic.

- Each pandemic or public health emergency poses different challenges and requires all to be flexible to adapt to those challenges.

DISCLOSURE

S.Y. Park is currently employed at Karius, Inc., but no financial assistance was received to support this article. E.M. Dufort has consulted with Hutton Health Consulting; however, no financial assistance was received to support this article. Otherwise, the authors have nothing to disclose. The authors are solely responsible for this document's contents and conclusions, which do not necessarily represent the views of their institutions.

REFERENCES

1. Qualls N, Levitt A, Kanade N, et al. Community mitigation guidelines to prevent pandemic influenza - United States, 2017. MMWR Recomm Rep (Morb Mortal Wkly Rep) 2017;66(1):1–34.
2. Park SY, Nakata MN, Elm JLM, et al. Outbreak of 2009 pandemic influenza A (H1N1) at a school - Hawaii, May 2009. MMWR Morb Mortal Wkly Rep 2010; 58(51):1440–4.
3. Martin B, DeWitt PE, Russell S, et al. Characteristics, outcomes, and severity risk factors associated with SARS-COV-2 infection among children in the US National COVID Cohort collaborative. JAMA Netw Open 2022;5(2):e2143151.
4. Ahmad FB, Cisewski JA, Xu J, et al. COVID-19 mortality update - United States, 2022. MMWR Morb Mortal Wkly Rep 2023;72(18):493–6.
5. da Costa VG, Saivish MV, Santos DER, et al. Comparative epidemiology between the 2009 H1N1 influenza and COVID-19 pandemics. J Infect Public Health 2020; 13(12):1797–804.

6. Feleszko W, Okarska-Napierała M, Buddingh EP, et al. Pathogenesis, immunology, and immune-targeted management of the multisystem inflammatory syndrome in children (MIS-C) or pediatric inflammatory multisystem syndrome (PIMS): EAACI Position Paper. Pediatr Allergy Immunol 2023;34(1):e13900.
7. Leonard MB, Pursley DM, Robinson LA, et al. The importance of trustworthiness: lessons from the COVID-19 pandemic. Pediatr Res 2022;91(3):482–5.
8. Nelson T, Kagan N, Critchlow C, et al. The danger of misinformation in the COVID-19 crisis. Mo Med 2020;117(6):510–2.
9. Rosenberg H, Shahbaz S, Rezaie S. The Twitter pandemic: The critical role of Twitter in the dissemination of medical information and misinformation during the COVID-19 pandemic. CJEM J Can Assoc Emerg Physicians 2020;22(4):418–21.
10. Turner KH, Jolls T, Hagerman MS, et al. Developing digital and media literacies in children and adolescents. Pediatrics 2017;140(Supplement_2):S122–6.
11. Krietsch Boerner L. The flu shot and the egg. ACS Cent Sci 2020;6(2):89–92.
12. Pardi N, Hogan MJ, Porter FW, et al. mRNA vaccines — a new era in vaccinology. Nat Rev Drug Discov 2018;17(4):261–79.
13. Verbeke R, Lentacker I, De Smedt SC, et al. The dawn of mRNA vaccines: The COVID-19 case. J Control Release 2021;333:511–20.
14. Institute of Medicine (US). Forum on medical, public health preparedness for catastrophic events. Available at:. Vaccine Supply. National Academies Press (US); 2010 . [Accessed 29 September 2023].
15. Quan NK, Anh NLM, Taylor-Robinson AW. The global COVID-19 vaccine surplus: tackling expiring stockpiles. Infectious Diseases of Poverty 2023;12(1):21.
16. Wiemken TL, Khan F, Puzniak L, et al. Seasonal trends in COVID-19 cases, hospitalizations, and mortality in the United States and Europe. Sci Rep 2023;13: 3886.
17. Effler PV, Chu C, He H, et al. Statewide school-located influenza vaccination program for children 5-13 years of age, Hawaii, USA. Emerg Infect Dis 2010;16(2): 244–50.
18. Benjamin-Chung J, Arnold BF, Mishra K, et al. City-wide school-located influenza vaccination: A retrospective cohort study. Vaccine 2021;39(42):6302–7.
19. Humiston SG, Schaffer SJ, Szilagyi PG, et al. Seasonal influenza vaccination at school: a randomized controlled trial. Am J Prev Med 2014;46(1):1–9.
20. Cauchemez S, Ferguson NM, Wachtel C, et al. Closure of schools during an influenza pandemic. Lancet Infect Dis 2009;9(8):473–81.
21. Chao DL, Halloran ME, Longini IM Jr. School opening dates predict pandemic influenza A(H1N1) outbreaks in the United States. JID (J Infect Dis) 2010;202(6): 877–80.
22. Ayouni I, Maatoug J, Dhouib W, et al. Effective public health measures to mitigate the spread of COVID-19: a systematic review. BMC Publ Health 2021;21(1):1015.
23. Viner R, Russell S, Saulle R, et al. school closures during social lockdown and mental health, health behaviors, and well-being among children and adolescents during the first COVID-19 wave: a systematic review. JAMA Pediatr 2022;176(4): 400–9.
24. Engzell P, Frey A, Verhagen MD. Learning loss due to school closures during the COVID-19 pandemic. Proc Natl Acad Sci U S A 2021;118(17). https://doi.org/10.1073/pnas.2022376118.
25. Collaborative TAS, Available at: https://abcsciencecollaborative.org/ (Accessed 10 August 2023).

Therapeutics Pipeline

Lauren Sauer, MSc[a], Alice Sato, MD, PhD[b],
Herbert Dele Davies, MD, MSc, MHCM[b,c,*]

KEYWORDS

- Medical countermeasures • Drug pipeline • Physiology • Formulations • Antivirals
- Therapeutics • Monoclonal antibodies • Polyclonal preparations

KEY POINTS

- Children have unique physiologic, developmental, and psychosocial needs and unique vulnerabilities, making them a challenging population for which to develop therapeutics. This is particularly apparent in the urgent and chaotic environment of a pandemic or outbreak.
- Pediatric populations have special ethics and consent consideration for participation in clinical trials and the development of pediatric medical countermeasures (MCMs). Special care should be taken in the development of consent and assent processes as well as considerations for communicating with parents and guardians.
- The development of MCMs for pediatric populations has historically been neglected, but advancements in trial design and regulatory modernization have created substantial advancements and opportunities clinicians should be aware of. In pandemics, it becomes particularly clear that variable disease manifestations can occur and that children often have different therapeutic needs than adults.
- A MCMs pipeline targeting specific therapeutic development for pediatric populations is essential to mitigating the impact of a pandemic on children. This article addresses the challenges inherent in these differences that must be taken into account.

INTRODUCTION AND BACKGROUND

Children have unique physiologic, developmental, and psychosocial needs and unique vulnerabilities, making them a challenging population for which to develop therapeutics.[1] This is particularly apparent in the urgent and chaotic environment of a pandemic or outbreak.[2] Advances in the development of medical countermeasures (MCM) for pediatric populations has grown substantially over the last decade, and the coronavirus disease 2019 (COVID-19) pandemic forced advancements in how we approach pediatric MCM

[a] GCHS, Special Pathogen Research Network, Department of Environmental, Agricultural and Occupational Health, UNMC College of Public Health, 984355 Nebraska Medical Center, Omaha, NE, USA; [b] Department of Pediatrics, Division of Pediatric Infectious Disease, University of Nebraska Medical Center, 987810, Nebraska Medical Center, Omaha, NE 68198-7810, USA; [c] Academic Affairs, University of Nebraska Medical Center, 987810 Nebraska Medical Center, Omaha, NE 68198-7810, USA
* Corresponding author. University of Nebraska Medical Center, 987810 Nebraska Medical Center, Omaha, NE 68198-7810.
E-mail address: dele.davies@unmc.edu

Pediatr Clin N Am 71 (2024) 481–498
https://doi.org/10.1016/j.pcl.2024.03.002
0031-3955/24/© 2024 Elsevier Inc. All rights reserved.

development.[3] In pandemics, it becomes particularly clear that variable disease manifestations can occur and that children often have different therapeutic needs than adults.[4] Consequently, a MCMs pipeline targeting this group is essential, and that the challenges inherent in these differences must be taken into account and addressed.

There are several unique aspects of children that make the development of therapeutics challenging, particularly in the abbreviated timelines required of a pandemic.

- Physiologic differences: Pediatric patients, from neonates to adolescents, have differences in absorption, distribution, metabolism, and excretion of drugs. Pharmacokinetics (PK) must be studied and cannot simply be assumed to have a linear relationship to adult dosing strategies. To further complicate matters, in utero or congenital infections may have significant morbidity and mortality, and therapeutics may need to be administered to pregnant persons, another highly vulnerable and physiologically unique population.
- Dosing and formulations: Pediatric populations often require vastly different dosages depending on age and weight, such that standard dose sizes may not apply or be easily met by available adult preparations.[5] Children may not be able to swallow adult tablets or capsules, so alternative formulations, such as liquids, or chewable or dispersible tablets may be required. Flavoring to improve or mask medication taste is generally needed.
- Limited clinical trials: Historically, children have been underrepresented in clinical trials due to ethical concerns and operational considerations, resulting in a paucity of pediatric-specific data for currently available therapeutic agents— even those which have been approved for adults for years.[6,7]
- Economic considerations: Pediatric populations represent a smaller market segment, which may deter some manufacturers from investing in pediatric-specific research.[8]

The regulations governing the pediatric drug development in the United States have evolved over several decades in response to a growing awareness of the unique therapeutic needs of children and the essential need for a better approach.[9] This evolution has emphasized the importance of novel approaches to studying therapeutics in pediatric populations to ensure their safety, efficacy, and appropriate dosing.

Novel approaches to the necessary pre-clinical work have improved the process for developing pediatric MCMs. These approaches include the use of modeling and simulations which can reduce (but not eliminate) the need for children to be directly involved in clinical studies.[10] Advancements in the use of juvenile animal models have also reduced the burden on children to participate in some clinical trials.[11]

In this article, we will describe the basics of the pediatric MCM development pipeline for various types of treatments that may be useful in pandemics, the ethical challenges associated with pediatric MCM development, and discuss opportunities for advancement as we continue to face twenty-first century pandemic threats.

TYPES OF THERAPEUTIC MEDICAL COUNTERMEASURES

There are several types of therapeutics that can be used to support the care of pediatric patients in a pandemic. These are described in the following sections, and **Table 1** provides an example of each type of therapeutic.

Antivirals

Viral outbreaks continue to be one of the greatest threats to humans, with the recent emergence of 3 coronaviruses (severe acute respiratory syndrome [SARS], Middle

Table 1
Example medical countermeasures

Type of Therapeutic	Example	Potential Use in a Pandemic
Antivirals	Oseltamivir (Tamiflu)	Used to treat and prevent influenza infections. In a pandemic, antivirals could be administered to reduce the severity and duration of the viral illness, decrease the spread of the virus, and possibly decrease mortality rates. New antivirals might be developed or existing ones repurposed depending on the nature of the pandemic-causing virus.
Monoclonal antibodies	Palivizumab (Synagis)	Originally developed for respiratory syncytial virus (RSV) in infants. During a pandemic, specific monoclonal antibodies could be developed or repurposed to target the pandemic-causing virus. They might be administered to provide passive immunity or reduce the severity of the infection.
Monoclonal antibody cocktails	Zmapp	ZMapp is a cocktail of 3 monoclonal antibodies. Used in the West Africa Ebola outbreak of 2013–2016, the cocktail was a promising treatment but exposed pitfalls in the emergency clinical trial regulatory processes. The approach led to reevaluation of the conduct of clinical trials and the compassionate use process in emergencies.
Polyclonal antibodies	Convalescent plasma	Used in multiple recent outbreaks and the COVID-19 pandemic, effectiveness of convalescent plasma has had with mixed results. While some studies indicated potential benefits, others showed limited or no benefit. The use of convalescent plasma in pediatrics requires careful consideration given the unique physiology and immune responses of children.
Immune stimulators	Bacillus Calmette-Guérin (BCG) vaccine	Although originally used for tuberculosis, some studies suggest BCG may boost the ability of the immune system to fight off pathogens. During a pandemic, immune stimulators could be used to bolster the immune response of the pediatric population, potentially offering broad-based defense until a specific vaccine or treatment becomes available.

East respiratory syndrome–related coronavirus, and SARS-related coronavirus 2) and the 2009 pandemic H1N1 ("swine flu") influenza occurring in just the past 20 years.[12] Over roughly the same time, spread of vector-borne illnesses such as West Nile virus and dengue have endangered the health of new populations around the globe. Primary Zika virus infection of pregnant persons revealed the unique susceptibility of fetal development to infection, with microcephaly, parenchymal calcifications, and other brain abnormalities.[13] The need to accelerate antiviral discovery remains the utmost priority in the wake of the COVID-19 pandemic.

The development of a new antiviral is generally stepwise and requires substantial investment in target identification and preclinical work.[14] Candidate antivirals must undergo in vivo screenings in order to understand their PK properties, metabolism, and toxicity.[15] Thus, the development of antiviral therapy is a tedious and time-consuming process and traditionally involves the following stages.

- Target identification and screening of antivirals: The goal of this phase is to develop and use in vitro assays to identify and validate specific biological molecules or pathways that the virus uses to infect, replicate, or cause disease, which can be intervened upon by potential drugs.[16]
- Lead generation and optimization (including modeling and simulation): The goal of this phase is to identify the most promising compounds (leads) from the initial phase and optimize them for better efficacy, safety, and druglike properties.[17]
- Preclinical and clinical studies: The goal of this phase is to evaluate the safety and efficacy of the optimized lead compounds in living organisms. They are tested in the in vitro setting and in animals during the pre-clinical phase to assess efficacy and establish safety profiles. Once these initial studies are completed and no significant concerns are found, compounds may be advanced to studies in humans during the clinical phase via a series of clinical trials to determine efficacy, effectiveness, safety, and best approaches to dosing and administration.[18] In public health emergencies, this phase may be bypassed for emergency use authorization (EUA) (process described in the following sections).
- Final registration of the antiviral: The goal of this phase is to obtain approval for the antiviral drug from regulatory agencies, allowing its sale and use in the general population. In public health emergencies, this phase may be bypassed for EUA.

Monoclonal and Polyclonal Antibody Preparations

The development of antibody-based therapeutics (either monoclonal single antibody or monoclonal antibody "cocktails," or polyclonal products derived from plasma from blood donors) for pediatric use mirrors the development process for adults, but with additional considerations specific to children. Both types of antibody treatment have unique properties, and their development processes differ in certain ways (**Table 2**). Both monoclonal and polyclonal antibody preparations have shown potential in various therapeutic areas, including infectious diseases, oncology, and autoimmunity.[19] As our understanding of these tools expands, they may play even more significant roles in pediatric care. Given that children are still growing and developing, understanding any long-term implications of an antibody therapy is critical.

Immune Modulators

The development of immune modulators, or immunomodulatory drugs, for pediatric use is a complex process. These drugs modulate or regulate the functioning of the

Table 2 Monoclonal antibodies versus polyclonal antibodies	
Monoclonal Antibodies	**Polyclonal Antibodies**
Refer to a homogenous population of antibodies that are produced by a single clone of plasma B cells.	Refer to a mixture of immunoglobulin molecules that are secreted against a particular antigen.
Produced by the same clone of plasma B cells.	Produced by different clones of plasma B cells.
Production requires hybridoma cell lines.	Production does not require hybridoma cell lines.
A homogenous antibody population.	A heterogeneous antibody population.
Interact with a particular epitope on the antigen.	Interact with different epitopes on the same antigen.

immune system and can be used to either enhance the immune response or suppress it, depending on the medical condition being treated. Immune stimulators play a crucial role in augmenting the body's natural defense mechanisms against pathogens of concern. Immune stimulators function by activating or modulating specific components of the immune system. Their working can be explained via various mechanisms, depending on the type of modulator.

- Toll-like receptor (TLR) activation: Some immune stimulators, including synthetic oligodeoxynucleotides or imiquimod, function by binding to specific TLRs, a class of proteins that play a key role in the innate immune system. Activation of TLRs can lead to the production of proinflammatory cytokines, type I interferons, and other mediators that enhance the body's defense mechanisms against pathogens.[20]
- Enhancement of antigen presentation: Certain immune stimulators enhance the ability of antigen-presenting cells, such as dendritic cells, to capture, process, and present antigens to T cells. This stimulation amplifies the adaptive immune response by facilitating the activation of T cells specific to the presented antigen.[21]
- Cytokine modulation: Some stimulators induce or augment the production of cytokines, proteins that mediate communication between cells in the immune system. For instance, interleukins or interferons might be upregulated, promoting an antiviral state in cells or stimulating the proliferation and function of immune cells.[22]
- Cell-mediated immunity enhancement: Some agents, like bacillus Calmette-Guérin (BCG) vaccine, stimulate cell-mediated immunity by enhancing the activity and proliferation of macrophages and T lymphocytes, providing improved defense against intracellular pathogens.[23]
- Stimulation of antibody production: Certain stimulators act on B cells to boost the production of antibodies against specific antigens, thereby enhancing humoral immunity.[24]
- Enhancement of phagocytosis: Some agents can boost the phagocytic activity of cells like macrophages and neutrophils, making them more efficient at engulfing and destroying pathogens.[25]
- Nonspecific immune activation (trained immunity): Certain stimulators, like BCG, can induce a state of heightened alertness or "memory" in innate immune cells, a phenomenon termed "trained immunity." Though the innate immune system

traditionally lacks specific memory (unlike the adaptive system), some stimulators can induce epigenetic changes in innate cells, leading them to respond more robustly upon subsequent encounters with pathogens.[26]

- Adjuvants in vaccines: Many vaccines contain adjuvant molecules, which are immune stimulators that alert and amplify the body's immune response to the vaccine's antigen. They might work by creating a depot effect (slow release of antigen), recruiting immune cells to the injection site, or activating innate immune pathways that augment the adaptive response to the vaccine antigen.[27] Vaccines will be discussed in more detail in chapter NN

APPROVAL OF PEDIATRIC THERAPEUTICS

The standard approach to approval of pediatric therapeutics as outlined by the US Food and Drug Administration (FDA) forms the basis for the regulatory pathway that will generally be used for the development of MCMs in and prior to a pandemic, as well. The FDA developed a pediatric study decision tree that serves as a framework for appropriately extrapolating adult data to pediatric populations (**Fig. 1**). This pathway can be applied to the development of MCMs. The general process is as follows:[18,28]

1. Research is conducted in the preclinical phase. This phase will have distinct research activities depending on the type of drug or biological product; however, the result is generally successful studies in animal models.
2. If the preclinical studies are promising, an investigational new drug (IND) application is submitted to the FDA. This application includes all information about the research on the drug, to date.[29]
3. If the IND application is approved, the drug enters into phase 1 trials. These are conducted in healthy volunteers and generally include less than 100 participants. The focus of this phase is on safety and toxicity of the drug, not efficacy or effectiveness. Routes of administration are also evaluated in this phase.
4. If the phase 1 trial is successful, the drug enters into phase 2, which focuses on effectiveness and appropriate dosing levels. These studies generally involve several hundred people who have the condition that the drug is designed to treat. These trials can last from several months to 2 years or more.
5. Phase 3 trials (**Fig. 2** for a description of the process for combining phase 2 and 3 clinical trials[30]) are large-scale randomized placebo-controlled trials. They are used to assess the drug's effectiveness, monitor for side effects, and may be used to compare the product to other drugs of similar purpose. This phase has several hundred to several thousand participants. Because of the large number of participants and the longer duration, these trials can be pivotal in the decision about whether a drug should be approved. They can last from 1 to 4 years.
6. Phase 4 trials are used to extrapolate data for additional populations or new uses. Often referred to as "postmarketing studies" or "postmarketing surveillance," phase 4 trials are studies that take place after a drug or medical device has received regulatory approval and is available for sale in the market. These trials are essential to understand the long-term safety, efficacy, and optimal use of the product in a broader population and real-world setting. Often, this is where the evaluation of pediatric applications occurs—based on safety and efficacy in adults. Additional safety and effectiveness data are collected in this phase. This phase can involve several thousand participants. The number and duration can vary greatly depending on the nature of the drug and its intended use, the purpose of the study, and regulatory requirements.

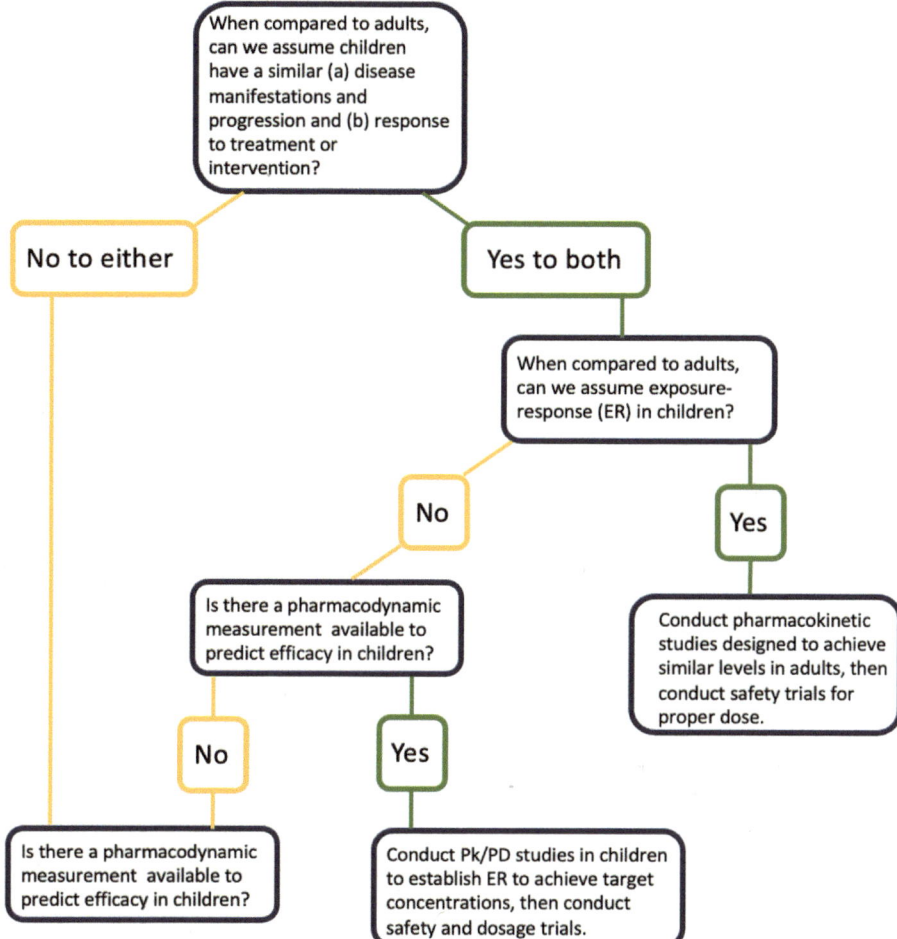

Fig. 1. Pediatric study decision tree. (Pediatric Science and Research Activities. *Adapted from*: https://www.fda.gov/ScienceResearch/SpecialTopics/PediatricTherapeuticsResearch/ ucm106614.htm)

Sub-Population Requirements

When conducting clinical trials in pediatric populations, special considerations are necessary due to the unique physiologic and developmental differences children present compared to adults. Carefully selecting pediatric subpopulations is essential to ensure the safety, efficacy, and ethical treatment of trial participants.[31] The following list is a summary of ways pediatric subpopulations can be selected for clinical trials.

1. Age-based grouping: Typically, pediatric patients are categorized based on age groups which reflect developmental changes:
   - Neonates (0–28 days)
   - Infants (29 days to<2 years)
   - Toddlers (2 years to<6 years)
   - Children (6 years to<12 years)
   - Adolescents (12 years to<18 years)

Combination Phase 2 and 3 Clinical Trials

Combining Phase 2 and Phase 3 clinical trials is a strategy sometimes employed to accelerate the development of a drug or treatment, especially when there is a pressing need, such as during an outbreak of a novel infectious disease. Combining the phases can save time and resources, as it avoids a pause between Phase 2 and Phase 3 trials and they are commonly refered to as phase 2/3 trials. This can be especially important in situations where there is an urgent need for new treatments.

There are novel approaches to study design and conduct that can be used to conduct phase 2/3 trials. One common approach in a combined Phase 2/3 trial is to use an adaptive or baysian trial design. This allows researchers to make changes to the trial procedures (like dose adjustments) based on interim results, without compromising the trial's integrity or validity. Unlike traditional (frequentist) statistical approaches, which rely on fixed sample sizes and p-values to assess treatment effects, Bayesian methods provide a flexible framework that can integrate prior information and real world data with current trial data to update the probability or belief about a treatment effect.

An alternative option is initiating the trial as a Phase 2 study, but including criteria in the protocol for progressing directly to Phase 3. This may involve predefined efficacy benchmarks, safety metrics, or other relevant measures.

At a predetermined point, an interim analysis is conducted. This is a crucial step that allows researchers to evaluate the data accumulated at pre-determined intervals, determine the appropriate progression of the trial, and facilitate modifications to the trial's next step based on the preliminary findings. If the criteria outlined in the protocol are met during the interim analysis, the trial can transition into Phase 3 without stopping. If the criteria are not determined to be met, the trial may be stopped due to inefficacy, or it might require modifications before proceeding. Upon transitioning to Phase 3, the trial typically expands to include a larger number of participants and may involve multiple trial sites, possibly across expanded regions and countries.

Even though the phases are combined, data collection remains rigorous. Safety and efficacy data continue to be monitored and collected. Additionally, because of the unique nature of combined trials, there's often more interaction with regulatory agencies (like the FDA in the US). This ensures that the design and progression of the trial meet the necessary standards and that any adaptations are well-justified and scientifically sound.

Fig. 2. Combining phase 2 and 3 clinical trials.

2. Weight stratification within age groups: Within each age category, participants may be further subdivided based on weight percentiles or categories. For drugs where weight significantly impacts the PK parameters (eg, volume of distribution), weight-based dosing or adjustments might be necessary even within the same age group. In these instances, studying weight stratifications can provide insights into dose adjustments.

3. Physiologic considerations: The age groupings described earlier are not just arbitrary divisions. Each group may metabolize or react to drugs differently based on organ maturity, enzyme activity, and other physiologic differences.

4. Disease characteristics: The progression, presentation, and pathophysiology of diseases may differ between children and adults, and among pediatric age groups. It is standard practice to select the appropriate subpopulation based on the disease or condition under investigation.

5. Developmental stage: This considers cognitive, emotional, and physical developmental stages. For instance, an intervention requiring complicated self-administration might not be appropriate for younger children.
6. Safety and ethical considerations: Ensure that the risk to benefit ratio is favorable. Often, trials start with older children first and, based on safety data, progressively include younger age groups.
7. Inclusion/exclusion criteria: These should be clear and specific for the pediatric population, considering comorbidities, previous treatments, and other factors relevant to children.
8. PK and pharmacodynamics (PD): Children might metabolize or respond to drugs differently than adults, which can affect dosing and therapeutic response. Trials might need to be stratified or designed differently for each subpopulation to gather relevant PK/PD data.
9. Prior data: Whenever possible, existing adult and pediatric data are used to hypothesize the drug's action in the targeted pediatric subpopulation. This can guide inclusion criteria and safety measures.

Safety Monitoring

In order to effectively track adverse events and incorporate real-world data into the understood safety profile of the therapeutics, the use of an adverse event reporting system may be used. In the United States, the US FDA has a system known as the FDA Adverse Event Reporting System (FAERS). This is similar to the well-known Vaccine Adverse Event Reporting System (VAERS).

FAERS is a database that contains information about adverse event and medication error reports submitted to the FDA. Its primary goal is to support the FDA's postmarketing surveillance program to identify new safety concerns or trends associated with marketed drugs and therapeutic biologics. The system collects data from health care professionals, consumers, and manufacturers. Manufacturers are required to submit reports to FAERS, but for health care professionals and consumers, reporting is voluntary. FAERS data is used by the FDA to identify potential safety concerns and might lead to changes in how a product is used or even its removal from the market. The FDA will conduct further evaluations if a potential safety concern is identified in FAERS.

The FDA provides quarterly FAERS data files to the public for the purpose of analysis. However, it is essential to interpret these data with caution. The mere reporting of an adverse event does not establish a causal relationship between the drug and the reported event. Like VAERS, FAERS has limitations, including potential underreporting, duplicate reporting, and the lack of a control group for comparison. It is a spontaneous reporting system, meaning it relies on individuals to report their observations and experiences, so it is susceptible to biases.

In addition to FAERS, the FDA also utilizes other methods and databases to monitor drug safety, like the Sentinel Initiative, which allows the FDA to actively query diverse health care databases to evaluate possible medical product safety issues quickly.

CONDUCTING PEDIATRIC MEDICAL COUNTERMEASURE RESEARCH

Children are historically thought of as vulnerable subjects which has created a protective approach to involving them in clinical studies. While important, that approach creates an environment where there is a paucity of safety or efficacy data in every type of therapeutic that may be used in pandemic response. The ethical imperative to improve this gap has been highlighted for over a decade.[32] The ethical foundation for including children in clinical research has evolved from one of exclusion to encouraged, but cautious, prioritization of their inclusion, owning primarily to the recognition of the gaps that exclusion as a principle creates.

Within the context of this reframing, considering children in clinical studies requires additional protections.

1. Participation of children must be "scientifically necessary" to even consider the risk-benefit analysis of participation.
2. The balance of risks associated with participation (and the associated procedures or interventions) to potential benefit to the participant must be evaluated and found to be appropriate.
3. The risk/benefit balance must be found to be appropriate *prior* to considering parental consent and child assent procedures.[33]

These protections must be prioritized, but in a pandemic may require a swift analysis to assess scientific necessity and the risk-benefit ratio.

The US FDA has long recognized the ethical and scientific complexities surrounding pediatric clinical trials. To ensure the protection and rights of children who participate in clinical trials, the FDA has established guidance documents and regulations. The welfare and rights of the participating child should always come first. Children should only be enrolled in clinical trials if the relevant scientific questions cannot be answered using adult participants or if the product is intended specifically for a pediatric population.

The FDA's guidance on pediatric clinical trials ensures that the unique physiologic, psychological, and developmental differences of children are considered. The regulations balance the need for rigorous scientific research with the heightened ethical considerations of studying this vulnerable population.

Risk and Informed Consent

Once the first 2 protections are met and clinical studies are approved to move forward, the processes of risk assessment and informed consent and assent can be considered.

In the United States, participation in research by children is regulated by the Common Rule (45 CFR 46) subpart D.[34] This section of the Common Rule places the burden of assessing the risks that the pediatric participants may face regarding their participation on the Institutional Review Board (IRB). The risk should be assessed and categorized (**Fig. 3**) and the study procedures should then detail how the process of obtaining informed consent from the child's parent or legally authorized representative (LAR) will occur. This process essentially mirrors the consent process requirements for adults

Research that is:

(1) not involving greater than minimal
(2) involving greater than minimal risk but presenting the prospect of direct benefit to the individual subjects (section 405);
(3) involving greater than minimal risk and no prospect of direct benefit to individual subjects, but likely to yield generalizable knowledge about the subject's disorder or condition (section 406)

Fig. 3. Categories of risk (from the Common Rule).

but is conducted with the parent or LAR. Additionally, whenever possible, assent to participate should be obtained by the child as well. This can be accomplished through use of developmentally appropriate language and resources to facilitate the child's understanding of what participation will mean at an age-appropriate and capacity-appropriate level.

There are ongoing challenges and lack of regulatory clarity regarding the process of obtaining informed consent in pediatric populations. Specific considerations for both consent and assent should be considered.

- Age of the pediatric patient/participant
- Cognitive ability of the pediatric patient/participant
- Maturity of the pediatric patient/participant
- Custodial relationship of the parent or LAR
- Ability to transfer study information to the parent/LAR and the child
- Age of the parent if the parent is a minor[35]

Additional Areas of Consideration

Pediatric study plans
For products that might be used in children, regulatory bodies often require sponsors to submit a pediatric study plan early in the development process. This plan outlines the proposed pediatric studies, their timelines, and justifications for the selected age groups and study designs.

Incorporating pediatric expertise
Pediatric clinical trials should ideally be designed and conducted by those with expertise in pediatric research. Additionally, IRBs reviewing pediatric trials should have members with pediatric expertise.

Remuneration
Remuneration for pediatric patients participating in clinical trials is a challenging landscape. While remuneration and compensation are essential aspects of clinical research, they must be managed with particular care in pediatric studies. Generally speaking, compensation for participation in clinical research is acceptable for covering costs of travel and time needed to participate in the study for the parent and possibly nominal amounts for the child.[36]

Recruitment
Recruitment for pediatric clinical trials requires careful considerations due to the unique and sensitive nature of involving children in research. Trial sites should be accessible to the target population. Offering transportation support can also enhance recruitment. Whenever possible, appointments should be flexible to accommodate school schedules and parents' work commitments.

Data safety monitoring
The FDA recommends that trials with children have a data monitoring committee or similar body, especially for studies with higher potential risks. This committee monitors patient safety and study data throughout the trial.

EMERGENCY USE AUTHORIZATION PROCESS

In public health emergencies such as a pandemic or outbreak, there are levers that can be used to expedite availability of drugs and biological products—including for pediatric populations. In these scenarios, therapeutics that do not currently hold

FDA approval can be accessed by leveraging the EUA mechanism. EUAs facilitate the availability and use of MCMs, including therapeutics, during public health emergencies by providing temporary authorization of medical products that may not have received regular FDA approval.

The following steps constitute the process for obtaining and using an EUA.[37]

- Determination of public health emergency: A public health emergency, which justifies the issuance of an EUA, must first be declared by the appropriate US authority. This can be declared by the Secretary of Health and Human Services based on a recommendation by the Director of the Centers for Disease Control and Prevention or the Director of the National Institutes of Health. Before applying for an EUA, the developer of the therapeutic will need to summarize and categorize as much data as possible regarding its safety and efficacy. This includes data from preclinical studies, clinical trials, or real-world use from other countries and will be used to assess the EUA application.
- Submission: The therapeutic's developer submits a request for EUA to the US FDA. The request typically includes
  - Data that demonstrate the therapeutic's safety and efficacy.
  - Information about the manufacturing process and facilities, ensuring that they can produce the therapeutic to a high quality.
  - The therapeutic's proposed labeling and fact sheets for health care providers and recipients.
  - FDA evaluation: The FDA reviews the submitted data to assess the therapeutic's safety, efficacy, and manufacturing quality. The FDA determines if the therapeutic's known and potential benefits outweigh its known and potential risks for the intended use during the public health emergency.
- Issuance of EUA: If the FDA finds that the criteria for issuance of an EUA are met, they can issue the EUA, which allows the therapeutic to be used for the duration of the public health emergency exclusively for its intended use that is specified in the EUA application.
- Conditions of EUA: The issuance of an EUA may come with certain conditions to ensure the continued protection of public health. This may include requirements for postmarketing data collection, monitoring for adverse events, and specific distribution and use restrictions.
- Communication: Once the EUA is issued, health care providers and the public need to be informed about the availability, benefits, and risks of the therapeutic. This typically involves distributing fact sheets and engaging in other communication efforts.
- Termination or revocation: The EUA remains in effect until the public health emergency declaration ends or the EUA is revoked by the FDA. If the therapeutic's developer wishes to continue marketing the product after the emergency is over, they must seek traditional FDA approval.
- Transition to full approval: Sometimes, following the issuance of an EUA, the manufacturer will continue to collect data to submit a biologics license application (BLA) or new drug application (NDA) to obtain full FDA approval.

It is important to note that the specifics of obtaining an EUA might vary depending on the specific regulatory framework of a country. The process described earlier is based on the US system, but other countries may have similar frameworks with different details. The EUA mechanism can be used to expedite delivery of MCMs approved by the FDA for adults to children.

PEDIATRIC STRATEGIC NATIONAL STOCKPILE

Once a product moves through clinical trials and into production, it may be included in the Strategic National Stockpile (SNS). The SNS is a US national repository of antibiotics, vaccines, chemical antidotes, antitoxins, and other critical medical supplies designed to supplement and resupply state and local public health agencies in case of emergencies.[38]

Regarding pediatric patients, the SNS is designed to be responsive to the needs of all populations, including children; however pediatric contents may be limited. While the specific contents of the SNS are considered sensitive information for national security reasons and may not be entirely disclosed, several items tailored to pediatric patient management include

1. Pediatric formulations of medications: This can include liquid formulations or easily dissolvable tablet forms of various medicines which might be too strong or unsuitable in adult formulations for children.
2. Pediatric medical supplies: This can encompass items such as pediatric-sized masks for protection against inhalation of contaminants, pediatric intravenous equipment, and other medical devices designed specifically for children.
3. Vaccines: In the case of certain outbreaks, vaccines suitable for children may be included in the stockpile.
4. Antidotes and antitoxins: The stockpile contains antidotes and antitoxins for a range of chemical, biological, radiological, and nuclear threats. For these agents, pediatric dosages or formulations might be available.
5. Equipment: Nebulizers, ventilators, and other essential equipment sized for pediatric patients might be included.
6. Guidance and training materials: Tied to the materials contained in the SNS are information and guidance for health care providers to ensure the correct use of stockpiled items. These materials would cover guidance on pediatric care during emergencies.

The SNS is intended to evolve based on the perceived threats and public health needs of the US population, so the exact contents changes over time. The emphasis, however, remains on ensuring that the health needs of all segments of the population, including pediatric patients, are addressed.

PEDIATRIC DRUG LANDSCAPE

In the United States, pediatric drug development has historically lagged behind drug development for adults. Recognizing the need for pediatric-specific medications and formulations, the US Congress and the FDA have established various incentives to encourage pharmaceutical companies to study and develop drugs for children (**Fig. 4**). These programs have fostered pediatric drug development, nationally and worldwide.[39,40]

1. Pediatric labeling requirement
   - FDA introduced a rule that required drug labels to state whether safety and effectiveness had been established in pediatric patients and, if not, to state that "safety and effectiveness in pediatric patients have not been established." This rule was one of the earliest efforts by the FDA to draw attention to the issue of pediatric drug testing.
2. Best Pharmaceuticals for Children Act
   - If a company voluntarily conducts pediatric studies based on FDA's specific requests (known as "Written Requests"), the company can qualify for an additional

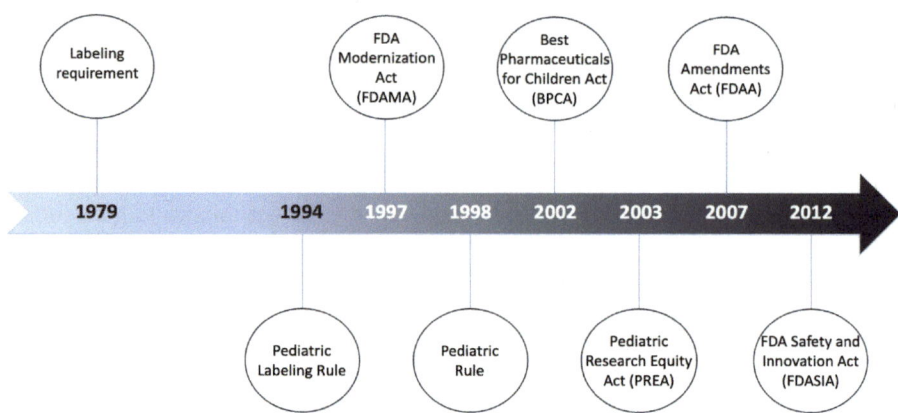

Fig. 4. Pediatric research regulatory timeline.

6 months of market exclusivity for the product, regardless of the study results. This can represent a significant financial incentive.

- The FDA may provide a priority review voucher for certain pediatric rare disease treatments. A priority review voucher entitles the holder to a 6-month review time by the FDA, rather than the standard 10 months.

3. Pediatric Research Equity Act (PREA)
   - PREA mandates that certain NDAs and BLAs include pediatric-specific data unless the FDA grants a waiver or deferral.
   - Results from pediatric studies can provide valuable information to health care providers, leading to clearer dosing recommendations and better understanding of drug effects in children.

4. Pediatric Priority Review Voucher Program
   - Transferable vouchers: For companies that develop a treatment for a rare pediatric disease, they can earn a pediatric priority review voucher, which can be used to expedite the review of a subsequent product. These vouchers are also transferable and can be sold to other companies. Their value can be significant due to the potential for faster product approval.

5. Pediatric Device Consortia Grant Program
   - While primarily focused on medical devices, this program provides funding and expertise to promote the development and availability of pediatric medical devices. This can assist companies in overcoming some of the financial and technical barriers associated with pediatric device development.

6. FDA's Pediatric Trial Network (PTN)
   - PTN collaborates with companies to design and conduct pediatric clinical trials, reducing the logistical and financial burdens on individual companies.

PEDIATRIC RESEARCH NETWORKS

In an outbreak or pandemic setting, coordinated approaches to pediatric research are essential to ensure enrollment criteria are met and promising therapeutics move through the pipeline efficiently. Pediatric clinical research networks have been established globally to promote and facilitate high-quality clinical research focused on conditions that affect children and may pivot or be leveraged in public health emergencies. These networks are collaborative efforts that involve multiple institutions, bringing together the expertise of clinicians, researchers, and other professionals to improve pediatric health outcomes. See **Fig. 5** for a few examples of pediatric networks that may be relevant for MCM development in a pandemic.

OPPORTUNITIES FOR INNOVATION

Pediatric clinical research in public health emergencies is a complex area that demands an agile, tailored response. Given the unique physiologic, psychological, and developmental needs of children, innovation in this field is essential. The research process for the pediatric MCM development pipeline poses unique challenges, in the regulatory, ethical, operational, and logistical spaces. Addressing these issues through innovation is crucial for the successful and timely completion of studies that can lead to safer and more effective treatments for children prior to the next pandemic.

- Strengthening basic and translational research: Investing in foundational research specific to pediatric populations, focusing on the unique pathophysiology of children using novel approaches to in vitro and animal research.
- Streamlining regulatory pathways: Simplifying and expediting regulatory pathways for pediatric MCMs without compromising safety. This can be achieved by providing clear guidance on study design and data requirements and fostering pre-pandemic activities such as templated protocols, collaborative recruitment plans, and pre-approved adaptive trial designs.
- Ethical considerations: Establishing clear ethical guidelines for conducting trials in children, especially during emergencies when standard protocols may be challenging to maintain.
- Collaborative research: Fostering pre-pandemic collaboration across global research networks dedicated to pediatric MCMs to pool resources, data, and expertise.
- Data sharing: Promoting open sharing of data and findings, which can accelerate the research process and provide richer datasets for analysis.
- Pediatric-specific formulations: Innovating child-friendly drug formulations such as chewable tablets, patches, or flavored solutions.
- Community engagement: Ensuring families and communities understand the importance of pediatric MCMs through outreach and education. Building trust can increase participation in trials and uptake of approved countermeasures.

Pediatric Trials Network (PTN): Funded by the Eunice Kennedy Shriver National Institute of Child Health and Human Development (NICHD), PTN focuses on the study of formulations, dosages, safety, and efficacy of drugs in children. https://pediatrictrials.org/

Pediatric Acute Lung Injury and Sepsis Investigators (PALISI) Network: This network focuses on pediatric critical care research, particularly around lung injury and sepsis. https://www.palisi.org/

Pediatric Emergency Care Applied Research Network (PECARN): Dedicated to pediatric emergency care research, PECARN aims to identify the best care practices for children in emergency care settings. https://www.pecarn.org/

Collaborative Pediatric Critical Care Research Network (CPCCRN): Funded by NICHD, this network aims to design and conduct multicenter trials and observational studies in pediatric critical care. https://www.cpccrn.org/

Pediatric Pandemic Network (PPN): While not explicitly a research network, the PPN is dedicated to empowering health care systems and communities to provide high-quality, equitable care to children every day and in crises and includes facilitation of pediatric research. https://pedspandemicnetwork.org

Fig. 5. Pediatric clinical research networks.

- Incentives for industry: Providing financial or regulatory incentives for pharmaceutical companies to invest in pediatric MCM research, which is traditionally less lucrative.
- Infrastructure and capacity building: Investing in health infrastructure, laboratories, and training to ensure regions most at risk have the capability to conduct essential research and deploy MCMs efficiently.
- Interdisciplinary collaboration: Fostering collaboration between clinicians, researchers, public health experts, ethicists, and industry to address the multifaceted challenges of pediatric MCM development in the most efficient way possible.

SUMMARY

The development of pediatric MCMs is vital for ensuring the health and safety of children during public health emergencies, such as pandemics, bioterror attacks, or natural disasters. Children have unique physiologic, psychological, and developmental needs, which can differ significantly from those of adults. There are opportunities to recognize and prioritize specific threats (biological, chemical, radiological, or nuclear) that may disproportionately impact children or require specialized interventions for this population which can be used to facilitate resource decision-making for pandemic MCM.

CLINICS CARE POINTS

- Separate planning and preparations are needed for pediatric populations to be able to access safe and effective therapeutics in outbreaks or pandemics, particularly those caused by emerging pathogens for which no established MCMs exist.
- Children have significantly different physiologic and immunologic responses to infections. Adult studies of new therapeutics do not address the safety and efficacy issues for children.
- Children are a vulnerable population for research. The risks in testing new agents in clinical trials in children need to be balanced with the risks of not having appropriately studied therapeutics available to children if not performed.
- The US Congress and US FDA have created multiple programs, guidance documents, and regulations to encourage development of pediatric therapeutics.

DISCLOSURE

The authors have no disclosures.

REFERENCES

1. Mulberg AE, Mathis L, Dunne J, et al. Introduction: pediatric drug development and therapeutics: continued progress for better drugs for children. In: Mulberg AE, Murphy D, Dunne J, et al, editors. Pediatric drug development. 2nd edition. Hoboken: Wiley-Blackwell; 2013. p. 3–5.
2. Connolly C, Golden J. Lessons ignored: children and pandemics. Am J Publ Health 2023;113(9):985–90.
3. Sanyaolu A, Okorie C, Marinkovic A, et al. Current advancements and future prospects of COVID-19 vaccines and therapeutics: a narrative review. Therapeutic Advances in Vaccines and Immunotherapy 2022;10. 25151355221097559.

4. Borio LL, Bright RA, Emanuel EJ. A national strategy for COVID-19 medical countermeasures: vaccines and therapeutics. JAMA 2022;327(3):215–6.

5. Ivanovska V, Rademaker CM, van Dijk L, et al. Pediatric drug formulations: a review of challenges and progress. Pediatrics 2014;134(2):361–72.

6. Bourgeois FT, Murthy S, Pinto C, et al. Pediatric versus adult drug trials for conditions with high pediatric disease burden. Pediatrics 2012;130:285–92.

7. Cohen E, Uleryk E, Jasuja M, et al. An absence of pediatric randomized controlled trials in general medical journals, 1985-2004. J Clin Epidemiol 2007; 60:118–23.

8. Li JS, Eisenstein EL, Grabowski HG, et al. Economic return of clinical trials performed under the pediatric exclusivity program. JAMA 2007;297(5):480–8.

9. Spadoni C. Pediatric drug development: challenges and opportunities. Curr Ther Res Clin Exp 2019;90:119.

10. Vinks AA, Emoto C, Fukuda T. Modeling and simulation in pediatric drug therapy: application of pharmacometrics to define the right dose for children. Clin Pharmacol Therapeut 2015;98(3):298–308.

11. Cappon GD, Bailey GP, Buschmann J, et al. Juvenile animal toxicity study designs to support pediatric drug development. Birth Defects Res B Dev Reprod Toxicol 2009;86(6):463–9.

12. Asif M, Nawaz S, Bhutta ZA, et al. Viral outbreaks: A real threat to the world. Advancements in Life Sciences 2020;8(1):08–19.

13. Bard D, Gubler DJ, Schaub B, et al. An update on Zika virus infection. Lancet 2017;390(10107):2099–109.

14. US Dept of Health and Human Services, Food and Drug Administration, Center for Drug Evaluation and Research. Guidance for Industry - antiviral product development - conducting and submitting virology studies to the agency. Available at: https://www.fda.gov/media/71223/download. Accessed April 1, 2024.

15. Al-Jabri AA, Wigg MD, Oxford JS. Initial in vitro screening of drug candidates for their potential antiviral activities. InVirology Methods Manual 1996;293–308. Academic Press.

16. Adamson CS, Chibale K, Goss RJ, et al. Antiviral drug discovery: preparing for the next pandemic. Chem Soc Rev 2021;50(6):3647–55.

17. De Clercq E. Antiviral drug discovery and development: where chemistry meets with biomedicine. Antivir Res 2005;67(2):56–7.

18. World Health Organization. Clinical trials. Available at: https://www.who.int/health-topics/clinical-trials#tab=tab_1. [Accessed 10 October 2023].

19. Berger M, Shankar V, Vafai A. Therapeutic applications of monoclonal antibodies. Am J Med Sci 2002;324(1):14–30.

20. Anwar MA, Shah M, Kim J, et al. Recent clinical trends in Toll-like receptor targeting therapeutics. Med Res Rev 2019;39(3):1053–90.

21. Li M, Itoh A, Xi J, et al. Enhancing antigen presentation and inducing antigen-specific immune tolerance with amphiphilic peptides. J Immunol 2021;207(8): 2051–9.

22. Deckers J, Anbergen T, Hokke AM, et al. Engineering cytokine therapeutics. Nature Reviews Bioengineering 2023;1(4):286–303.

23. Zahavi D, AlDeghaither D, O'Connell A, et al. Enhancing antibody-dependent cell-mediated cytotoxicity: a strategy for improving antibody-based immunotherapy. Antibody Therapeutics 2018;1(1):7–12.

24. Hoffman W, Lakkis FG, Chalasani G. B cells, antibodies, and more. Clin J Am Soc Nephrol: CJASN 2016;11(1):137.

25. Hübel K, Dale DC, Liles WC. Therapeutic use of cytokines to modulate phagocyte function for the treatment of infectious diseases: current status of granulocyte colony-stimulating factor, granulocyte-macrophage colony-stimulating factor, macrophage colony-stimulating factor, and interferon-γ. JID (J Infect Dis) 2002; 185(10):1490–501.
26. Nica V, Popp RA, Crişan TO, et al. The future clinical implications of trained immunity. Expet Rev Clin Immunol 2022;18(11):1125–34.
27. Kim JH, Kim DH, Jo S, et al. Immunomodulatory functional foods and their molecular mechanisms. Exp Mol Med 2022;54(1):1.
28. Dunne J, Rodruguez WJ, Murphy D, et al. Extrapolation of adult data and other data in pediatric drug development programs. Pediatrics 2011;128(5):e1242–9.
29. U.S. Food and Drug Administration. Investigational new drug (IND) application. Available at: https://www.fda.gov/drugs/types-applications/investigational-new-drug-ind-application. [Accessed 10 October 2023].
30. Sato A, Shimura M, Gosho M. Practical characteristics of adaptive design in phase 2 and 3 clinical trials. J Clin Pharm Therapeut 2018;43(2):170–80.
31. Neville KA, Kaufmann RE, Abdel-Rahman S. Development and clinical trial design. In: Mulberg AE, Murphy D, Dunne J, et al, editors. Pediatric drug development. 2nd edition. Hoboken: Wiley-Blackwell; 2013. p. 281–91.
32. Shaddy RE, Denne SC, Committee on Drugs and Committee on Pediatric Research. Clinical report – guidelines for the ethical conduct of studies to evaluate drugs in pediatric populations. Pediatrics 2010;125(4):850–60.
33. Roth-Cline MD, Nelson RM. Ethical considerations in pediatric research. In: Mulberg AE, Murphy D, Dunne J, et al, editors. Pediatric drug development. 2nd edition. Hoboken: Wiley-Blackwell; 2013. p. 83–93.
34. Office of the Assistant Secretary for Health. Subpart A of 45 CFR part 46: Basic HHS policy for protection of human subjects. Available at: https://www.hhs.gov/ohrp/sites/default/files/revised-common-rule-reg-text-unofficial-2018-requirements.pdf. (Accessed April 1, 2024).
35. Available at: https://link.springer.com/article/10.1007/s40272-014-0108-y.
36. Kimberly MB, Hoehn KS, Feudtner C, et al. Variation in standards of research compensation and child assent practices: a comparison of 69 institutional review board-approved informed permission and assent forms for 3 multicenter pediatric clinical trials. Pediatrics 2006;117:1706–11.
37. US Food and Drug Administration. Emergency use authorization. Available at: https://www.fda.gov/emergency-preparedness-and-response/mcm-legal-regulatory-and-policy-framework/emergency-use-authorization. [Accessed 12 October 2023].
38. US Government Accountability Office. HHS Should Address Strategic National Stockpile Requirements and Inventory Risks. GAO-23-106210. Available at: https://www.gao.gov/products/gao-23-106210. 2022. Accessed October 12, 2023.
39. Ward RM, Hirschfeld S. History of children and the development of regulations at the FDA. In: Mulberg AE, Murphy D, Dunne J, et al, editors. Pediatric drug development. 2nd edition. Hoboken: Wiley-Blackwell; 2013. p. 6–15.
40. Dunn A, Jung D, Bollinger LL, et al. Accelerating the availability of medications to pediatric patients by optimizing the use of extrapolation of efficacy. Therapeutic Innovation & Regulatory Science 2022 Nov;56(6):873–82.

Vaccine Confidence as Critical to Pandemic Preparedness and Response

Shannon H. Baumer-Mouradian, MD[a],
Annika M. Hofstetter, MD, PhD, MPH[b], Sean T. O'Leary, MD, MPH[c],
Douglas J. Opel, MD, MPH[d],*

KEYWORDS

• Pandemic • Vaccine • Child • Preventive health services

KEY POINTS

• Vaccine confidence is a belief that vaccines work, are safe, and are part of a trustworthy medical system. Vaccine confidence was in decline prior to the onset of the COVID-19 pandemic and was further exacerbated by several pandemic-related factors, including expedited vaccine development, the politicization of the vaccine authorization process, and the expansion of antivaccine activism.

• Critical to the success of pandemic mitigation efforts is to build and maintain public trust in vaccines and the vaccine enterprise as well as to leverage existing infrastructure, collaborations between key stakeholders, and learnings from past pandemics.

• Strengthening vaccine confidence requires constant attention that will prove its worth in any emerging public health crisis. Pediatric clinicians should identify opportunities to collaborate with public health officials to build and maintain vaccine confidence among parents and the public.

BACKGROUND

In the aftermath of the COVID-19 pandemic, the director of the US Centers for Disease Control and Prevention described the need to better prepare the United States for the

[a] Department of Pediatrics, Medical College of Wisconsin, 9000 W. Wisconsin Avenue, Milwaukee, WI 53226, USA; [b] Department of Pediatrics, University of Washington School of Medicine and Center for Clinical and Translational Research, Seattle Children's Research Institute, M/S CURE-4, PO Box 5371, Seattle, WA 98145, USA; [c] Department of Pediatrics and Adult and Child Center for Health Outcomes Research and Delivery Science, University of Colorado Anschutz Medical Campus, 1890 North Revere Court, Aurora, CO 80045, USA; [d] Department of Pediatrics, University of Washington School of Medicine and Treuman Katz Center for Pediatric Bioethics and Palliative Care, Center for Clinical and Translational Research, Seattle Children's Research Institute, M/S: JMB-6; 1900 Ninth Avenue, Seattle, WA 98101, USA
* Corresponding author. M/S: JMB-6; 1900 Ninth Avenue, Seattle, WA 98101.
E-mail address: douglas.opel@seattlechildrens.org

Pediatr Clin N Am 71 (2024) 499–513
https://doi.org/10.1016/j.pcl.2024.01.017   **pediatric.theclinics.com**

next large scale infectious disease outbreak, highlighting the need to restore eroded public trust, develop sustainable investments in public health, and shield science from partisanship.[1] These themes, among others, resonate globally.[2–8] The task we face is both important and immense: "Now is the time to truly transform the international system for pandemic preparedness and response and not merely tinker with it."[9]

A critical component of this needed transformation in pandemic preparedness and response is restoring vaccine confidence. Vaccine confidence is a belief that vaccines work, are safe, and are part of a trustworthy medical system.[10] The COVID-19 pandemic exposed the fragility of the public's confidence in vaccines and the vaccine enterprise, limiting the public health impact of vaccination. In this study, we will review the state of vaccine confidence and hesitancy in the United States prior to the COVID-19 pandemic, identify factors that emerged during the COVID-19 pandemic that exacerbated this pre-existing milieu, review learnings from past pandemics, and offer recommendations for improving vaccine confidence in time for future pandemics.

Concepts and Definitions

There has been a collection of constructs used in research aiming to understand and improve vaccine uptake. These constructs include vaccine attitudes, confidence, hesitancy, intentions, refusal, acceptance, coverage, and delay, among others. Little attention, however, has been paid to defining these constructs, determining how they relate to each other, and describing their antecedents. The result has often been a conflation and interchangeable use of these constructs.[11] As a result, it is often difficult to understand how to apply findings from existing literature to vaccine policy and programs.

Recently, consensus has developed around a behavioral model for vaccination (**Fig. 1**).[10,12] Central to this model is the premise that attitudes inform intentions which shape behavior.[13] Attitudes reflect how individuals think and feel about vaccination and include vaccine confidence. Intentions are one's motivation to get vaccinated and include willingness and vaccine hesitancy. Vaccine hesitancy is defined as a motivational state of being conflicted about, or opposed to, getting vaccinated. Behavior is what one does and includes vaccine refusal, acceptance, delay, uptake, and coverage.

This model appropriately highlights the numerous factors that influence vaccine uptake. While all of these factors deserve consideration, vaccine confidence and hesitancy have an arguably outsized level of importance. In 2019, the World Health Organization named vaccine hesitancy as 1 of the top 10 public health threats globally.[14] In 2022, the Vaccine Confidence Subcommittee of the National Vaccine

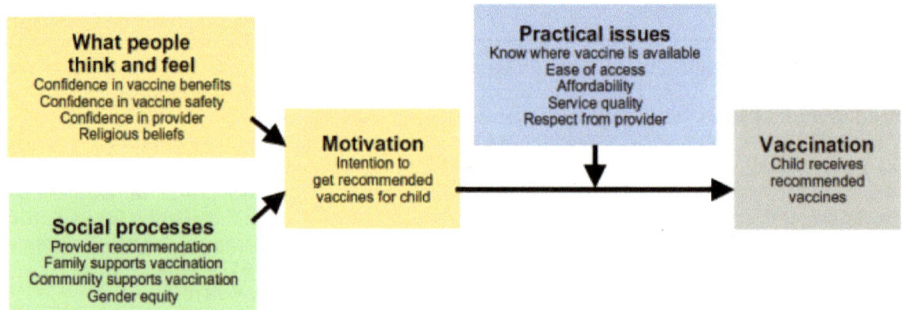

Fig. 1. Behavioral model for vaccination. *Adapted from* Bussink-Voorend D, Hautvast JLA, Vandeberg L, Visser O, Hulscher M. A systematic literature review to clarify the concept of vaccine hesitancy. Nat Hum Behav. 2022;6(12):1634-1648.

Advisory Committee at the US Department of Health and Human Services stated in their report on Sustaining and Increasing Confidence in Vaccination across the Lifespan that vaccine confidence is "important beyond uptake for maintaining trust in vaccination recommendations and fostering a more resilient public, with that resiliency reflected in willingness to accept new information, new vaccines, and evolving science."[10] For these reasons, we focus on vaccine confidence and hesitancy in the context of the COVID-19 pandemic to help inform current and future pandemic planning, response, and recovery.

DISCUSSION
Vaccine Confidence and Hesitancy in the United States Before and During the COVID-19 Pandemic

Childhood vaccination coverage in the United States prior to the COVID-19 pandemic was high.[15,16] However, there were indications that parent vaccine attitudes were shifting, parent intentions to vaccinate their child were waning, and vaccination behaviors were changing. For example, there was evidence that public trust in vaccines was eroding,[17] nonmedical exemptions from kindergarten-entry vaccine requirements were rising,[18,19] and the proportion of parents refusing or delaying childhood vaccines was growing.[20,21] What emerged was a growing threat to individual and public health from large clusters of unvaccinated individuals that facilitated the transmission of vaccine-preventable disease.[22,23] By 2019, the United States experienced the greatest number of measles cases since 1992 as a result of outbreaks within these clusters.[24]

Efforts to counter these trends were introduced, such as the CDC's Vaccinate with Confidence campaign to strengthen public trust in vaccines and reduce the burden of a vaccine preventable outbreaks.[25] Progress, however, would take time. Upon arrival of the COVID-19 pandemic and the prospect of a vaccine being central to mitigation efforts, several factors converged to exacerbate this pre-existing milieu of vaccine attitudes, intentions, and behaviors.[26]

Expedited vaccine development
Operation Warp Speed was a US government-funded partnership between the Department of Health and Human Services and the Department of Defense that aimed to produce 300 million doses of a safe and effective COVID-19 vaccine by January 2021. Efforts to expedite vaccine development included a large influx of government funding, initiation of large-scale manufacturing during clinical trials, and combining clinical trial phases or running them concurrently.[27] The first COVID-19 vaccine received an Emergency Use Authorization (EUA) from the US Food and Drug Administration (FDA) for individuals aged 16 years and above on December 11, 2020, with authorization expanded to all children greater than 6 months old within the subsequent 24 months.[28,29]

Despite the CDC director citing this historic achievement as an "important step forward in our nation's fight against COVID-19,"[30] segments of the public were more wary. The Pfizer and Moderna vaccines were the first vaccines developed using messenger-RNA technology and the first vaccines made available to the broader public through an EUA. These firsts had an impact on people's willingness to accept a COVID-19 vaccine: vaccine novelty was quickly identified as a common reason for caregivers to report not wanting to vaccinate their child for COVID-19.[26,31,32] One parent's perspective captured these sentiments succinctly: "I am hesitant to take a vaccine or have my child injected with a vaccine that is so new. I would be afraid of complications in future years that are now unknown."[33]

This issue of newness brought renewed attention among the public to the vaccine development and authorization processes.[34,35] In fact, the core issue underlying an authorization for emergency use—is the vaccine safe and effective enough given the data available and given the costs of the pandemic?—was widely aired and debated.[36–38] To have confidence and trust in an EUA, transparency was critical so that parents and the public could see how their individual health, their child's health, and the public's health were the primary interests driving decision-making. Transparency, however, was lacking early in the COVID-19 pandemic.[39,40] This seriously compromised public trust and confidence in the FDA, in the government, and in public health authorities.[41,42] Perhaps not surprisingly, parental concerns about COVID-19 vaccine safety, potential for serious side effects, and uncertainty about long-term side effects have lingered and been central contributors to suboptimal vaccine uptake throughout the pandemic.[31–33,43–49]

Politicization of COVID-19 vaccine authorization

In addition to compromising public trust, the politicization of the COVID-19 pandemic and vaccine authorization process subjected vaccines to partisanship: it halted long-standing endorsements by bipartisan political leaders of vaccines and the processes to ensure vaccine safety and effectiveness.[50] Vaccine confidence and vaccine uptake quickly became associated with political affiliation.[32,51] More broadly, this transformation of vaccines into a political issue carried with it the potential to undermine public health and science. It has long been appreciated that science must drive public health, which, in turn, must drive policy.[52] When this is reversed, the credibility of public health agencies is undercut, and their ability to effectively control a pandemic is weakened.

Concerns over vaccine necessity and the perceived risk of COVID-19 illness

Early in the COVID-19 pandemic, children were observed to have lower rates of COVID-19 infection and a milder disease course.[53–55] The role of children in viral transmission was also not initially clear.[56] For many parents, these observations translated into a low perceived threat of COVID-19 for their child, with vaccination against COVID-19 perceived as unnecessary.[44,49,57] A common reason cited by parents who had not yet vaccinated their eligible children against COVID-19 was not being worried about the disease.[58]

Strong evidence supports the relationship between risk perception and vaccination behavior.[59] It is not a pandemic per se that will drive behavior to receive a vaccine developed to protect against the disease causing the pandemic. Rather, it is parents' perceptions of their child's susceptibility to the disease along with other factors, such as the ability of the vaccine against the antigen to protect their child against disease. In the end, the COVID-19 pandemic did not result in high uptake of COVID-19 childhood vaccines by US parents.[60] It may also not have had a positive impact on how parents viewed other vaccines. For instance, while some investigators found parents more willing to vaccinate their child against influenza since the onset of the COVID-19 pandemic,[61] others found that an initial positive effect of the COVID-19 pandemic on parent general vaccine attitudes quickly dissipated.[62]

Evolution and expansion of antivaccine activism and vaccine misinformation

Antivaccine activism has existed since the advent of vaccines themselves. Though historically relegated to the fringe, antivaccine activism had become more organized and mainstream prior to the COVID-19 pandemic. With the pandemic's onset, antivaccine activism evolved and expanded further, strengthening its network, broadening its identity with right-wing ideology,[63] and adopting tactics that involved directly targeting and harassing public health officials and vaccine supporters.[64]

This more organized antivaccine network amplified conspiratorial rhetoric during the pandemic, working to discredit the vaccine development and evaluation process[65] and to promote the narrative that COVID-19 vaccines are harmful.[66] These misinformation and disinformation campaigns had a negative effect on COVID-19 vaccine attitudes, intentions, and behaviors. For instance, investigators found that a third of US adults believed in one or more conspiracy theories regarding COVID-19.[67] Among parents, beliefs in COVID-19 conspiracy theories were associated with a lower intent to vaccinate their children.[68,69]

A renewed strain on the social contract

If the social contract, at its core, means citizens giving up some individual freedoms in exchange for the state or government maintaining social goods, like security and public health, then the pandemic once again exposed that the social contract has rarely been reciprocal for many Americans. People of color, including children, bore disproportionate risks for COVID-19-associated illnesses, hospitalizations, and deaths,[70] and particularly early in the pandemic, bore disproportionate access to COVID-19 vaccines.[71-73] Given this, COVID-19 vaccine confidence and hesitancy among people of color was not only about vaccine newness and safety, but also about systemic social injustice.[74] Freedoms had been given up, but little security or health had been gained in return. As James Baldwin wrote in the 1960s, that is unfortunately still true today, "Allegiance, after all, has to work two ways; and one can grow weary of an allegiance which is not reciprocal."[75]

Lessons from Past Pandemics

The historian Charles Rosenberg, in his book *The Cholera Years*, argued that the cholera epidemics of the 1800s in the United States were not solely public health events, but also social events influenced by the cultural, religious, and economic debates at the time.[76] In this way, the cholera epidemics, like smallpox before it and influenza since, reshaped society's relationship with public health. These past epidemics, for instance, forced a reckoning with how societal inequities translated to disparities in disease burden and access to treatment. They compelled a revisiting of the balance between individual freedoms and the common good. And they influenced re-examinations of the processes and policies invoked during public health crises. Each remains relevant today and has implications for vaccine confidence, hesitancy, and uptake: what would the impact on vaccine confidence and uptake be with use of an expedited process for authorizing a vaccine against the antigen causing the epidemic? With a vaccine mandate? With a vaccine prioritization and distribution plan that does not account for social vulnerability and susceptibility to disease?

Critical to the success of pandemic mitigation efforts that involve vaccination is to have an infrastructure in place to facilitate collaboration between key stakeholders that leverages learnings from past pandemics and their impact on vaccine confidence and uptake. These stakeholders ought to include behavioral and social scientists,[77] disaster preparedness and public health policymakers, and front-line clinicians. As Ankomah and colleagues state, "during [pandemic vaccine] planning, a careful consideration of the underlying factors that influence vaccine acceptance or hesitancy, effective risk communication, and education strategies have the advantage of building public confidence in vaccination."[78] The novel 2009 influenza A (H1N1) pandemic, in which vaccines were approved within 3 to 6 months of declaring the pandemic in June 2009, offers some specific insights into how this infrastructure could be beneficial in the roll-out of a vaccine in the context of a pandemic.[78]

First, though an EUA was ultimately not utilized for an H1N1 vaccine, investigations into the potential impact of an EUA on H1N1 vaccine uptake found that an EUA would have been negatively associated with vaccine acceptability.[79] Second, common barriers to H1N1 vaccine uptake included concerns over vaccine side effects, media conspiracy, misinformation, and the speed in which the vaccine was developed.[78] However, there was also evidence that those who did receive the H1N1 vaccine were willing to promote H1N1 vaccination in their community.[80] Third, there were problems in the equitable distribution of H1N1 vaccines despite attempts by local health jurisdictions to prioritize vaccine access among underserved and underinsured populations.[81] Early identification of disparities in vaccine uptake through mechanisms such as a national race/ethnicity reporting requirement could have improved public health response efforts.[81] In these ways, the H1N1 pandemic foreshadowed several issues and opportunities experienced during the COVID-19 pandemic that, with increased coordination and connection between stakeholders involved in both, could have helped improve COVID-19 vaccine confidence, uptake, and equity.

Recommendations for Improving Vaccine Confidence in Time for the Next Pandemic

We present 3 recommendations to improve vaccine confidence during routine and crisis times. Strengthening vaccine confidence is work requiring constant attention that will prove its worth in any emerging public health crisis. These recommendations are aligned with existing recommendations from the Centers for Disease Control and Prevention,[25] the World Health Organization,[82] the National Vaccine Advisory Committee at the US Department of Health and Human Services,[10] and the National Academies of Sciences, Engineering, and Medicine.[83]

Build trust in the government and vaccine enterprise

To promote trust in the science behind vaccines, the institutions that authorize vaccines, and the clinicians that administer vaccines, transparency is key. It is essential that the role of federal vaccine committees not be politicized and that a unified, proactive, highly visible communication structure is used to regularly inform the American public about vaccine development, safety processes, approval, and recommendation criteria.[82,84] This communication must be interpretable, context and culture specific, and accurate.[82,84,85] These qualities are especially critical when expedited vaccine development and an EUA for vaccine approval will be utilized.

Since concerns about vaccine safety are highly associated with vaccine intentions and behavior, it is essential to assuage vaccine safety concerns by rapidly deploying and coordinating vaccine safety monitoring resources. Transparency in vaccine safety data reporting must also be achieved to instill trust and promote vaccine confidence and uptake. Public health messaging must offer clear and understandable information about vaccine risks and their likelihoods[43,84] and explain the scientific standards utilized throughout vaccine development, approval, and distribution process.[51] The 5 principles for effective risk communication are essential (**Fig. 2**).[83]

Transparency and accountability are also key to ensuring that information conveyed can be trusted as accurate. Policy makers and professional organizations should monitor media platforms for false vaccine information, expose networks of false information, and consider holding publishers of false information liable.[50,85] During COVID-19, programs such as the Virality Project established a nonpartisan, multistakeholder model composed of health sector leaders, federal health agencies, state and local health officials, social media platforms, and civil society organizations focused on

1. Do not wait.
2. Be credible.
3. Be clear.
4. Express empathy and show respect.
5. Acknowledge uncertainty and
    manage expectations.

Fig. 2. Five principles for effective risk communication.[1] National Academies of Sciences, Engineering, and Medicine. 2021. Strategies for Building Confidence in the COVID-19 Vaccines. Washington, DC: The National Academies Press. https://doi.org/10.17226/26068

monitoring and analyzing emerging misinformation and disinformation. Similar programs are needed to combat misinformation and disinformation for emerging public health issues.[86] Public forums to address safety concerns as well as to discuss the complexities of approval processes and post-roll out safety monitoring provide scientists and decision-makers another opportunity to improve understanding and promote confidence in a novel vaccine.[43,84] Utilizing social media channels and having an online presence to provide reliable sources of information are also important to dispel myths and counteract false information.[43]

Maintaining trust in the vaccine enterprise will also require population resilience against vaccine myths as well as strong state and local vaccine programs that are prepared to respond to any event that may erode vaccine confidence.[82] To achieve this, there needs to be ongoing communication with parents and the public "to build awareness and knowledge of risks and benefits of immunization and diseases."[82] In part, this can be achieved through the promotion of routine vaccines by clinicians. Indeed, those intending to vaccinate their child against COVID-19 were more likely to have a history of being up to date with routine vaccinations or have received the influenza vaccine for the child and parent.[31,32] Engaging with parents regarding routine vaccines recommended for their child has the potential to positively shape their vaccine attitudes, overall vaccine confidence, and trust in the vaccine enterprise.

Educate and empower clinicians

Clinicians continue to play an influential role in promoting vaccine uptake. Foremost, clinicians remain the most trusted source of vaccine information for parents.[84,87–90] During COVID-19, 75% of parents reported clinicians to be the top source of information regarding COVID-19,[90] with trust in clinicians being the most consistent driver of vaccine uptake.[43]

To maintain this trustworthiness, clinicians themselves must be knowledgeable and confident in the safety and efficacy of a vaccine to engage with parents regarding their vaccine concerns and to provide a strong recommendation for the vaccine.[87] Politicization of the COVID-19 vaccine authorization process undermined the confidence of a significant minority of clinicians in COVID-19 vaccines and the processes and institutions meant to ensure their safety. In one survey study conducted immediately before the first COVID-19 vaccine was authorized for emergency use, 34% of health care worker respondents did not trust the FDA to oversee vaccine development and safety, and 46% did not trust information from the government about COVID-19.[91]

Clinicians ought to be integrated into pandemic preparedness teams long before a pandemic to build partnership, trust, and to leverage their expertise.[82] Strong partnerships between clinicians, health authorities, and policymakers that facilitate ongoing information exchange can help health authorities and policymakers, for instance, understand barriers to reaching priority groups in communities in which clinicians practice. These partnerships can also help clinicians align with health authorities and policymakers on vaccine messaging, with clinicians able to disseminate information and develop communication plans in their practices and the broader community.[92] Additionally, this information exchange may help clinicians keep up to date on the latest scientific evidence supporting vaccine recommendations amidst dynamic pandemic conditions.

It is also critical to support and advise clinicians in how to adjust their vaccine communication during a pandemic. For instance, the standard communication approach for routine vaccines that involves initiating the vaccine conversation with a presumptive format required revision during the COVID-19 pandemic. This presumptive approach is justifiable when there is high degree of certainty that the vaccine is of high benefit and low risk.[93] Routine vaccines meet this threshold: they have been comprehensively studied over many decades, and based on this comprehensive data showing high benefit and low risk, have received full approval by federal oversight agencies and are universally recommended by federal advisory committees. COVID-19 vaccines authorized for emergency use, while still deserving of a strong

Table 1
Six community engagement strategies to build COVID-19 vaccine confidence

Engagement Strategy	Rationale
Form partnerships with community organizations	Strong existing community relationships bring organizations closer to their audiences, can help facilitate tailoring of information to those communities, and can develop trusted leaders who can be effective spokespersons
Engage with and center the voices and perspectives of trusted messengers who have roots in the community	Mobilizing members of communities who value vaccination can effectively counter vaccine hesitancy
Engage across multiple accessible channels	Effective community engagement requires use of a variety of channels to reach marginalized populations, including messaging in multiple languages, in different settings (eg, town halls, faith-based gatherings, community events), and across different media
Begin or continue working toward racial equity	Elevating racial equity when talking about vaccines, that is, by recognizing how systemic racism has disadvantaged specific communities, avoids obscuring the structural factors that impact health
Allow and encourage public ownership of COVID-19 vaccination	Public ownership of COVID-19 Vaccination initiatives through public oversight, such as actively seeking engagement with the public, listening to feedback and adapting accordingly, and establishing local public oversight committees, can improve confidence in COVID-19 vaccination
Measure and communicate inequities in vaccine distribution	Measurement of the effect of vaccine distribution schema on specific communities and communication of those findings to the public is critical to building trust

Adapted from National Academies of Sciences, Engineering, and Medicine. 2021. Strategies for Building Confidence in the COVID-19 Vaccines. Washington, DC: The National Academies Press.

recommendation in support of uptake, did not meet this threshold. In this circumstance, separate communication strategies were initially needed to promote vaccine confidence and uptake. For COVID-19 vaccines, clinicians were advised to lead with listening, use an open-ended invitation for the patient or parent to share their perspective, and incorporate motivational interviewing (MI) techniques into their vaccine conversations.[94] MI and invitational rhetoric (an invitation to understanding as a means of creating a relationship rooted in equality, value, and self-determination) were, in fact, demonstrated on small scales to be successful in improving COVID-19 vaccine intentions among parents.[25,95,96]

Foster equity and community engagement

Simply put, "there may be no better ballast for maintaining trust in the childhood vaccine enterprise than by achieving equity in childhood vaccine delivery and coverage."[97] Socially vulnerable communities must be prioritized in vaccine distribution schemes[51] and community stakeholders must be involved in the development and dissemination of pandemic vaccine-related policies. Six community engagement strategies designed to combat mistrust and build confidence in COVID-19 vaccines have broad appeal beyond COVID-19 (**Table 1**).[83]

Bidirectional dialog should be sought with community members and leaders regarding their unique needs and vaccine concerns, particularly among those communities that have been historically marginalized. Community partners should be invited to help craft specific culturally appropriate messages to help inform communities about disease specifics (eg, disease rates in local communities that include personal stories from community members[57]), vaccine availability, and vaccine safety and efficacy. Public health officials should also facilitate collaboration between community partners and the media to highlight how the pandemic has affected their community as well as barriers and successes in vaccine uptake.[82,84] Vaccine ambassadors—community members trained to disseminate health or vaccine information in their communities—can be an effective and powerful mechanism to frame vaccination as the social norm.[25,98]

SUMMARY

Emerging infectious diseases, such as Ebola, Zika, and COVID-19, offer an alarming reminder of the impact of scourges of old as well as the promise of vaccines to maintain health. Perhaps the most important lesson from the COVID-19 pandemic was the fragility of the public's trust in the vaccine enterprise.[97] To be prepared for the next pandemic, we must work to restore and retain trust and confidence in vaccines and the vaccine enterprise.

CLINICS CARE POINTS

- Pediatric clinicians have been consistently cited as the most important influence on parental vaccine decision-making. This held true during the COVID-19 pandemic. Given this influence, pediatric clinicians should continue to engage with, educate, and strongly recommend vaccines to parents to not only promote uptake but foster trust and vaccine confidence.

- The fields of pediatrics and public health have a shared commitment to disease prevention. Pediatric clinicians should identify opportunities where they can collaborate with health authorities and public health policy-makers to advocate for child health and improve vaccine confidence and uptake.[92]

DISCLOSURE

The authors have no conflicts of interest, whether financial or other.

REFERENCES

1. Walensky RP, What I Need to Tell America Before I Leave the C.D.C. *The New York Times*, Available at: https://www.nytimes.com/2023/06/27/opinion/rochelle-walensky-cdc-pandemic-despair.html, 2023. Accessed July 12, 2023.
2. Sirleaf HEEJ and Clark H, A road map for a world protected from pandemic threats. The independent pandel for pandemic preparedness and response, Available at: https://live-the-independent-panel.pantheonsite.io/wp-content/uploads/2023/05/Final-Road-Map-Report_May-2023_Interactive.pdf, 2023. Accessed July 12, 2023.
3. Sirleaf HEEJ and Clark H, Transforming or tinkering? Inaction lays the groundwork for another pandemic. The independent panel for pandemic preparedness and response, Available at: https://live-the-independent-panel.pantheonsite.io/wp-content/uploads/2022/05/Transforming-or-tinkering_Report_Final.pdf, 2022. Accessed July 12, 2023.
4. Sirleaf HEEJ and Clark H, COVID-19: make it the last pandemic.Independent Panel for Pandemic Preparedness and Response, Available at: https://theindependentpanel.org/wp-content/uploads/2021/05/COVID-19-Make-it-the-Last-Pandemic_final.pdfhttps://theindependentpanel.org/, 2021. Accessed July 12, 2023.
5. World Health Organization, Strengthening WHO preparedness for and response to health emergencies proposal for amendments to the International Health Regulations. 2005, Available at: https://apps.who.int/gb/ebwha/pdf_files/WHA75/A75_18-en.pdf, 2022. Accessed July 12, 2023.
6. World Health Organization, First meeting of the intergovernmental negotiating body to draft and negotiate a WHO convention, agreement or other international instrument on pandemic prevention, preparedness and response. A/INB/1/2 Rev.1, Available at: https://apps.who.int/gb/inb/pdf_files/inb1/A_INB1_2Rev1-en.pdf, 2022. Accessed July 12, 2023.
7. G20 High level independent panel on financing the global commons for pandemic preparedness and response. A global deal for our pandemic age, Available at: https://pandemic-financing.org/, 2021. Accessed July 12, 2023.
8. Global Preparedness Monitoring Board, From worlds apart to a world prepared: global Preparedness Monitoring Board report 2021, Available at: https://www.gpmb.org/annual-reports/annual-report-2021, 2021. Accessed July 12, 2023.
9. Clark H, Cárdenas M, Dybul M, et al. Transforming or tinkering: the world remains unprepared for the next pandemic threat. Lancet (London, England) 2022; 399(10340):1995–9.
10. National Vaccine Advisory Committee, Sustaining and increasing confidence in vaccination across the lifespan: recommendations from the national vaccine advisory committee U.S. Department of Health and Human Services, Available at: https://www.hhs.gov/sites/default/files/sustaining-increasing-confidence-vaccination-across-lifespan-recommendations-national-vaccine-advisory-committee.pdf, 2022. Accessed July 12, 2023.
11. Bussink-Voorend D, Hautvast JLA, Vandeberg L, et al. A systematic literature review to clarify the concept of vaccine hesitancy. Nat Human Behav 2022;6(12): 1634–48.
12. Brewer NT. What Works to Increase Vaccination Uptake. Acad Pediatr 2021; 21(4s):S9–16.

13. Fishbein M, Ajzen I. Predicting and changing behavior: the reasoned action approach. New York: Psychology Press; 2009.
14. World Health Organization. Ten threats to global health. 2019. Available at: https://www.who.int/news-room/spotlight/ten-threats-to-global-health-in-2019. [Accessed 24 April 2020].
15. Hill HA, Elam-Evans LD, Yankey D, et al. Vaccination Coverage Among Children Aged 19-35 Months - United States, 2015. MMWR (Morb Mortal Wkly Rep) 2016; 65(39):1065-71.
16. Seither R, Calhoun K, Mellerson J, et al. Vaccination Coverage Among Children in Kindergarten - United States, 2015-16 School Year. MMWR (Morb Mortal Wkly Rep) 2016;65(39):1057-64.
17. Sciences AAoAa. Public trust in vaccines: defining a research agenda. Cambridge: Mass; 2014.
18. Omer SB, Richards JL, Ward M, et al. Vaccination policies and rates of exemption from immunization, 2005-2011. N Engl J Med 2012;367(12):1170-1.
19. Richards JL, Wagenaar BH, Van Otterloo J, et al. Nonmedical exemptions to immunization requirements in California: a 16-year longitudinal analysis of trends and associated community factors. Vaccine 2013;31(29):3009-13.
20. Hough-Telford C, Kimberlin DW, Aban I, et al. Vaccine Delays, Refusals, and Patient Dismissals: A Survey of Pediatricians. Pediatrics 2016;138(3).
21. Kempe A, O'Leary ST, Kennedy A, et al. Physician response to parental requests to spread out the recommended vaccine schedule. Pediatrics 2015;135(4): 666-77.
22. Atwell JE, Van Otterloo J, Zipprich J, et al. Nonmedical vaccine exemptions and pertussis in California, 2010. Pediatrics 2013;132(4):624-30.
23. Omer SB, Enger KS, Moulton LH, et al. Geographic clustering of nonmedical exemptions to school immunization requirements and associations with geographic clustering of pertussis. Am J Epidemiol 2008;168(12):1389-96.
24. Patel MK, Goodson JL, Alexander JP Jr, et al. Progress Toward Regional Measles Elimination - Worldwide, 2000-2019. MMWR (Morb Mortal Wkly Rep) 2020;69(45): 1700-5.
25. Centers for Disease Control and Prevention. Vaccinate with confidence. 2019. Available at: https://www.cdc.gov/vaccines/partners/vaccinate-with-confidence. html. [Accessed 22 August 2023].
26. Hammershaimb EA, Campbell JD, O'Leary ST. Coronavirus Disease-2019 Vaccine Hesitancy. Pediatr Clin 2023;70(2):243-57.
27. Olive JK, Hotez PJ, Damania A, et al. The state of the antivaccine movement in the United States: A focused examination of nonmedical exemptions in states and counties. PLoS Med 2018;15(6):e1002578.
28. Woodworth KR, Moulia D, Collins JP, et al. The advisory committee on immunization practices' interim recommendation for use of pfizer-BioNTech COVID-19 vaccine in children aged 5–11 Years — United States. 2021. Available at: https://www.cdc. gov/mmwr/volumes/70/wr/mm7045e1.htm#suggestedcitation. [Accessed 17 February 2022].
29. Wallace M, Woodworth KR, Gargano JW, et al. The Advisory Committee on Immunization Practices' Interim Recommendation for Use of Pfizer-BioNTech COVID-19 Vaccine in Adolescents Aged 12–15 Years — United States. Available at: MMWR (Morb Mortal Wkly Rep) 2021;70:749-52 https://www.cdc.gov/mmwr/ volumes/70/wr/mm7020e1.htm#suggestedcitation.
30. CDC recommends COVID-19 vaccines for young children [press release]. Online Centers for Disease Control and Prevention, Available at: https://www.cdc.gov/

media/releases/2022/s0618-children-vaccine.html, 2022. Accessed August 28, 2023.

31. Goldman RD, Yan TD, Seiler M, et al. Caregiver willingness to vaccinate their children against COVID-19: Cross sectional survey. Vaccine 2020;38(48):7668–73.

32. Szilagyi PG, Shah MD, Delgado JR, et al. Parents' Intentions and Perceptions About COVID-19 Vaccination for Their Children: Results From a National Survey. Pediatrics 2021;148(4).

33. Hetherington E, Edwards SA, MacDonald SE, et al. SARS-CoV-2 vaccination intentions among mothers of children aged 9 to 12 years: a survey of the All Our Families cohort. CMAJ Open 2021;9(2):E548–55.

34. Kaiser Family Foundation. KFF health tracking poll - September 2020. 2020. Available at: https://www.kff.org/coronavirus-covid-19/report/kff-health-tracking-poll-september-2020/. [Accessed 21 January 2022].

35. Opel DJ, Diekema DS, Ross LF. Should We Mandate a COVID-19 Vaccine for Children? JAMA Pediatr 2021;175(2):125–6.

36. McGinley L, Johnson CY. Debate rages over whether FDA should use emergency powers to clear a coronavirus vaccine early. Washington Post; 2020.

37. Avorn J, Kesselheim AS. Up Is Down - Pharmaceutical Industry Caution vs. Federal Acceleration of Covid-19 Vaccine Approval. N Engl J Med 2020;383(18): 1706–8.

38. Schwartz JL. Evaluating and deploying covid-19 vaccines - the importance of transparency, scientific integrity, and public trust. N Engl J Med 2020;383(18): 1703–5.

39. Stolberg SG. Trump may reject tougher F.D.A. Vaccine Standards, Calling Them 'Political'. N Y Times 2020.

40. Dawsey J, Sonmez F and Kane P. Trump acknowledges he intentionally downplayed deadly coronavirus, says effort was to reduce panic, *Wash Post*, 2020. Available at: https://www.washingtonpost.com/politics/trump-reaction-woodward-interview-coronavirus/2020/09/09/fc21e67e-f2ca-11ea-b796-2dd09962649c_story.html. Accessed September 3, 2021.

41. Kaiser Family Foundation. KFF health tracking poll – october 2020. 2020. Available at: https://files.kff.org/attachment/Topline-KFF-Health-Tracking-Poll-October-2020.pdf. [Accessed 21 January 2022].

42. Robert Wood Johnson Foundation, Harvard TH. Chan school of public health. The public's perspective on the United States public health system. 2021. Available at: https://cdn1.sph.harvard.edu/wp-content/uploads/sites/94/2021/05/RWJF-Harvard-Report_FINAL-051321.pdf. [Accessed 23 January 2022].

43. Majid U, Ahmad M, Zain S, et al. COVID-19 vaccine hesitancy and acceptance: a comprehensive scoping review of global literature. Health Promot Int 2022;37(3).

44. Schilling S, Orr CJ, Delamater AM, et al. COVID-19 vaccine hesitancy among low-income, racially and ethnically diverse US parents. Patient Educ Counsel 2022; 105(8):2771–7.

45. Ruggiero KM, Wong J, Sweeney CF, et al. Parents' Intentions to Vaccinate Their Children Against COVID-19. J Pediatr Health Care 2021;35(5):509–17.

46. Suran M. Why Parents Still Hesitate to Vaccinate Their Children Against COVID-19. JAMA 2022;327(1):23–5.

47. Bell S, Clarke R, Mounier-Jack S, et al. Parents' and guardians' views on the acceptability of a future COVID-19 vaccine: A multi-methods study in England. Vaccine 2020;38(49):7789–98.

48. Hamel LL, L, Kearney A, Stokes M, et al. KFF COVID-19 vaccine monitor: winter 2021 update on parent's views of vaccine for kids 2021, Available at: https://www.

kff.org/coronavirus-covid-19/poll-finding/kff-covid-19-vaccine-monitor-winter-2021-update-on-parents-views-of-vaccines/, 2021. Accessed August 28, 2023.

49. Garbin A, Chiba EK, Garbin CAS, et al. Systematic review: Impact of parental decision on paediatric COVID-19 vaccination. Child Care Health Dev 2023;49(5):787–99.

50. Sharfstein JM, Callaghan T, Carpiano RM, et al. Uncoupling vaccination from politics: a call to action. Lancet 2021;398(10307):1211–2.

51. Lin C, Tu P, Beitsch LM. Confidence and Receptivity for COVID-19 Vaccines: A Rapid Systematic Review. Vaccines (Basel) 2020;9(1).

52. Koplan JP, McPheeters M. Plagues, public health, and politics. Emerg Infect Dis 2004;10(11):2039–43.

53. Lu X, Zhang L, Du H, et al. SARS-CoV-2 Infection in Children. N Engl J Med 2020;382(17):1663–5.

54. Zhang M, Zhang P, Liang Y, et al. A systematic review of current status and challenges of vaccinating children against SARS-CoV-2. J Infect Public Health 2022;15(11):1212–24.

55. Mehta NS, Mytton OT, Mullins EWS, et al. SARS-CoV-2 (COVID-19): What Do We Know About Children? A Systematic Review. Clin Infect Dis 2020;71(9):2469–79.

56. Rajmil L. Role of children in the transmission of the COVID-19 pandemic: a rapid scoping review. BMJ Paediatr Open 2020;4(1):e000722.

57. Baumer-Mouradian SH, Hart RJ, Visotcky A, et al. Understanding Influenza and SARS-CoV-2 Vaccine Hesitancy in Racial and Ethnic Minority Caregivers. Vaccines (Basel) 2022;10(11).

58. Kaiser Family Foundation. COVID-19 vaccine monitor. 2022. Available at: https://www.kff.org/coronavirus-covid-19/dashboard/kff-covid-19-vaccine-monitor-dashboard/#parents. [Accessed 28 July 2022].

59. Brewer NT, Chapman GB, Gibbons FX, et al. Meta-analysis of the relationship between risk perception and health behavior: the example of vaccination. Health Psychol 2007;26(2):136–45.

60. Kaiser Family Foundation. KFF COVID-19 vaccine monitor: parents and kids. 2023. Available at: https://www.kff.org/coronavirus-covid-19/dashboard/kff-covid-19-vaccine-monitor-dashboard/#parents. [Accessed 19 September 2023].

61. Goldman RD, McGregor S, Marneni SR, et al. Willingness to Vaccinate Children against Influenza after the Coronavirus Disease 2019 Pandemic. J Pediatr 2021;228:87–93 e82.

62. Opel DJ, Furniss A, Zhou C, et al. Parent attitudes towards childhood vaccines after the onset of SARS-CoV-2 in the United States. Academic pediatrics 2022.

63. Hotez PJ. COVID19 meets the antivaccine movement. Microb Infect 2020;22(4–5):162–4.

64. Carpiano RM, Callaghan T, DiResta R, et al. Confronting the evolution and expansion of anti-vaccine activism in the USA in the COVID-19 era. Lancet 2023;401(10380):967–70.

65. Hotez P, Batista C, Ergonul O, et al. Correcting COVID-19 vaccine misinformation: Lancet Commission on COVID-19 Vaccines and Therapeutics Task Force Members. EClinicalMedicine 2021;33:100780.

66. Nazar S, Pieters T. Plandemic Revisited: A Product of Planned Disinformation Amplifying the COVID-19 "infodemic". Front Public Health 2021;9:649930.

67. Earnshaw VA, Eaton LA, Kalichman SC, et al. COVID-19 conspiracy beliefs, health behaviors, and policy support. Transl Behav Med 2020;10(4):850–6.

68. Iannello P, Colautti L, Magenes S, et al. Black-and-white thinking and conspiracy beliefs prevent parents from vaccinating their children against COVID-19. Appl Cognit Psychol 2022. https://doi.org/10.1002/acp.3999.

69. Allen JD, Fu Q, Nguyen KH, et al. Parents' Willingness to Vaccinate Children for COVID-19: Conspiracy Theories, Information Sources, and Perceived Responsibility. J Health Commun 2023;28(1):15–27.

70. Centers for Disease Control and Prevention. Risk for COVID-19 infection, hospitalization, and death by race/ethnicity. Available at: 2021 https://stacks.cdc.gov/view/cdc/107296. [Accessed 17 June 2023].

71. Hughes MM, Wang A, Grossman MK, et al. County-Level COVID-19 Vaccination Coverage and Social Vulnerability - United States, December 14, 2020-March 1, 2021. MMWR (Morb Mortal Wkly Rep) 2021;70(12):431–6.

72. Goyal MK, Simpson JN, Boyle MD, et al. Racial and/or Ethnic and Socioeconomic Disparities of SARS-CoV-2 Infection Among Children. Pediatrics 2020;146(4).

73. Lee EH, Kepler KL, Geevarughese A, et al. Race/Ethnicity Among Children With COVID-19-Associated Multisystem Inflammatory Syndrome. JAMA Netw Open 2020;3(11):e2030280.

74. Boyd R. Black People Need Better Vaccine Access, Not Better Vaccine Attitudes. New York Times; 2021.

75. Baldwin J. Nobody knows my name: more notes of a native son. New York: Dial Press; 1961.

76. Rosenberg CE. The cholera years: the United States in 1832, 1849, and 1866. Chicago, IL: The University of Chicago Press; 1962.

77. Schoch-Spana M, Brunson EK, Long R, et al. The public's role in COVID-19 vaccination: Human-centered recommendations to enhance pandemic vaccine awareness, access, and acceptance in the United States. Vaccine 2021;39(40): 6004–12.

78. Ankomah AA, Moa A, Chughtai AA. The long road of pandemic vaccine development to rollout: A systematic review on the lessons learnt from the 2009 H1N1 influenza pandemic. Am J Infect Control 2022;50(7):735–42.

79. Quinn SC, Kumar S, Freimuth VS, et al. Public willingness to take a vaccine or drug under Emergency Use Authorization during the 2009 H1N1 pandemic. Biosecur Bioterrorism Biodefense Strategy, Pract Sci 2009;7(3):275–90.

80. Frew PM, Hixson B, del Rio C, et al. Acceptance of pandemic 2009 influenza A (H1N1) vaccine in a minority population: determinants and potential points of intervention. Pediatrics 2011;127(Suppl 1):S113–9.

81. Plough A, Bristow B, Fielding J, et al. Pandemics and health equity: lessons learned from the H1N1 response in Los Angeles County. J Publ Health Manag Pract 2011;17(1):20–7.

82. World Health Organization. Vaccination and Trust. 2017. Available at: https://www.who.int/publications/i/item/vaccination-and-trust. [Accessed 28 August 2023].

83. National Academies of Sciences. Engineering, and Medicine. Strategies for building confidence in the COVID-19. Washington, DC: Vaccines; 2021.

84. Salmon D, Opel DJ, Dudley MZ, et al. Reflections On Governance, Communication, And Equity: Challenges And Opportunities In COVID-19 Vaccination. Health affairs (Project Hope) 2021;40(3):419–25.

85. Lazarus JV, Romero D, Kopka CJ, et al. A multinational Delphi consensus to end the COVID-19 public health threat. Nature 2022;611(7935):332–45.

86. The virality Project. *Mems, magnets, and microchips: Narrative dynamics around COVID-19 vaccines* stanford digital repository, Available at: https://purl.stanford.edu/mx395xj8490, 2022. Accessed August 28, 2023.
87. Paterson P, Meurice F, Stanberry LR, et al. Vaccine hesitancy and healthcare providers. Vaccine 2016;34(52):6700–6.
88. de Albuquerque Veloso Machado M, Roberts B, Wong BLH, et al. The Relationship Between the COVID-19 Pandemic and Vaccine Hesitancy: A Scoping Review of Literature Until August 2021. Front Public Health 2021;9:747787.
89. Smith PJ, Kennedy AM, Wooten K, et al. Association between health care providers' influence on parents who have concerns about vaccine safety and vaccination coverage. Pediatrics 2006;118(5):e1287–92.
90. Shen AK, Browne S, Srivastava T, et al. Persuading the "Movable Middle": Characteristics of effective messages to promote routine and COVID-19 vaccinations for adults and children - The impact of COVID-19 on beliefs and attitudes. Vaccine 2023;41(12):2055–62.
91. Shekhar R, Sheikh AB, Upadhyay S, et al. COVID-19 Vaccine Acceptance among Health Care Workers in the United States. Vaccines (Basel) 2021;9(2).
92. Kuo AA, Thomas PA, Chilton LA, et al. Pediatricians and Public Health: Optimizing the Health and Well-Being of the Nation's Children. Pediatrics 2018; 141(2).
93. Blumenthal-Barby J, Opel DJ. Nudge or Grudge? Choice Architecture and Parental Decision-Making. Hastings Cent Rep 2018;48(2):33–9.
94. Opel DJ, Lo B, Peek ME. Addressing Mistrust About COVID-19 Vaccines Among Patients of Color. Ann Intern Med 2021;174(5):698–700.
95. Ryan GW, Goulding M, Borg A, et al. Development and Beta-Testing of the CONFIDENCE Intervention to Increase Pediatric COVID-19 Vaccination. J Pediatr Health Care 2023;37(3):244–52.
96. Make J, Lauver A. Increasing trust and vaccine uptake: Offering invitational rhetoric as an alternative to persuasion in pediatric visits with vaccine-hesitant parents (VHPs). Vaccine X 2022;10:100129.
97. Opel DJ, Brewer NT, Buttenheim AM, et al. The legacy of the COVID-19 pandemic for childhood vaccination in the USA. Lancet (London, England) 2023;401(10370):75–8.
98. Schoeppe J, Cheadle A, Melton M, et al. The Immunity Community: A Community Engagement Strategy for Reducing Vaccine Hesitancy. Health Promot Pract 2017;18(5):654–61.

Pandemic Planning, Response, and Recovery for Pediatricians
A Focus on Health Equity and Social Determinants of Health

Joelle N. Simpson, MD, MPH[a,b,*], Joseph L. Wright, MD, MPH[a,c]

KEYWORDS

- Health equity • Pediatric readiness • Disaster preparedness
- Social determinants of health • Pandemic preparedness

KEY POINTS

- The COVID-19 pandemic amplified health inequities and placed tremendous strain on our society, economy, education systems, and health care infrastructure.
- Building on pediatric readiness frameworks is a recommended approach to creating a pediatric pandemic plan.
- Health equity considerations need to be built into all policies, processes, and systems at the outset.
- The evolving national discourse on racism and inequities across communities including social injustices faced by minoritized groups is important framing for pandemic planning across all phases of disaster including preparedness, response, and recovery.

INTRODUCTION

The advent of the COVID-19 pandemic in the United States and, indeed, around the world, has led to unprecedented examination, consideration, and reckoning of the impact of inherent and explicit societal inequities on differential population health outcomes. As such, specific attention has been rendered to recognizing and addressing

[a] Department of Pediatrics and Emergency Medicine, George Washington University School of Medicine, Washington, DC, USA; [b] Emergency Medicine & Trauma Center, Children's National Hospital, 111 Michigan Avenue, Northwest, Washington, DC 20010, USA; [c] Department of Health Policy and Management, George Washington University School of Public Health, Washington DC 20052
* Corresponding author. Emergency Medicine & Trauma Center, Children's National Hospital, 111 Michigan Avenue, Northwest, Washington, DC 20010.
E-mail address: jnsimpso@childrensnational.org

Pediatr Clin N Am 71 (2024) 515–528
https://doi.org/10.1016/j.pcl.2024.02.001
0031-3955/24/© 2024 Elsevier Inc. All rights reserved.
pediatric.theclinics.com

the longstanding drivers of underlying health status that disproportionately impact historically marginalized and minoritized people, and that confer unique vulnerabilities in the face of acute emergencies such as a pandemic. The authors of this article, both active protagonists at the nexus of equity, social justice, emergency and disaster preparedness, and everyday readiness, have collaborated to introduce a focus on health equity and the social determinants of health as applied to an overarching framework of pandemic preparedness. Dr. Wright presents an overview of the intertwined context of societal inequities and health disparities, supported by important definitions, including those that are historically aligned with structural and institutional racism. Dr. Simpson follows with a comprehensive analysis of the three phases of pediatric pandemic preparedness; planning, response and recovery, articulated through an equity lens with an emphasis on critical lessons learned, and with thought leadership from an emerging national infrastructure designed to be specifically attendant to the unique needs of children and families.

CONTEXT
Inequities, Disparities, and Social Determinants of Health

Health Equity is the state in which everyone has a fair and just opportunity to attain their highest level of health. Achieving this requires ongoing societal efforts that; address historical and contemporary injustices; overcome economic, social, and other obstacles to health and health care; and eliminate preventable health disparities. Achieving health equity requires changing the systems and policies that have resulted in the generational injustices that give rise to racial and ethnic health disparities.[1] It is important to clarify the distinction between inequities and disparities, terminology that is often conflated. *Inequities* are characterized by differences that are the result of systemic, preventable, avoidable, and unjust policies and practices that create barriers to the achievement of optimal health status.[1] *Disparities* represent the outcomes that adversely affect groups of people who have systematically experienced greater social or economic obstacles to health based on their racial or ethnic group or other characteristics historically linked to discrimination, exclusion or other inequities.[2] Finally, the *Social Determinants of Health* collectively represent the array of economic, political, and social resources and opportunities that comprise the conditions in which people are born, grow, live, work, play, worship and age, and the wider set of forces and systems shaping the conditions of daily life that strongly influence health.[3]

While the national attention drawn to the impact of the COVID-19 pandemic on children and families has seemingly revealed new and profound disparities, in actuality, deleterious outcomes that disproportionately affect marginalized populations are emblematic of inequities that are broadly manifest and have always been present just below the surface.[4] The longstanding nature of many contemporary inequities is historically rooted in racist practices and policies, such as redlining in which minoritized groups have been subject to environmental injustices due to housing discrimination.[5] Such community-level inequity can be categorically defined as *Structural Racism* in which local, state, and/or national policies, laws, and regulations systematically create differential access to services and opportunities based on race.[6] *Institutional Racism* is more narrowly defined when such bias and discrimination is experienced in business or organizational settings, such as hospitals or schools, in which racially minoritized groups may be unfairly disadvantaged.[6] See **Box 1** for definitions.

These types of pre-existing inequities have been documented to be a major source of vulnerability in past public health emergencies and natural disasters such as

Box 1 Terminology	
Term	Definition
Health Equity	The state in which everyone has a fair and just opportunity to attain their highest level of health. Achieving this requires ongoing societal efforts that; address historical and contemporary injustices; overcome economic, social, and other obstacles to health and health care; and eliminate preventable health disparities. Achieving health equity requires changing the systems and policies that have resulted in the generational injustices that give rise to racial and ethnic health disparities.[1]
Inequities	Differences that are the result of systemic, preventable, avoidable, and unjust policies and practices that create barriers to the achievement of optimal health status.[1]
Disparities	Outcomes that adversely affect groups of people who have systematically experienced greater social or economic obstacles to health based on their racial or ethnic group or other characteristics historically linked to discrimination, exclusion or other inequities.[2]
Social Determinants of Health	Array of economic, political, and social resources and opportunities that comprise the conditions in which people are born, grow, live, work, play, worship and age, and the wider set of forces and systems shaping the conditions of daily life that strongly influence health.[3]
Structural Racism	When local, state, and/or national policies, laws, and regulations systematically create differential access to services and opportunities based on race.[6]
Institutional Racism	When bias and discrimination is experienced in business or organizational settings, such as hospitals or schools, in which racially minoritized groups may be unfairly disadvantaged.[52]
Minoritized	Social groups (eg, race, religion, sex, gender identity, sexual orientation) that are systematically devalued and unfairly disadvantaged in society. This devaluing includes how the group is represented and what resources they have access to. Although these groups have traditionally been referred to as *minorities,* replacing this language with the term *minoritized* better captures the forces that create the lower status in society. Furthermore, since people of color represent the global majority, it helps signal that a group's status is not necessarily related to their proportion of the population.[52]

Hurricane Katrina in 2005, the 2009 H1N1 pandemic, as well as, a factor in the long-term health consequences of children during the influenza pandemic of 1921.[7–9] As the complexity of pandemic preparedness is considered in the context of health equity and social drivers, it is essential that pediatric professionals further overlay the unique physical, mental health, behavioral, and developmental needs foundational to the care of children that must be addressed and met in all aspects of everyday readiness, disaster preparedness, response, and recovery.[10]

A vital component of leveling the playing field for all populations, that is, in the vein of "a rising tide floats all boats," is ensuring that data collection, analysis, and reporting through all phases is uniformly stratified by race, ethnicity, and language. For hospitals and health systems, this competency vis-a-vis quality and safety data is now an expected performance standard under the recent elevation by The Joint Commission of health equity to a National Patient Safety Goal (NPSG).[11,12] As an NPSG, structural and institutional inequities are considered "never events" and must be addressed at the highest levels of organizational leadership for health systems. Further, the Residency Review Committee of the Accreditation Council on Graduate Medical Education and the American Board of Pediatrics has identified training requirements and professional activities relevant to addressing health disparities as certification competencies.[13,14] Such regulatory emphasis, coupled with a commitment to a transparent and granular understanding of differential lived experiences at baseline, is not only essential to the pandemic planning, response, and recovery process, but also charts a public health path to social justice. Predictive community-based modeling tools such as the Social Vulnerability Index and the Child Opportunity Index will only be as useful in preparedness, resource allocation, and mitigation strategy decision-making as the validity and accuracy of the stratified metrics that proactively populate them.[15]

HEALTH EQUITY AND THE COVID-19 PANDEMIC

The COVID-19 pandemic amplified health inequities and placed tremendous strain on our society, economy, education systems, and health care infrastructure. The global lockdown measures to "flatten the curve" of the pandemic including physical distancing and social isolation inevitably created disruptions in routines for children and their families which will have long lasting implications for a child's development and mental health. Further, heightened focus on issues of racism and injustices faced by individuals of color, particularly in the aftermath of the George Floyd murder in May 2020, intensified during the pandemic as media coverage gained the attention of a public that was mostly socially isolated and working from home.[16] The evolving national discourse on racism and inequities across communities, including social injustices faced by minoritized groups, is important to the framing of pandemic planning across all phases of disaster including preparedness, response, and recovery.

According to the American Academy of Pediatrics (AAP) state level data report, children represented 15.6 million or 17.9%, of total cumulated cases of COVID-19 since the pandemic began in March 2020 through May 2023, the period during which publicly reported case numbers for children were consistently available at the state level.[17] COVID-19 has become a leading cause of death for children and young people aged 0 to 19 years in the US since 2021, ranking eighth among all causes of death for that age group.[18] Given that the pandemic had such a profound impact on society, it is difficult to assess the degree to which mitigation strategies prevented poor outcomes specifically for children and adolescents. A helpful framework within which to set a benchmark for disaster planning can be found in pediatric readiness assessments. The National Pediatric Readiness Project (NPRP), led by the Emergency Medical Services for Children (EMSC) program in partnership with the American Academy of Pediatrics (AAP), the American College of Emergency Physicians (ACEP), and the Emergency Nurses Association (ENA) is an assessment of an emergency department's (ED) capability to provide high quality care for children based on the latest guidelines in pediatric emergency practice. High pediatric readiness in EDs is associated with a 76% lower mortality rate in ill children and a 60% lower mortality rate in injured children.[19,20] Further, pediatric readiness is demonstrated to be associated with an elimination of disparity in mortality for Black children with traumatic injuries.[21,22] The guiding principles of pediatric readiness includes ensuring every emergency medical system, fire-rescue agency, and emergency department has pediatric-specific champions, competencies, policies, equipment, and other resources needed to provide high-quality emergency care for children.[23,24] Pandemic and disaster planning, response, and recovery efforts can build on these NPRP measures by identifying key areas of greatest need for health care teams and communities to be prepared to care for ill and injured children.

The pandemic had a significant impact on both inpatient and outpatient health care practices, including a rapid transition to virtual care, new and rapidly evolving clinical guidelines, and deployment of medical countermeasures such as vaccines. Pediatricians are uniquely positioned to mitigate the long-term trajectory of COVID-19 on the health and wellness of pediatric patients. Chokshi and colleagues best summarized the pediatricians' role during the pandemic with the following guidance, "To effectively care for children during COVID-19 pediatricians need to appreciate the stress and potential traumatic effect of the pandemic."[25] Early in the pandemic, reports of the disproportionate impact of COVID-19 on racial and/or ethnic and socioeconomic groups noted up to six-fold differences in the positivity rates of Hispanic children relative to white children.[26] These disparities have been attributed to recognized health inequities that existed before the pandemic.[27] The societal shifts imposed by a pandemic, most notably the emphasis on social isolation, school closures, and the deployment of new and evolving clinical and public health guidelines, increase psychological stress and take an emotional toll on all. Health inequities stem from social factors, including education, employment status, income level, gender, and ethnicity. Although children were relatively spared from the serious consequences of COVID-19 illness relative to older adults, the impact of limited access to care, less frequent developmental and mental health screening, learning loss from missed school days, reduced immunization uptake, and increased food and housing insecurity could have longer term consequences for a child's life. To eliminate health inequities, we would have to overcome the economic, social, and other nonmedical drivers of health, which we refer to as the social determinants of health.

ADDRESSING HEALTH EQUITY AND RECOGNIZING SOCIAL DETERMINANTS OF HEALTH IN PEDIATRIC PANDEMIC PLANNING

Black, indigenous, and people of color (BIPOC) communities experienced the highest rates of infection, hospitalization, and death during the COVID-19 pandemic.[28] The Centers for Disease Control and Prevention reported between February and July 2020, the first 5 months of the pandemic, Hispanic, Black, and American Indian and Alaska Native (AIAN) youth <21 years of age accounted for approximately 75% of deaths due to COVID-19, despite representing 41% of the US population in that age bracket.[29] In a cross-sectional study of COVID-19 deaths in US adults, the initial proportion of non-Hispanic black adults compared with non-Hispanic white adults was three-fold greater in mortality rates. This difference decreased substantially during the course of the pandemic and has been attributed to the geographic shift of the pandemic to nonmetropolitan areas over time.[30] While a similar analysis has not been published for mortality rates in pediatric populations across the span of the pandemic, some extrapolations can be made on the impact of the disparities highlighted in adult studies on children from minoritized populations who may have been more likely to lose a family member to COVID-19. In a multicenter cohort study of the clinical manifestations of COVID-19 illness in the pediatric population, patients with the severe subset of COVID-19 infections, namely MIS-C (Multisystem Inflammatory Syndrome in Children), were mostly non-Hispanic black suggesting a disproportionate burden of the disease on these patients and their families.[31] Ongoing studies are needed to quantify and qualify the impact of the pandemic on children and adolescents particularly with regard to disparities in health outcomes. For example, the early data on a three-fold difference in mortality rates in certain racial and ethnic groups, or the time-line for observations in metropolitan versus non-metropolitan populations for disease spread or vaccination rates is helpful to guide planning at the local, regional, and national levels of pediatric practice.[30] Three key drivers of disparate pediatric health outcomes noted during the COVID-19 pandemic are highlighted for consideration in future pediatric pandemic planning: (1) risk of unemployment and economic disruption, (2) access to mental and behavioral health services, and (3) capability to support telehealth and distance learning. Each of these observations are areas where focused planning and mitigation efforts could aid in closing the gap in health outcomes and facilitate pandemic response and recovery planning.

Unemployment and Economic Disruption

The COVID-19 pandemic has been associated with significant financial hardship and economic disruption to a disproportionate degree for lower-wage workers who identify as other than white, non-Hispanic.[32] Mass layoffs and unemployment further destabilized people who were already struggling to afford basic needs such as housing, food, childcare, and medical care. According to the Bureau of Labor Statistics, the unemployment rate peaked at 14.7% in April 2020; the highest rate in the past decade.[33] Studies conducted during the pandemic found that Black and Hispanic respondents were much less likely to receive unemployment insurance than White respondents despite their identical locations and similar work histories.[32] Current literature also links job loss and unemployment to worse mental health.[34] People of color and those from other marginalized groups are over-represented in jobs that may expose individuals to higher risk of infection, with limited options to work remotely. Most of these at-risk jobs during the pandemic were front-line workers employed in lower-wage positions that are essential to maintaining the operations and infrastructure of communities, such as jobs related to building sanitation, food production, transportation, and municipal services. Fear of lost wages due to unpaid sick leave or inability to quarantine or isolate because of family housing or limited access to health insurance coverage and the ability to pay for medical care creates a crisis of limited options to protect oneself and family members and is therefore a significant driver of health outcomes.[35]

Mental and Behavioral Health

The proportion of pediatric ED visits for mental health concerns increased by 8% compared with general pediatric ED visits, which increased by 1.5% annually according to data from the 2015 to 2020 Pediatric Health Information System, a database reflecting 49 tertiary care US children's hospitals.[36] The reduction in psychiatric care facilities nationwide and the diminished availability of pediatric mental health outpatient services, especially during the early months of the COVID-19 pandemic, made the ED an important access point for acute and critical mental health needs for many children and adolescents.[37] Notably, the American Academy of Pediatrics, American Academy of Child and Adolescent Psychiatry, and Children's Hospital Association declared a National State of Emergency in Children's Mental Health based on the crisis of increasing mental health problems among children and adolescents, which were made worse by the COVID-19 pandemic.[38] Factors such as bias and discrimination based on race, gender, immigration status, and socioeconomic status further complicate adequate and equitable access to mental and behavioral health services.[39] The highest rates of suicidal ideation are in American Indian and Alaskan Native high school students and along with youth in other racial and ethnic minority groups, who have known inequities in mental and behavioral health outcomes.[40]

Pediatricians should be aware of higher-risk populations for mental and behavioral health screening, including LGBTQ + children and adolescents because they are at increased risk for higher anxiety, depression, suicidality, and substance use.[41,42] Mental and behavioral concerns often increase during specific times of crisis, such as after natural disasters, pandemics, or other events affecting population-level stress, and are therefore an important consideration in disaster planning.[43]

Telehealth and Distance Learning

Telehealth emerged early as an important tool to provide clinical care during the COVID-19 pandemic. Variability in the adoption of telehealth services across pediatric and pediatric subspecialty practices may be attributed to the reliance on physical examinations versus history taking for visits; where the telemedicine modality may be more of a challenge than a tool; and limitations in caregiver access to reliable devices and Internet services.[44] The communities most devastated by COVID-19 are often also the same communities with inadequately resourced schools. An expected public health response to a pandemic is to take measures to curb the spread of infection, thus K–12 schools are among the first institutions to close their buildings, changing access to and modalities of the delivery of education for children.[35] These school closures, while necessary to mitigate infection risk, may further contribute to the differential learning loss for children from under-resourced school systems and communities.

Pediatrician's Role in Promoting Child Health During Pandemics

Three specific areas whereby children are likely to feel the burden of the pandemic are: (1) due to economic disruption likely due to changes in their families' socioeconomic status, which may contribute to food and housing insecurity; (2) worsened mental health associated with a lack of access to care services, removal from social support networks, and loss of a caregiver; and (3) a change in their access to education due to school closures, staff shortages or isolation mandates.[4] A variety of resources have been developed since the beginning of the COVID-19 pandemic to help pediatricians support patients and the pediatric workforce from reputable authorities such as the American Academy of Pediatrics and federally funded programs focused on pediatric readiness and pandemic or disaster preparedness to include the Emergency Medical Services for Children program, the Pediatric Disaster Centers of Excellence and the Regional Pediatric Pandemic Network.[45–47]

Millions of children from low-income families did not get vaccinations, screenings, mental health care, and dental services in the early months of the pandemic. Pediatricians can screen for social determinants of health such as food insecurity and housing stability, especially for families who may be disproportionately impacted. Pediatricians can help children and youths with special health care needs and children with behavioral challenges obtain access to needed services. Pediatricians can proactively engage and work with LGBTQ + youths and their families, given the higher rates of anxiety, depression, suicidality, and substance use in this patient population, to educate, counsel, and provide appropriate referrals for resources as needed. Similarly, a proactive strategy to support adolescents in the juvenile justice system who may experience increased isolation, stress, anxiety, and depression; and children in the child welfare system who have unique needs with complex trauma and loss should be a component of system-wide and community-based pandemic preparedness, response, and recovery planning.

Pediatricians can ask parents and caregivers about their own well-being, which could impact the ability to support their child. Pediatricians can use their expertise in providing surveillance, screening, assessment, and guidance around developmentally appropriate behaviors and remind parents their child's behavior may be a way of expressing emotional distress. Pediatricians are valuable leaders in their communities because they have the most experience of any physician when it comes to navigating vaccine communications, addressing patients' concerns, and promoting follow up on booster doses. Incorporating health equity perspectives in planning communications and developing strategies for community engagement is essential. Opportunities to collaborate with and learn from structured networks focused on pandemic or disaster preparedness for children have fortunately increased since the pandemic and can be found in the Emergency Medical Services for Children state programs, the Pediatric Disaster Centers of Excellence, and the Regional Pediatric Pandemic Network.[45–47]

ADDRESSING HEALTH EQUITY AND THE PEDIATRICIAN'S ROLE IN PANDEMIC RESPONSE

There are a number of steps pediatricians can take to support their practice and patients during a pandemic. Safeguarding the medical home to maintain continuity of practice within the community is essential. Measures that support the medical home include participating within networks, collaboratives, and coalitions. Every state has one or more health care coalitions that may serve as a mechanism to rapidly deploy information and resources at the state or local level. Health care coalitions are groups of local health care and responder organizations such as EMS, hospitals, and primary care networks, that work together to improve emergency preparedness at a local and regional level. Pediatricians are seen as a trusted entity for patients and for other health care professionals as experts in the care of pediatric patients. As leaders in the health care coalitions, pediatricians can establish intentional strategies to reach marginalized populations and advocating for diverse communication tools and services, such as mobile health or digital health. Federal funding issued by the Administration for Strategic Planning and Response within the Department of Health and Human Services created three Pediatric Disaster Centers of Excellence that serve as demonstration projects to improve disaster response capabilities for children in the United States. These three centers are: Region V for Kids, Western Regional Alliance for Pediatric Emergency Management (WRAP-EM) and Gulf 7- Pediatric Disaster Network and work closely with the respective health care coalitions in their regions. Resources can be found within these networks specific to understanding pediatric disaster planning frameworks in different regions of the country.[45–47]

Medical countermeasures are also key to pandemic response; most notably vaccines. A key to mitigating the disproportionate impact of pandemics is equilibrating access to vaccines. Vaccination hesitancy and refusal are often shaped by multilevel factors including perceived disease risk and vaccine confidence which can be influenced by religious and political beliefs at the individual level, a lack of effective communication and engagement strategies at the community level, and social inequities, including availability, affordability, and access at the structural level. Additionally, individuals who have experienced bias and discrimination and/or racism from health care systems or governmental agencies may feel increased mistrust toward the same structures that have contributed to their experiences of marginalization and discrimination.

During the COVID-19 pandemic, who conveys information about the risks and benefits of vaccines is as essential as the content of the message itself. Studies have shown that a strong recommendation from a trustworthy source, such as a pediatrician, can heavily influence a parent's motivation to immunize their children.[48] A top-down approach without community engagement could reinforce distrust and fear among marginalized communities. Some opportunities realized during the COVID-19 pandemic include the National Institutes of Health Rapid Acceleration of Diagnostics Underserved Populations (RADx-UP) and the Return to School Initiative that created a consortium of research projects studying COVID-19 testing patterns in communities across the United States, its territories and tribal nations.[49] Lessons learned from this community engaged based research included the use of school settings as a unique context for understanding family and school culture-based concerns for implementing vaccination programs.[50] Coordinating with school systems is a natural fit for pediatricians and could be both a planning and recovery strategy implemented in the aftermath of the COVID-19 pandemic. Children with disabilities, those from lower-income homes, and those from racial and ethnic minority groups are more likely to be hospitalized and have poor outcomes in a pandemic. For many of these same children, a wide range of social, economic, and environmental disadvantages have made it more difficult for them to access COVID-19 vaccines.[51] Pediatricians have been champions for pediatric readiness across health care systems to support everyday readiness in caring for the pediatric patient and can also use the lessons learned in the aftermath of the pandemic to reinforce pediatric disaster planning for these populations.

ADDRESSING SOCIAL DETERMINANTS OF HEALTH IN PEDIATRIC PANDEMIC RECOVERY

Pediatricians who have been at the forefront of anti-vaccine campaigns and other assaults on science and science communication are often experienced with focusing on scientific facts and advocating with a singular mission of doing what is best for children. Engaging parents and caretakers and pediatric patients and being an effective communicator of preventive measures with public health information and anticipatory guidance are routine calls to action for pediatricians. These skills are especially important in combatting the surge of *mis*-information; that is, false information that is spread, regardless of intent to mislead; during the pandemic. An even greater threat may be the increased anti-science propaganda mostly on social media as a form of *dis*-information with an intentional focus on being misleading or biased. Social, cultural, religious, or political influences that influence skepticism in science often exist in communities where inequities in science literacy and/or mis-trust of health systems is prominent. Community engagement and serving as a trusted messenger and committed partner in health is critical in the process of recovery.

Regaining pre-pandemic vaccination schedule compliance, particularly among children, is also of utmost importance in the recovery phase. Global advocacy to accelerate catch up immunizations has been a focus of the World Health Organization recognizing that unvaccinated communities place all children at risk as viruses, such as measles, do not recognize borders. Ongoing support for continuity of care for chronic diseases and preventive services including screening for mental health is also essential. In the aftermath of the COVID-19 pandemic, advocacy for policy changes and health care reform particularly for policies that help close the gap in care for children from under resourced populations is paramount.

An emerging national infrastructure that can serve as a resource for pediatricians and pediatric health networks in all phases of pandemic planning is the Regional Pediatric Pandemic Network (RPPN) – a federally funded program supported by the Health Resources and Services Administration (HRSA) of the US Department of Health and Human Services (HHS) and an example of a resource born out of advocacy during the COVID-19 pandemic. Launched in 2021, the RPPN is a network of ten children's hospitals representing diverse regions across the US with five goals in its charter: (1) increase children's hospitals partnerships with local, state, regional, and national emergency preparedness systems; (2) collaborate with community partners to address disparities and ensure health equity; (3) improve the pediatric emergency readiness of health care systems, including hospital and prehospital systems; (4) increase the capability of telehealth systems to address the unique needs of children and families; and (5) accelerate the real-time dissemination of research-informed pediatric care.[47]

Future planning efforts must also consider the possibility of a pandemic that might have had greater morbidity or mortality in youth, in contrast to the COVID-19 experience, with a more urgent call to develop earlier mitigation strategies and countermeasures focused on children. The call to action is substantial in the aftermath of a pandemic. Many physicians may experience feelings of guilt related to an exaggerated sense of responsibility. These factors play a role in the exhaustion and burnout of clinical teams in the aftermath of a pandemic. While significant investments are needed on a national level to reinforce and reinvigorate the health care workforce, it is worthwhile to note that shared experiences among pediatricians builds community and may be protective against secondary trauma and post-traumatic stress from an event such as the pandemic.

SUMMARY

Important lessons learned from the COVID-19 pandemic include integrating a health equity strategy that is data informed, engages communities, and builds upon everyday readiness needs in caring for the pediatric population in all phases of disaster/pandemic planning. Health equity considerations need to be built into all policies, processes, and systems at the outset. Ultimately, health disparities will persist until structural issues contributing to inequity, including the social determinants of health, are addressed. Understanding communities and drivers of health disparities at the local level is a first step to tackling this issue. Next, building on pediatric readiness frameworks is a recommended approach to creating a pediatric pandemic plan. Importantly, engaging communities and partnering with established networks or coalitions can amplify efforts for more effective outcomes.

CLINICS CARE POINTS

- The unique physical, mental health, behavioral and developmental needs foundational to the care of children must be addressed in all phases of disaster planning.
- Disparities noted during public health emergencies and disasters have been attributed to historic inequities that stem from social drivers of health such as education, employment status, income level, gender and ethnicity.
- Higher pediatric readiness in emergency departments is associated with lower mortality rates in ill and injured children.

DISCLOSURE

The authors have no relevant financial or non-financial interests to disclose.

FUNDING

Dr Simpson serves as a Principal Investigator for the Pediatric Pandemic Network. The Pediatric Pandemic Network is supported in part by the Health Resources and

Services Administration (HRSA) of the U.S. Department of Health and Human Services (HHS) as part of cooperative agreements U1IMC43532 and U1IMC45814 with 0 percent financed with nongovernmental sources.

REFERENCES

1. What is health equity? Centers for Disease Control and Prevention. Available at: https://www.cdc.gov/healthequity/whatis/index.html. [Accessed 18 December 2023].
2. Healthy people 2020 overview of health disparities. HealthyPeople.gov. Available at: http://www.healthypeople.gov/2020/about/disparitiesAbout.aspx. [Accessed 18 December 2023].
3. Social determinants of health. World Health Organization. Available at: https://www.who.int/health-topics/social-determinants-of-health. [Accessed 18 December 2023].
4. National Academies of Sciences, Engineering, and Medicine. Addressing the long-term effects of the COVID-19 pandemic on children and families. 2023. Washington, DC: The National Academies Press; 2023. https://doi.org/10.17226/26809. Available at: . [Accessed 20 December 2023].
5. Lane HM, Morello-Frosch R, Marshall JD, et al. Historical redlining is associated with present-day air pollution disparities in U.S. cities. Environ Sci Technol Lett 2022;9(4):345–50.
6. Wright JL, Johnson TJ. Child health advocacy: the journey to antiracism. Pediatr Clin North Am 2023;70(1):91–101.
7. Zoraster R. Vulnerable populations: Hurricane Katrina as a case study. Prehosp Disast Med 2010;25(1):74–8.
8. Quinn SC, Kumar S, Freimuth VS, et al. Racial disparities in exposure, susceptibility, and access to health care in the US H1N1 influenza pandemic. Am J Public Health 2011;101(2):285–93.
9. Beach B, Clay K, Saavedra M. The 1918 influenza pandemic and its lessons for COVID-19. J Economic Literature 2022;60(1):41–84.
10. Needle S, Wright JL, Fagbuyi DB, et al. AAP Disaster Preparedness Advisory Council; Committee on Pediatric Emergency Medicine. Ensuring the health of children in disasters. Pediatrics 2015;136(5):e1407–17.
11. National Patient Safety Goal to improve health equity. Joint Commission. Available at: https://www.jointcommission.org/-/media/tjc/documents/standards/r3-reports/r3_npsg-16.pdf. [Accessed 19 December 2023].
12. Perlin J, Plough A. Health systems need to transform data collection to advance health equity. Popul Health Manag 2023;26(2):128–31.
13. ACGME Program for Graduate Medical Education Requirements for Pediatrics, 2022. ACGME. Available at: https://www.acgme.org/globalassets/pfassets/reviewandcomment/320_pediatrics_rc_022023.pdf. [Accessed 19 December 2023].
14. Unaka NI, Winn A, Spinks-Franklin A, et al. An entrustable professional activity addressing racism and pediatric health inequities. Pediatrics 2022;149(2). https://doi.org/10.1542/peds.2021-054604. e2021054604.
15. Ramgopal S, Jaeger L, Cercone A, et al. The Child Opportunity Index and pediatric emergency medical services utilization. Prehosp Emerg Care 2022;27:1–8.
16. Dreyer BP, Trent M, Anderson AT, et al. The death of George Floyd: bending the arc of history toward justice for generations of children. Pediatrics 2020;146(3). e2020009639.

17. COVID-19 pandemic. AAP News; 2023. Available at: https://publications.aap.org/aapnews/news/1362/COVID-19. [Accessed 20 December 2023].

18. Flaxman S, Whittaker C, Semenova E, et al. Assessment of COVID-19 as the underlying cause of death among children and young people aged 0 to 19 years in the US. JAMA Netw Open 2023;6(1):e2253590.

19. Ames SG, Davis BS, Marin JR, et al. Emergency department pediatric readiness and mortality in critically ill children. Pediatrics 2019;144(3):e20190568. Erratum in: Pediatrics. 2020 May;145(5).

20. Newgard CD, Lin A, Malveau S, et al, Pediatric Readiness Study Group. Pediatric Readiness Study Group. Emergency department pediatric readiness and short-term and long-term mortality among children receiving emergency care. JAMA Netw Open 2023;6(1):e2250941. Erratum in: JAMA Netw Open. 2023 Feb 1;6(2):e231365.

21. Jenkins PC, Lin A, Ames SG, et al, Pediatric Readiness Study Group. Emergency department pediatric readiness and disparities in mortality based on race and ethnicity. JAMA Netw Open 2023;6(9):e2332160.

22. Gutman CK, Hall JE, Lion KC. Emergency department pediatric readiness and the search for solutions that promote child health equity. JAMA Netw Open 2023;6(9):e2332168.

23. Remick K, Gausche-Hill M, Joseph MM, et al, American Academy of Pediatrics, Committee on Pediatric Emergency Medicine, Section on Surgery, American College of Emergency Physicians, Pediatric Emergency Medicine Committee, Emergency Nurses Association, Pediatric Committee, Pediatric Readiness in the Emergency Department, Policy Statement, Organizational Principles to Guide and Define the Child Health Care System and/or Improve the Health of All Children. American Academy of Pediatrics, Committee on Pediatric Emergency Medicine, Section on Surgery; American College of Emergency Physicians, Pediatric Emergency Medicine Committee; Emergency Nurses Association, Pediatric Committee. Pediatric readiness in the emergency department: organizational principles to guide and define the child health care system and/or improve the health of all children. Ann Emerg Med 2018;72(6):e123–36. Epub 2018 Nov 1.

24. Moore B, Shah MI, Owusu-Ansah S, et al, Committee on Pediatric Emergency Medicine, Section on Emergency Medicine, EMS Subcommittee, Section on Surgery. American Academy of Pediatrics, Committee on Pediatric Emergency Medicine and Section on Emergency Medicine EMS Subcommittee; American College of Emergency Physicians, Emergency Medical Services Committee; Emergency Nurses Association, Pediatric Committee; National Association Of Emergency Medical Services Physicians, Standards and Clinical Practice Committee; National Association of Emergency Medical Technicians, Emergency Pediatric Care Committee. Pediatric readiness in emergency medical services systems. Pediatrics 2020;145(1):e20193308.

25. Chokshi B, Pletcher BA, Strait JS. A trauma-informed approach to the pediatric COVID-19 response. Curr Prob Pediatr Adolesc Health Care 2021;51(2):e100970.

26. Goyal MK, Simpson JN, Boyle MD, et al. Racial and/or ethnic and socioeconomic disparities of SARS-CoV-2 infection among children. Pediatrics 2020;146(4). e2020009951.

27. Sharma SV, Chuang R-J, Rushing M, et al. Social determinants of health-related needs during COVID-19 among low-income households with children. Prevent Chronic Dis 2020;17:E119.

28. Andraska EA, Alabi O, Dorsey C, et al. Health care disparities during the COVID-19 pandemic. Semin Vasc Surg 2021;34(3):82–8.

29. Bixler D, Miller AD, Mattison CP, et al, Pediatric Mortality Investigation Team. Pediatric Mortality Investigation Team. SARS-CoV-2-associated deaths among persons aged <21 years - United States, February 12-July 31, 2020. MMWR Morb Mortal Wkly Rep 2020;69(37):1324–9. Available at: https://www.cdc.gov/mmwr/volumes/69/wr/mm6937e4.htm?utm_source=mp-fotoscapes. [Accessed 20 December 2023].

30. Lundberg DJ, Wrigley-Field E, Cho A, et al. COVID-19 mortality by race and ethnicity in US metropolitan and nonmetropolitan areas, March 2020 to February 2022. JAMA Netw Open 2023;6(5):e2311098.

31. Fernandes DM, Oliveira CR, Guerguis S, et al, Tri-State Pediatric COVID-19 Research Consortium. Tri-State Pediatric COVID-19 Research Consortium. Severe acute respiratory syndrome coronavirus 2 clinical syndromes and predictors of disease severity in hospitalized children and youth. J Pediatr 2021;230:23–31.e10.

32. Ananat EO, Daniels B, Fitz-Henley Ii J 2nd, et al. Racial and ethnic disparities in pandemic-era unemployment insurance access: implications for health and well-being. Health Aff 2022;41(11):1598–606.

33. Labor force statistics from the current population survey. United States Bureau of Labor Statistics. Available at: https://www.bls.gov/cps/. [Accessed 1 December 2023].

34. Gassman-Pines A, Ananat EO, Fitz-Henley J. COVID-19 and parent-child psychological well-being. Pediatrics 2020;146(4). e2020007294.

35. National Academies of Sciences, Engineering, and Medicine; Division of Behavioral and Social Sciences and Education; Board on Children, Youth, and Families; Board on Science Education; Standing Committee on Emerging Infectious Diseases and 21st Century Health Threats; Committee on Guidance for K-12 Education on Responding to COVID-19. Reopening K-12 schools during the COVID-19 pandemic: prioritizing health, equity, and communities. National Academies Press (US); 2020. Available at: http://www.ncbi.nlm.nih.gov/books/NBK564017/. [Accessed 20 December 2023].

36. Cushing AM, Liberman DB, Pham PK, et al. Mental health revisits at US pediatric emergency departments. JAMA Pediatr 2023;177(2):168–76.

37. Cree RA, So M, Franks J, et al. Characteristics associated with presence of pediatric mental health care policies in emergency departments. Pediatr Emerg Care 2021;37(12):e1116–21.

38. American Academy of Pediatrics. AAP, AACAP, CHA declare national emergency in children's mental health. 2021. Available at: https://www.aap.org/en/advocacy/child-and-adolescent-healthy-mental-development/aap-aacap-cha-declaration-of-a-national-emergency-in-child-and-adolescent-mental-health/. [Accessed 18 December 2023].

39. Trent M, Dooley DG, Dougé J, American Academy of Pediatrics Section on Adolescent Health, Council on Community Pediatrics, & Committee on Adolescence. The impact of racism on child and adolescent health. Pediatrics 2019;144(2):e20191765.

40. Saidinejad M, Duffy S, Wallin D, et al, American Academy of Pediatrics Committee on Pediatric Emergency Medicine, American College of Emergency Physicians Pediatric Emergency Medicine Committee, Emergency Nurses Association Pediatric Committee. American Academy of Pediatrics, Committee on Pediatric Emergency Medicine and Section on Emergency Medicine EMS

Subcommittee; American College of Emergency Physicians, Emergency Medical Services Committee; Emergency Nurses Association, Pediatric Committee. The management of children and youth with pediatric mental and behavioral health emergencies. Pediatrics 2023;152(3). https://doi.org/10.1542/peds.2023-063255. e2023063255.

41. Ferlatte O, Salway T, Rice S, et al. Perceived barriers to mental health services among canadian sexual and gender minorities with depression and at risk of suicide. Commun Mental Health J 2019;55(8):1313–21.

42. Hottes TS, Bogaert L, Rhodes AE, et al. Lifetime prevalence of suicide attempts among sexual minority adults by study sampling strategies: a systematic review and meta-analysis. Am J Publ Health 2016;106(5):e1–12.

43. Banerjee D, Kosagisharaf JR, Sathyanarayana Rao TS. The dual pandemic" of suicide and COVID-19: a biopsychosocial narrative of risks and prevention. Psychiatr Res 2021;295:113577.

44. Uscher-Pines L, McCullough C, Dworsky MS, et al. Use of telehealth across pediatric subspecialties before and during the COVID-19 pandemic. JAMA Netw Open 2022;5(3):e224759.

45. Emergency Medical Services for Children (EMSC). Health Resources and Services Administration. Available at: https://mchb.hrsa.gov/programs-impact/emergency-medical-services-children-emsc. [Accessed 1 December 2023].

46. Pediatric Disaster Care Centers of Excellence. Administration for Strategic Preparedness and Response. Available at: https://aspr.hhs.gov/NDMS/Pages/PDCCOE.aspx. [Accessed 1 December 2023].

47. Regional Pediatric Pandemic Network. Health Resources and Services Administration. Available at: https://mchb.hrsa.gov/programs-impact/pediatric-pandemic. [Accessed 1 December 2023].

48. Ignacio M, Oesterle S, Mercado M, et al. Narratives from African American/Black, American Indian/Alaska Native, and Hispanic/Latinx community members in Arizona to enhance COVID-19 vaccine and vaccination uptake. J Behav Med 2023; 46(1–2):140–52.

49. National Institutes of Health. Rapid Acceleration of Diagnostics Underserved Populations. Available at: https://radx-up.org/. [Accessed 2 January 2024].

50. Pulgaron ER, D'Agostino EM, Johnson SB, et al. Reflections from school communities in underserved populations on childhood COVID-19 vaccination. Pediatrics 2023;152(Supp 1). e2022060352M.

51. Oliveira CR, Feemster KA, Ulloa ER. Pediatric COVID-19 health disparities and vaccine equity. J Pediatr Infect Dis 2022;11(Supp_4):S141–7.

52. Sensoy O, DiAngelo R, Banks JA. Is everyone really equal?: an introduction to key concepts in social justice education. 1st edition. New York, NY: Teacher's College Press; 2012. p. 5.

Vaccine Development

Elizabeth A.D. Hammershaimb, MD, MS[a,b,*],
James D. Campbell, MD, MS[a,b]

KEYWORDS

- Pediatric vaccines • Smallpox • Influenza • Anthrax • Ebola • COVID-19 • Mpox
- Emerging infections

KEY POINTS

- This article considers ethical considerations surrounding pediatric vaccine development for pandemic preparedness.
- It examines some historical cases of pediatric vaccines developed during past smallpox, influenza, and 2019 coronavirus disease pandemics.
- It discusses the current state of vaccine development for pandemic preparedness, including vaccines against smallpox/mpox, influenza, anthrax, and Ebola that are included in the US Strategic National Stockpile and vaccines being developed against priority pathogens identified by the World Health Organization.

INTRODUCTION

Decade after decade, ever since their advent, vaccines have been touted as one of the greatest public health achievements. Alongside sanitation and antibiotics, vaccines are a tool for the mitigation—and, in some cases, eradication—of morbidity and/or mortality due to infectious diseases. As such, vaccines have been an essential pillar of mankind's strategic response to infectious diseases.

Whether intentional or unintentional, outbreaks and pandemics pose a particular threat to biosecurity. The need for vaccines against biothreats is well established, but there are special considerations around the development of vaccines against biothreat agents for use in pediatric populations. This review discusses some of the theoretic arguments surrounding pediatric vaccine development in the setting of a pandemic versus biothreat preparedness, historical examples of pediatric vaccine development to combat pandemics, the state of vaccine development for pandemic (and on a smaller scale, biothreat) preparedness, and conclusions.

---

[a] Center for Vaccine Development and Global Health, University of Maryland School of Medicine, 685 West Baltimore Street, Room 480, Baltimore, MD 21201, USA; [b] Department of Pediatrics, University of Maryland School of Medicine, Baltimore, MD, USA
* Corresponding author.
E-mail address: ehammershaimb@som.umaryland.edu

Pediatr Clin N Am 71 (2024) 529–549
https://doi.org/10.1016/j.pcl.2024.01.018
0031-3955/24/© 2024 Elsevier Inc. All rights reserved.

ETHICAL CONSIDERATIONS
Introduction

Preparation and response to pandemics and biothreats that may affect children highlight a spectrum of ethical issues for consideration. Vaccines can provide protection from pandemic pathogens and are optimally administered to susceptible persons before exposure. As pandemics may erupt and spread quickly and are, by their nature, not completely predictable, ethical concerns and themes may be more prominent in considerations of vaccines against pandemic pathogens than with vaccines directed against nonpandemic pathogens. These topics include the following: (1) when is it acceptable or preferable to test experimental vaccines against pandemic pathogens in the pediatric population? and (2) what constitutes just and equitable distribution of vaccines and related products, particularly when products are scarce and how do children fit into prioritization schemes for allocation? Although many other ethical themes may also be important to consider, the authors highlight these concerns.

Timing of Clinical Trials of Pediatric Vaccines Directed Against Pathogens Causing Pandemics or of Pandemic Potential

Children, in large part due to their inability to provide fully informed consent and inability to fully comprehend discussions related to participation in research, are considered vulnerable. Vulnerable persons who participate in medical research, including clinical trials of experimental vaccines, are given special protections to minimize the harm that may occur if such additional protections were not in place. When considering the testing of vaccines to combat pathogens that are causing or are deemed likely to cause a pandemic, in children, these vulnerable population protections remain important. Parents or legal guardians of children must play an integral role in deciding whether to give permission for their child to participate in a study of a vaccine or other proposed biomedical countermeasure.

When considering whether to provide permission for their child to participate in a study of a vaccine against a pandemic pathogen and whether participation is in the best interest of their child, certain pieces of information will be important for a parent/legal guardian. For a potential pandemic pathogen, how likely is it to emerge and spread? If it causes a pandemic, how contagious is it expected to be, and are there alternate means of protection? Is there reason to believe that children will have differential risk of becoming infected or, among those persons infected, differential risk of severe morbidity or mortality? Will children likely drive transmission? Has the vaccine been tested in adults yet, and what is known about adverse effects and beneficial outcomes, such as immune responses that predict protection or actual protection from illness? If the exact vaccine formulation proposed in the study has not been tested previously, what is known about similar vaccines, for example, ones made by the same manufacturing platform, or using the same vector or technology?

When considering initiating clinical studies of vaccines against pandemic pathogens, in distinction to vaccines against nonpandemic pathogens, there is a heightened emphasis on the balance between speed and increasingly complete knowledge to inform study design and individual decisions to enroll. For endemic diseases, the scales tend to tip toward gathering greater information before deciding to execute studies in children. Often, for nonpandemic infections, many years pass, and many trials are completed in adults, before children are included. This approach seems the prudent one when developing vaccines for some nonpandemic pathogens, but for pandemic pathogens, particularly those with high infectivity or high severity in children, if the public waits until a vast amount of adult data are available, large numbers of children may already have been infected and suffered the consequences of those infections before ever testing the vaccine in their age group.

Deciding when it is acceptable to begin trials in children is a discussion that should be undertaken before a pandemic begins. Persons with expertise in vaccinology, pediatrics, ethics, pandemics, and other fields should provide parameters for acceptable initiation. These parameters are not likely the same for each pathogen, but determining which characteristics of pandemic pathogens are key to defining "tripwires" to move from adult studies to children and from older to younger child age brackets is a crucial step toward rational and ethical study timing. Regulatory bodies and public health authorities should consider these contingencies beforehand and provide written guidance on how to apply them.

Consider the following scenario: experts predict that a particular pathogen is likely to cause a pandemic soon, and children and adults are anticipated to suffer equally. A vaccine against this pathogen, one that uses a technology already used for other licensed vaccines, has undergone early phase testing in adults and been found to be safe in small numbers of volunteers, and to lead to immune responses predicted to provide protection. A putative optimal adult dose and regimen have been determined by balancing reactogenicity (local and systemic vaccine-related adverse events) and immune responses. Should such a vaccine now be tested in children? If not, what is the bar that needs to be passed to allow for pediatric trials?

Institutional review boards (IRBs), in the United States, when reviewing a human subject research trial that involves children, must determine whether the study is (1) no greater than minimal risk; (2) greater than minimal risk but with the prospect of individual direct benefit; (3) a minor increase over minimal risk but without the prospect of individual direct benefit; or (4) more than a minor increase over minimal risk and without the prospect of individual direct benefit.[1,2] In the above scenario, as the pathogen has not yet led to a pandemic, but is only predicted to do so, is it acceptable for individual IRBs to determine that a study of the vaccine in children is greater than minimal risk with the prospect of direct benefit or a minor increase over minimal risk but with no prospect of direct benefit? To meet the former risk category level, the IRB would be stating that the unknown risk of adverse effects of the vaccine, and any other risk inherent to participation, is of greater probability and magnitude than encountered in daily life (greater than minimal risk), but that potential protection from a future pandemic, one that is predicted, but not actually yet happening, constitutes the prospect of direct benefit for the participating child. To meet the latter risk category, the IRB would be stating that, as the vaccine has been studied in a small number of adults and similar vaccines are already licensed and in use, the anticipated risks are only a minor increase over minimal, meaning that they are, perhaps, not dissimilar to the risks of getting one of the licensed vaccines that uses the same platform. In addition, for the latter determination, the IRB would be stating that there is no prospect of individual benefit because there is no current circulation of the pathogen predicted to cause the pandemic. These decisions are weighty and difficult.

It is not unreasonable to expect that different IRBs, drug authorities, manufacturers, and investigators would have different approaches to interpreting these risk categories when applied to vaccines directed against pandemic pathogens and potential pandemic pathogens and when applied with different amounts of knowledge about both the pandemic disease and the vaccine risks and benefits. Additional guidance and considerations for these contingencies would help as we prepare for future pandemics and in response to emerging pandemics.

During the recent 2019 coronavirus disease (COVID-19) pandemic, a team of ethicists, led by members of the Department of Bioethics at the National Institutes of

Health (NIH), reviewed the ethical ramifications of the timing of pediatric studies, vis-à-vis data available from trials enrolling adults, when evaluating vaccines against COVID-19.[3] They stated that "Waiting too long to enroll minors could unjustly deny minors and their families the benefits of a vaccine and has the potential to delay an effective response to the pandemic by a year or longer. At the same time, enrolling minors too soon runs the risk of exposing them to excessive risks." They suggest a set of guidelines on when to enroll children in COVID-19 vaccine trials. These guidelines, or principles, could be extrapolated to other vaccines directed against pandemic pathogens. They describe the advantages and disadvantages of enrolling children with "standard" (nonpandemic) timing (waiting to start pediatric trials until there is considerable safety and efficacy known in adults), "earlier" timing (when safety but not efficacy is established in adults), and "earliest" (when neither safety nor efficacy is established). Pathways and rationale for IRB-allowable approval under existing federal regulations are provided. Importantly, they highlight community engagement and partnerships. Careful review of these tenets, before the next pandemic, with more specific, operational guidance and assistance to industry, academia, and regulators, would facilitate our choice of appropriate pediatric vaccine trial timing and structure and avoid forcing those discussions to be had exclusively during the pandemic. It would also be beneficial if guidance on the rapidity of age de-escalation in pediatric vaccine trials for pandemic pathogens was proposed and available before the next pandemic and then improved or updated with each new pandemic experience.

The Pediatric Research Equity Act of 2003 requires that manufacturers who are requesting permission to market and distribute pharmaceuticals, including vaccines, must "assess the safety and effectiveness of the drug or the biological product for the claimed indications in all relevant pediatric subpopulations" with few exceptions.[4] There is, however, no specified timeframe by which these assessments must be accomplished. This Act and other initiatives have led to more and more studies of products in children and better understanding of age-related doses, regimens, and side effects. It would be beneficial to children if additional guidance with relation to this Act were published and adherence to such guidance could help to protect children from pandemic pathogens.

Allocation of Vaccines When Scarce and Including Children When Prioritization Is Necessary

Emanuel and colleagues remind us that many of the challenges encountered during pandemics involve not only technical and logistical issues but also value-laden issues.[5] These concerns include enforcing requirements, allocation of scarce resources, and others. The investigators make explicit the decision nodes that keenly involve values, including equity in access to protection, choice of approaches to policies, making decisions in the absence of strong data, and choosing between conflicting objectives. They posit 5 values that are fundamental to making decisions on allocating scarce resources, such as vaccine for distribution early in a pandemic: (1) maximizing benefit and minimizing harm; (2) mitigating disadvantage; (3) reciprocity for those who have faced a disproportionate burden; (4) instrumental value (prioritizing those whose protection will benefit others); and (5) treating all persons as moral equals. Others have also provided guidance on principles guiding allocation of scarce resources during pandemics.[6] Although such principles do not forge policy, they can be used as guiding values for blueprints that can be used for pandemic preparedness. A practical implementable framework that takes advantage of these thoughtful reviews on the undergirding of ethical policies will benefit all. Children may not have a strong voice at the time of a pandemic; how they will be valued and afforded protection should be established before any pandemic arises.

HISTORICAL CASES

The history of vaccine development in the setting of pandemics illustrates the delicate balance that must be struck between exposing children to greater risk from the disease at hand versus from a potential countermeasure.

Smallpox

Variolation was the practice of immunizing patients against smallpox (variola major) by inoculating them with material from the pustules of patients with a milder form of the infection (variola minor). A practice that had long been in place in Asia and subsequently Africa and the Middle East, variolation was introduced into the United Kingdom and the American colonies in 1721. The procedure ran the risk not only of precipitating fatal illness in the patient but also of spreading from the patient to others.[7] Another form of immunization was desperately needed.

In 1796, Edward Jenner tested a theory that exposure to cowpox could protect against smallpox. In his very first experiment, he inoculated his gardener's 8 year old child, James Phipps, with fluid from human cowpox lesions collected from the hands of milkmaid Sarah Nelmes. Jenner later intentionally repeatedly exposed Phipps to variola virus, but Phipps never developed smallpox.[8] Although Jenner was not the first to attempt this (English cattle-breeder Benjamin Jesty inoculated his family with cowpox in 1774),[9] he was the first to publicize his work and gain the attention of the medical community. Jenner sought to conduct larger studies, but he could not find volunteers; after the publication of his work *Variolae Vaccinae* in 1798, vaccination took off across Europe, and by 1802, it had reached Massachusetts—without systematic studies demonstrating safety or efficacy in children or adults.[10]

Over time, smallpox vaccination was achieved using different orthopoxviruses, including cowpox, horsepox, and ultimately, vaccinia. Vaccinia became the standard that was used in vaccine manufacturing, with different countries producing vaccines from different vaccinia strains. In 1931, the US Food and Drug Administration (FDA) licensed Dryvax, a vaccine that was derived from the New York City Board of Health strain of vaccinia. Dryvax was subsequently used in the global eradication campaign but is no longer manufactured.[11,12] Dryvax was not without adverse effects; the most common adverse effects were those that are seen after administration of other types of vaccines—injection site pain or swelling, fever, fatigue, lymphadenopathy, myalgias, arthralgias, itching, and abdominal pain or nausea. However, there are also some serious rare side effects not associated with other vaccines, including eczema vaccinatum, progressive vaccinia, contact vaccinia, encephalitis, and myopericarditis.[13] Some of these adverse effects were so severe as to warrant administration of vaccinia immune globulin to treat the reactions. Studies in the 1950s to 1960s found that there were higher rates of postvaccination complications in children less than 1 year of age, and in 1968, the American Academy of Pediatrics recommended that primary vaccination of children against smallpox should be deferred until after the first birthday.[14] Routine childhood immunization against smallpox in the United States ultimately ended in 1972, decades after the last outbreak in the United States.[10] Smallpox was declared eradicated by the World Health Organization (WHO) in 1980, but recommendations for vaccinating laboratory and health care personnel at an increased risk of occupational exposure to smallpox and other orthopoxviruses have remained in place.

Influenza

Pandemics of influenza are caused by viral strains that have not previously been commonly circulating in current human populations. Over the past one and a quarter centuries, there have been 4 influenza pandemics of varying scope and severity.[15] Strains of influenza that may lead to future pandemics are tracked by the United States and worldwide surveillance of both human and animal strains, particularly, but not exclusively, strains isolated from pigs and birds.

Influenza virus was first isolated in 1933, and by the 1940s, vaccines were available, but their use in the United States was largely limited to military personnel until the 1960s after the 1957 to 1958 influenza pandemic changed public health strategies.[16] In contrast to the 1918 influenza pandemic, a larger proportion of excess deaths during the 1957 pandemic were among persons greater than 65 years of age with more than 60% of excess deaths occurring in the older age group.[17] After 1960, routine seasonal vaccination against influenza included the elderly and those with high-risk medical conditions in addition to the military.[18] In 1968, however, a new strain of influenza, H3N2 (Hong Kong) brought about another pandemic.[15] Multiple small studies tested the 1968 H3N2 influenza vaccine in children, some as young as less than 2 years of age, concurrently with its administration to adults.[19-24] It was not until the 1970s that large, controlled clinical trials of influenza vaccines were conducted in children.[25] It was another quarter-century before the Centers for Disease Control and Prevention (CDC) Advisory Committee on Immunization Practices (ACIP) recommended that in 2004, seasonal influenza vaccination in children ages 6 to 23 months due to their high risk of morbidity and mortality, and in 2008, that recommendation was expanded to all children ages 6 months and older.[26,27]

In March 2009, a new H1N1 influenza strain caused severe outbreaks in Mexico and the United States that evolved into a global pandemic by June 2009.[28,29] The spread of the novel H1N1 around the Northern Hemisphere set off a race to develop both monovalent and, eventually, polyvalent vaccines against the newly emerged strain. Large-scale multicenter clinical trials included both adults and children.[30,31] By September 2009, 4 new monovalent vaccines against H1N1 2009 received FDA approval and ACIP recommendation for use; of the 4, 3 had pediatric indications with one product having been approved for use in children as young as 6 months.[32,33]

COVID-19

Shortly after SARS-CoV-2 was identified in China in 2019, the global scientific community raced to create, manufacture, and test a vaccine against SARS-CoV-2. At the time, COVID-19 (the disease caused by SARS-CoV-2) was ripping through the elderly population such that the emphasis was on protecting the elderly and middle-aged adults with comorbidities, but it was also causing excess mortality among people of all ages without comorbidities. Vaccines against COVID-19 were developed, manufactured, tested, authorized, and made available for US adults 338 days from the original release of the viral genetic sequence.[34]

Because early reports of the epidemiology of the disease indicated that morbidity and mortality were greatest in older adults and in adults with underlying medical problems, emphasis was placed on testing, authorizing, and deploying vaccines for adults. Early on, there was considerable focus on comparing symptomatic illness rates, hospitalization rates, and deaths between older persons and children, and because the hospitalization and case fatality rates were lower in children than in adults, there was less concern about studying and deploying medical countermeasures, including vaccines, in children.

As time passed, the focus for evaluating severity for children began to shift from comparisons with adults to comparisons with other childhood infections and other causes of pediatric illness, hospitalization, and death. Although death rates in US children attributable to COVID-19 were considerably lower than in older adults and adults with underlying chronic medical conditions, deaths due to COVID-19 and multisystem inflammatory syndrome in children (MIS-C), a postinfectious inflammatory syndrome triggered by SARS-CoV-2, exceeded the prevaccine death rates for almost all vaccine-preventable infectious diseases before the introduction of their respective vaccines.[35,36] In fact, during the time period from August 1, 2021 to July 31, 2022, COVID-19 was the eighth leading cause of death in US children; the fifth leading cause when unintentional injuries, assault, and suicide were excluded; and the most common cause of death in which the etiology was infectious or due to a respiratory disease.[37]

Although there was some groundswell to initiate pediatric COVID-19 vaccines earlier in the pandemic following more preliminary adult vaccine trial data, the general sentiment was that the disease was too mild and the data on the leading vaccine candidates (namely mRNA vaccines) were too sparse to initiate pediatric trials before large numbers of adults were vaccinated and definitive safety and efficacy were established.[3,36] As we prepare for future pandemics and consider medical countermeasures, including vaccines, it will be important to consider what was learned from recent pandemics, particularly with regard to consideration of children.

THE STOCKPILE

In 1998, the US Government established the National Pharmaceutical Stockpile, collecting antibiotics and vaccines to respond to biothreats. In the aftermath of the 2001 anthrax attacks, as other biomedical supplies (such as ventilators and N95 respirators) were amassed, it was renamed as the Strategic National Stockpile (SNS) in 2003. The SNS has been deployed in response to national emergencies such as the 9/11 attacks and Hurricane Katrina, but from the beginning, it has had a major focus on preparation for pandemic influenza.[38,39] As discussed earlier, pandemic H1N1 swine influenza swept the globe in 2009, and the race to develop an updated influenza vaccine was supported, in large part, by the US Government.

Today, the SNS contains few vaccines relative to the other medical countermeasures and medical equipment that are housed therein. Aside from influenza vaccines, which are updated annually based on globally circulating strains of influenza, the only publicly known vaccines that are stocked in the SNS include vaccines against anthrax, Ebola virus, and smallpox/mpox.[38–40] Most vaccines in the SNS have not been rigorously studied in pediatric populations, and the dosage of each that confers the greatest protection balanced against the least risk has not been established in pediatric populations, except for the Ebola virus vaccines.[41,42]

Influenza

Preparedness for influenza epidemics occurs every year. In the United States, in addition to other resources, we have the Pandemic Vaccines and Adjuvants Program in the Influenza and Emerging Infectious Diseases section of the Biomedical Advanced Research and Development Authority (BARDA). This program is tasked with accelerating pandemic response times and managing and implementing strategic use of the US National Pre-Pandemic Influenza Vaccine Stockpile. They manage production, assure vaccine implementation response, purchase vaccines against influenza viruses and strains with pandemic potential, and provide supports to improve influenza vaccines.[43]

Our current platforms for influenza vaccines in the United States include inactivated viruses that have been grown in embryonated chicken eggs or in cell culture, recombinant influenza antigens expressed in another organism, and live attenuated (cold-adapted) influenza viruses administered by spray into the nares. Potentially promising new technologies include other means to attenuate live influenza viruses, such as removal of an essential gene; mRNA products, packaged in lipid nanoparticles that express key influenza antigens; and numerous avenues of research that are exploring more broadly protective influenza vaccines or even universally protective vaccines.[44–46] These approaches include multivalent vaccines and vaccines that use antigens that are more conserved across influenza strains, such as the hemagglutinin stalk/stem. The US Government has established a consortium, the Collaborative Influenza Vaccine Innovation Centers, to advance influenza vaccine science. It is a network of research centers that evaluate improvements in immune responses in seasonal influenza vaccines, develop and test innovative influenza vaccine platforms, and perform preclinical animal studies, early phase clinical trials, and healthy volunteer human challenge studies.[47]

Anthrax

Although the pandemic potential of *Bacillus anthracis*, the causative agent of anthrax, is limited by the lack of person-to-person spread, sporadic outbreaks occur, and a large epidemic in Zimbabwe in 1978 to 1980 resulted in more than 17,000 human cases and more than 200 human deaths.[48] *B anthracis* is ubiquitous in the environment, affecting livestock and cattle worldwide, making it easy to obtain, and when aerosolized spores are inhaled, highly lethal.[49]

The first anthrax vaccine was developed by Louis Pasteur in 1881 and had only veterinary applications. Anthrax was used as a bioweapon against livestock in World War I and was tested as a bioweapon against humans during World War II.[49] Anthrax vaccines for human use were developed by the Soviet Union beginning in the 1930s, by the United Kingdom in the 1950s, and by the United States in the 1960s with the first US anthrax vaccine, Anthrax Vaccine Adsorbed (AVA or BioThrax), being licensed by the FDA in the early 1970s.[50,51] Despite AVA having been licensed for more than 50 years, it has never been studied in children or adolescents less than 18 years of age.

Soviet efforts to weaponize anthrax resulted in an accidental release of *B anthracis* spores in the city of Sverdlovsk in 1979, killing more than 60 civilians.[49] A failed attempt to deploy anthrax by the Japanese cult Aum Shinrikyo in 1993 further heightened concerns about the potential for an anthrax attack on the United States.[52] In 1998, the Department of Defense instituted the Anthrax Vaccine Immunization Program in which military and select civilian personnel were mandated to receive AVA for pre-exposure prophylaxis (PrEP).[50] Between 1998 and 2008, about 2 million adults received AVA through the program, which was temporarily halted at various times due to complaints about side effects, objection to the mandate, and arguments about the risk–benefit ratio for service members who were not deployed to combat zones.[53]

As early as October 2000, AVA was recommended by the ACIP for postexposure prophylaxis (PEP) vaccination (PEP-Vx) in combination with antibiotics after exposure to aerosolized *B anthracis* spores.[54,55] A different dosing regimen for AVA as PrEP was approved in 2008 that changed the regimen from 6 subcutaneous doses to 5 intramuscular doses.[56] Since then, another 2 million military service members have received AVA PrEP, some of whom were pregnant women who were inadvertently vaccinated. In 2010, the ACIP recommended that AVA could be used in children and pregnant women for PEP-Vx following exposure to aerosolized *B anthracis* spores, and a 2012 ACIP review of pregnancy outcomes after vaccination with AVA found no concerning safety patterns in either the infants or their mothers.[57,58] Despite a 2011 report by the National Biodefense Science Board urging pediatric anthrax vaccine trials, a 2013 bioethics commission ruled that age de-escalation studies could only be conducted if certain conditions were met and if data in young adults ages 18 to 20 years demonstrated safety in that age group.[53,59] In 2015, the FDA formally expanded BioThrax's licensure to include a 3 dose regimen over 28 days for PEP-Vx in nonpregnant adults.[60] A 2019 ACIP review of data surrounding AVA found no significant safety concerns in either nonpregnant or pregnant recipients of the vaccine, including recipients ages 18 to 20 years, and affirmed ACIPs recommendation that AVA could be used as PEP in children and pregnant women under emergency use regulatory provisions.[61]

A newer formulation, AV7909 (Cyfendus), which contains the original AVA plus a CpG-oligonucleotide adjuvant, CpG7909, was licensed by the FDA in July 2023 and is expected to replace AVA in the SNS given its ability to produce a protective immune response after only 2 doses given 14 days apart.[62] To date, despite a great amount of clinical data collected on vaccines and monoclonal antibodies against anthrax in adults, no trials have been conducted in children, and as such, there are no data on the safety, immunogenicity, or optimal dosing or route of administration of either AVA or CpG7909 in humans less than 18 years of age.

Ebola

In contrast to anthrax, *Ebolaviruses* do spread from person to person after an initial spillover event from an infected animal to a susceptible human and, after infection, may persist in immunologically privileged sites within the body. Person-to-person spread is via bodily fluids (including not only blood, urine, vomitus, and feces but also saliva, sweat, semen, breast milk, and amniotic fluid) or contact with items contaminated with infected bodily fluids.[63]

Ebola first emerged in 1976 in 2 concurrent outbreaks, one in Zaïre (now the Democratic Republic of the Congo) and one in Sudan (now South Sudan). Six species of *Ebolavirus* have been identified, four of which cause human disease: Zaïre, Sudan, Taï Forest, and Bundibugyo. Case fatality rates vary by outbreak but have ranged from 25% to 90% depending on the circumstances of the outbreak and of the response that followed. *Zaïre ebolavirus,* commonly referred to as Ebola virus, is the deadliest of the species and has the highest mortality rates in young children.[63]

The degree to which Ebola poses a threat to the North American public is a controversial topic. Almost all infections occur in the context of local epidemics in sub-Saharan Africa, though some cases of forward transmission by infected travelers have been reported. Rather than a naturally occurring Ebola pandemic, concerns about Ebola as a biothreat center on attempts to weaponize the virus by foreign states and nefarious entities. In the 1980s and into the early 1990s, the Soviet Union had a bioweapon program that sought to weaponize Ebola by inserting *Ebolavirus* genes into vaccinia and smallpox—a so-called "Ebolapox." In the mid-1990s, the Japanese cult Aum Shinrikyo, whose attempted anthrax attack mentioned above failed, was believed to also be attempting to weaponize Ebola, though it is unclear whether they possessed *Ebolavirus* cultures. In 2008, an al-Qaeda operative was arrested in Afghanistan in possession of plans for the weaponization of Ebola using dirty bombs.[64] Around the same time, there were also concerns that suicide terrorists might infect themselves with Ebola and move through the population infecting unwitting members of the public.

In 2014 to 2016, a large Ebola epidemic tore through West Africa killing more than 11,000 people in Liberia, Sierra Leone, and Guinea. In response to the outbreak and with fears of weaponized Ebola looming in the background, the US Government invested in programs to detect, treat, and prevent Ebola. Multiple vaccines for the prevention of Ebola were studied during this time, including the live attenuated recombinant vesicular stomatitis virus vectored *Zaïre ebolavirus* virus glycoprotein vaccine (rVSV-ZEBOV, or ERVEBO), which began as a project of the Public Health Agency of Canada's National Microbiology Laboratory and received funding from BARDA, was first approved by the FDA in 2019 for use in adults $\geq$18 years of age.[65] A pediatric study had been planned as part of the initial biologics licensure application (BLA) but was deferred in order to expedite rollout of the vaccine to adults. A supplemental BLA was later approved in 2023 that extended the use of ERVEBO down to age 12 months.[66] The vaccine is given as a single intramuscular (IM) dose; it is unclear at this time at what cadence boosters will be required to prevent Ebola virus infection.

In addition to ERVEBO, the WHO has prequalified another Ebola vaccine regimen that has been licensed by the European Medical Agency. This regimen consists of 2 heterologous doses of vaccines: Zabdeno (Ad26.ZEBOV, a monovalent recombinant, replication-incompetent human adenovirus type 26 vectored Ebola virus glycoprotein vaccine) followed by Mvabea (MVA-BN-Filo, a polyvalent filovirus vaccine using a modified vaccinia Ankara-Bavarian Nordic vector) separated by 8 weeks. Additional boosters are recommended if 4 months have passed since the second dose and there is a risk of exposure. The Zabdeno + Mvabea regimen is licensed for use down to 1 year of age and was found to be safe, well tolerated, and immunogenic in a phase 2 clinical trial in infants 4 to 11 months of age.[67,68] A third vaccine in advanced stages of testing is ChAd3.EBOZ, a replication defective chimpanzee adenovirus type 3 vectored Ebola virus glycoprotein vaccine; a phase 2 clinical trial found that ChAd3.EBOZ was immunogenic and well tolerated in children 1 to 17 years of age.[69] Ongoing studies are evaluating the combination of a ChAd3.EBOZ prime with versus without a Mvabea boost. At this time, ERVEBO is the only Ebola vaccine licensed in the United States and contained in the SNS, but Zabdeno/Mvabea and ChAd3.EBOZ may follow suit.

Smallpox and Mpox

Variola virus (the causative agent of smallpox) and mpox (formerly known as monkeypox) are 2 distinct orthopoxviruses in the same genus as vaccinia virus, cowpox virus, horsepox virus, camelpox virus, *Akhmeta virus*, and *Alaskapox virus*.[70] Despite the global eradication of smallpox in 1980, variola has remained a pathogen of concern for its pandemic potential and its potential use as a bioweapon. After the virus was declared eradicated by the WHO, 2 stores of the virus were maintained: one at the CDC in Atlanta, GA, and one at the Russian State Centre for Research on Virology and Biotechnology in Koltsovo, Novosibirsk Region, Russian Federation. Although these stores are thought to be secure, questions remain about the security of stores of variola that were in other locations before a 1979 agreement to destroy remaining stores or send them to the 2 designated locations. On the dissolution of the Soviet Union, sites that were previously under the control of the USSR and were used to test smallpox bioweapons fell under the jurisdiction of the newly sovereign state of Kazakhstan, raising concerns about the accessibility of these sites to nefarious actors.[71] Similarly, multiple "forgotten" samples have been discovered at sites around the United States, including the NIH laboratories in Bethesda, MD.[72] Debate has raged over the ethics and strategic implications of destroying all known remaining stores; more recent arguments in favor of maintaining the stores cite global warming as a factor to consider, noting that thawing human bodies in the permafrost may provide additional opportunities to obtain variola virus.[73,74] The coupling of unsecured stores of variola with a population that is largely nonimmune (as a result of the cessation of routine smallpox vaccination after 1972 in the United States) to a highly virulent and transmissible pathogen has fueled efforts to ensure preparedness should smallpox re-emerge.

As such, the SNS includes 3 vaccines against smallpox: ACAM2000, Aventis Pasteur Smallpox Vaccine (APSV), and MVA-BN (Jynneos). ACAM2000 is a live, replication-competent vaccinia virus vaccine licensed for use in adults at risk of smallpox.[75] Similarly, APSV is a live, replication-competent vaccinia virus vaccine that is investigational but could potentially be deployed as an investigational new drug or under emergency use authorization (EUA) in an emergency situation if the supply of licensed smallpox vaccine was exhausted.[76] MVA-BN, on the other hand, is a nonreplicating, live virus vaccine licensed not only for the prevention of smallpox but also for the prevention of mpox.[77] ACAM2000 was first approved in 2007, and by early 2008, it had completely replaced DryVax in the SNS on the basis of noninferior immunogenicity in adults, but ACAM2000 has never been given to children, leaving its safety and tolerability profile unknown.[75] APSV also has never been administered to children.

MVA-BN was initially authorized, in 2019, for use in adults 18 years or above to prevent both smallpox and mpox.[77] In 2022, clusters of cases of mpox began appearing outside of West and Central Africa, where mpox is endemic, ultimately erupting into a global mpox pandemic and affecting not only persons engaging in high-risk behaviors but also children and close contacts of infected persons.[78] In the United States, the SNS deployed MVA-BN vaccine to Americans at heightened risk of mpox, including to children and adolescents for PEP under EUA issued on August 9, 2022.[79] This public health decision was informed, in part, by safety data about the use of MVA-BN-vectored vaccines in children, including the studies of MVA-BN-Filo mentioned above. As part of the response to the mpox outbreak, MVA-BN has been administered to children as young as 4 months of age in the United States, and as of September 26, 2023, more than 1500 children had received one or more doses of MVA-BN, including more than 800 children under the age of 12 years.[80] A study is ongoing to evaluate the safety, tolerability, and immunogenicity of MVA-BN in adolescents 12 to 17 years of age.[81(p2)]

Between June 1 and November 30, 2022, 87 children 0 to 16 years of age in the United Kingdom received a dose of MVA-BN for mpox PEP. None of them had serious adverse events or developed mpox postvaccination. Forty-five children completed their 7 day follow-up questionnaire, and of these, 36% reported no reactions, 40% reported local reactions (swelling and pain), and 24% reported systemic reactions (rash, fever, or feeling hot). Seven children provided blood samples, and it was confirmed that they mounted robust antibody responses against mpox virus B2, B6, and vaccinia virus B5 as well as cellular immune responses to an MVA vector similar to MVA-BN that were maintained more than 3 months after vaccination.[82] The study provides the first data about the immunogenicity of MVA-BN as a stand-alone vaccine in children.

FUTURE DIRECTIONS

Experts review the pathogens and pathogen groups predicted to cause future pandemics. These include hemorrhagic fevers such as Ebola and Lassa fever, vector-transmitted pathogens such as Zika, and others. The WHO and individual countries have garnered the expertise of pandemic preparedness scientists to prioritize the needs of research and development for those diseases they believe are most likely to emerge or reemerge as pathogens. The diseases currently listed by the WHO are those caused by coronaviruses (SARS CoV-1, SARS CoV-2, and Middle East respiratory syndrome coronavirus), hemorrhagic fevers (Crimean-Congo, Ebola, Marburg, and Lassa fever), and vector-borne or reservoir-transmitted pathogens (Nipah and henipaviral diseases, Rift Valley fever, and Zika).[83] In addition, there is what is referred to as "Disease X." This concept refers to a serious pandemic caused by a pathogen that is not yet causing human disease. Given that the pathogen or even type of pathogen for Disease X is not known, it is the one that requires access to the broadest number and types of vaccine platforms to prepare for its arrival.[83]

For each pathogen of pandemic potential and for Disease X, their effect on children must be included in plans for preparedness. The WHO has set a "Blueprint" for research and development for such pathogens. It has recognized that research and development of medical products, including vaccines, is market-driven unless there are other sources of encouragement, funding, and prioritization. They identified 9 elements to guide priorities: (1) human transmissibility, (2) severity, (3) spillover potential, (4) evolutionary potential, (5) available countermeasures, (6) difficulty of detection or control, (7) public health context, (8) potential geographic scope, and (9) potential societal impacts.[84]

The US Government has multiple agencies involved in pandemic preparedness, including the National Institute of Allergy and Infectious Diseases (NIAID) at the NIH. They publish the NIAID Pandemic Preparedness Plan. The goals of this plan are to extensively characterize pathogens of concern, shorten the time from onset of emergence to authorization of countermeasures, including vaccines, and eliminate gaps in research, infrastructure, and technology. For vaccines, the agency supports identifying antigenic targets, solving structures of surface proteins, characterizing the immune response, supporting structure-guided vaccine design, and studying adjuvants.[85] Support for all of these prepandemic scientific endeavors will likely bring us closer to having vaccines for pandemics that can be deployed even faster than the approximately 1 year it took for COVID-19 vaccines. Some believe 100 days from pandemic identification to vaccine readiness is an attainable target, including the Coalition for Epidemic Preparedness Initiative.[86] If that goal is to be met for future pandemics, numerous efficiencies must be preset, including in the areas of regulatory affairs, manufacturing, clinical trial design, and others.

Although one will find a less than exhaustive list of vaccine research for pathogens of pandemic concern, the following descriptions will show that progress continues to be made for these kinds of vaccines, across multiple platforms.

Vaccines Against Coronavirus Diseases

We now have multiple vaccine options available for protection against SARS-CoV-2 and the technologies used to make them are likely amenable to production of vaccines against other coronaviruses that could emerge as the cause of a pandemic. Still, there are important gaps, including improved temperature stability, protection against mutated variants, and use in the youngest children. Attempts to develop vaccines against coronaviruses that could protect against multiple strains or even a "pan-coronavirus" vaccine are underway.[87,88]

Vaccines Against Crimean-Congo Hemorrhagic Fever

The Crimean-Congo Hemorrhagic Fever (CCHF) virus, a bunyavirus, causes severe viral hemorrhagic fever outbreaks in Africa, the Balkans, the Middle East, and Asia. CCHF has a high case fatality rate. It is transmitted by ticks and livestock. Human-to-human transmission can also occur when there is contact with infected blood or other body fluids.[89]

There are no vaccines for CCHF in use for people or animals other than one derived from mouse brain tissue that was used in Bulgaria. There is, though, a vaccine in pre-clinical trials. It uses glycoproteins from the CCHF virus expressed in MVA-BN. It protected mice in one study but failed to protect mice in another.[90,91] No human studies have been performed, but the platform (MVA-vectored antigens) has been studied in children for a number of pathogen targets.

Vaccines Against Marburg

Marburg is a filovirus, similar to Ebola virus, and it causes a disease similar to Ebola. Unlike Ebola, though, there are no approved vaccines. There is a WHO-guided initiative to develop Marburg vaccines, and a number of vaccines have been tested.[92] A vaccine that uses vesiculo-stomatitis virus (VSV) as a vector and expresses a Marburg surface glycoprotein showed promise in a nonhuman primate (NHP) model when used as either PrEP or PEP.[93,94] A vaccine that is VSV-based but expresses antigens for Marburg, Ebola, and Lassa also conferred very high protection in NHPs.[95,96] These vaccines have not been tested in humans.

In addition, adenoviruses and MVA have been tested as vectors and have shown promise in NHPs. An Ad26/MVA combination vaccine against Marburg and Ebola has been tested in adults in the United Kingdom and in children in Sierra Leone.[97,98] ChAd3 has also been used as a vector in a study in adults in the United States and a trial in Uganda is expected to begin soon.[99,100]

Vaccines Against Lassa Fever

Lassa fever is another acute viral hemorrhagic fever and is caused by Lassa virus, an arenavirus. People are typically infected by exposure to food or household items contaminated with urine or feces of infected rats. It can also be spread person-to-person and in the laboratory. The disease is found in parts of West Africa. About 20% of those infected have severe disease. There are no vaccines authorized for use against Lassa fever. Preclinical studies of vaccines that are inactive, viral-like particles, peptide epitope vaccines, and DNA vaccines have not been promising. The use of alphavirus vectors, which are single-cycle replication defective, and the use of MVA, VSV, the yellow fever vaccine strain, and others has been more encouraging in the laboratory and in animals.[101]

SUMMARY

Although we have the ability to make predictions about pathogens that are likely to cause pandemics and pathogens that could be used as agents of bioterror or biowarfare, it is difficult to estimate the likelihood of any single event or pathogen, and thus dangerous to focus preparedness efforts too narrowly. Biothreats, by their nature, may not always give us warning, and they can quickly overwhelm our capacity to respond to them. When we consider how to invest our resources for pandemic preparedness, we need to include children proactively rather than reactively. Cross-cutting issues and items that can be anticipated to lead to roadblocks in our efficient and timely response to a pandemic can be tackled prepandemic. The breadth of options for vaccine construction and development has expanded tremendously over the last few decades. We need to take advantage of that by continuing to explore the optimal way to protect ourselves and our children from future threats. Traditional and more novel vaccine platforms, adjuvants, and antigens must be studied in children as well as adults. Even when vaccine products for pathogens of concern, which have not yet caused a pandemic, are not ready for study in children, the more extensively the technologies are used to develop and test vaccines that are currently a threat to children, the more knowledge we will gain on appropriate doses and regimens, expected adverse reactions, and important immunologic outcome measures.

We currently rely, globally, on a limited number of large-scale manufacturers of vaccines. Their combined capacity to supply a new vaccine or vaccines to the entire globe, early in a pandemic, while continuing to manufacture and deliver currently recommended vaccines, is tenuous. For true global preparedness, the capacity of manufacturers in low and middle resource countries to make vaccines must be enhanced. Once established, such infrastructure would be expected to be able to produce vaccines that are relatively inexpensive and can increase the timeliness of adequate supply of vaccines for persons living in poorly resourced countries. These manufacturing capabilities must already be in place, making vaccines against nonpandemic pathogens, before any pandemic emerges. In addition, continued investment in the infrastructure and capacity of sites in low and middle resource countries to nimbly perform clinical trials will greatly expedite the introduction of new vaccines for pandemics. All of these initiatives will require capital investment at times when other significant public health problems remain to be solved.

In summary, much has been learned about vaccines and their use against pandemic pathogens from historical outbreaks and campaigns as well as recent experiences, such as influenza A H1N1, COVID-19, and mpox. These types of pathogens and a number of others may cause pandemics in the future, and prepandemic preparedness and investment is the key to successfully mitigating the effects of any future pandemic. It is important that the needs of children are included in all preparedness plans, that we carefully consider how and when children should be included in research involving medical countermeasures, including vaccines, and that we include the topic of children in the discussions and decisions regarding equitable distribution of vaccines during a pandemic.

CLINICS CARE POINTS

- Pediatricians can be assured that vaccines against influenza, COVID-19, Ebola, and to some extent smallpox/mpox have been shown to be safe in children and are valuable tools in pandemic response.
- In the event of an anthrax exposure, pediatricians should be prepared to counsel parents about post exposure prophylaxis with a vaccine and antibiotics.
- Pediatricians can help prepare for emerging pandemics by advocating for children to be included in vaccine development studies and at all stages of vaccination planning and implementation.

DISCLOSURES

E.A. Hammershaimb and J.D. Campbell are investigators on clinical trials of COVID-19 vaccines developed by Moderna and Novavax and of an anthrax vaccine developed by Emergent. Their institution receives funds for the conduct of these trials; the authors have no direct financial interests in any of these companies.

FUNDING

E.A. Hammershaimb and J.D. Campbell are supported in part by the Infectious Diseases Clinical Research Consortium through the National Institute for Allergy and

Infectious Diseases of the National Institutes of Health, under award number UM1AI148684. The content is solely the responsibility of the authors and does not necessarily represent the official views of the National Institutes of Health.

REFERENCES

1. 45 CFR Part 46 – Protection of Human Subjects. Available at: https://www.ecfr.gov/current/title-45/part-46. [Accessed 10 November 2023].
2. 21 CFR Part 50 – Protection of Human Subjects. Available at: https://www.ecfr.gov/current/title-21/part-50. [Accessed 10 November 2023].
3. Mintz K, Jardas E, Shah S, et al. Enrolling Minors in COVID-19 Vaccine Trials. Pediatrics 2021;147(3). e2020040717.
4. Institute of Medicine (US). Forum on Drug Discovery D. Regulatory Framework. In: Addressing the barriers to pediatric drug development: workshop summary. National Academies Press (US); 2008. Available at: https://www.ncbi.nlm.nih.gov/books/NBK3997/. [Accessed 1 September 2023].
5. Emanuel EJ, Upshur REG, Smith MJ. What Covid Has Taught the World about Ethics. N Engl J Med 2022;387(17):1542–5.
6. Lawrence C, Vick DJ, Maryon T, et al. Ethical allocation of COVID-19 vaccine in the United States: an evaluation of competing frameworks for the current pandemic and future events. J Publ Health Pol 2022;43(2):234–50.
7. Radetsky M. Smallpox: a history of its rise and fall. Pediatr Infect Dis J 1999; 18(2):85.
8. Jenner Institute. About Edward Jenner. Available at: https://www.jenner.ac.uk/about/edward-jenner. [Accessed 10 November 2023].
9. Pead PJ. Benjamin Jesty: new light in the dawn of vaccination. Lancet 2003; 362(9401):2104–9.
10. Smallpox. Available at: https://historyofvaccines.org/history/smallpox/timeline. [Accessed 12 October 2023].
11. Esparza J, Lederman S, Nitsche A, et al. Early smallpox vaccine manufacturing in the United States: Introduction of the "animal vaccine" in 1870, establishment of "vaccine farms", and the beginnings of the vaccine industry. Vaccine 2020; 38(30):4773–9.
12. Center for Biologics Evaluation and Research. ACAM2000 (Smallpox Vaccine) Questions and Answers. Available at: FDA 2022; https://www.fda.gov/vaccines-blood-biologics/vaccines/acam2000-smallpox-vaccine-questions-and-answers. [Accessed 31 August 2023].
13. Neff JM, Lane JM, Pert JH, et al. Complications of smallpox vaccination. I. National survey in the United States, 1963. N Engl J Med 1967;276(3):125–32.
14. Neff JM, Lane JM. smallpox vaccination: before or after one year of age? Pediatrics 1968;42(6):986–9.
15. History of Flu (Influenza): Outbreaks and Vaccine Timeline. Mayo Clinic. Available at: https://www.mayoclinic.org/coronavirus-covid-19/history-disease-outbreaks-vaccine-timeline/flu. [Accessed 6 December 2023].
16. Barberis I, Myles P, Ault SK, et al. History and evolution of influenza control through vaccination: from the first monovalent vaccine to universal vaccines. J Prev Med Hyg 2016;57(3):E115–20.
17. Simonsen L, Clarke MJ, Schonberger LB, et al. Pandemic versus epidemic influenza mortality: a pattern of changing age distribution. J Infect Dis 1998;178(1): 53–60.

18. Surgeon General. Surgeon General's Advisory Committee on Influenza Research Report of February, 1960. Publ Health Rep 1960;(75):944.
19. Foy HM, Cooney M, McMahan R, et al. A field trial of Hong Kong-strain influenza vaccine in Seattle schoolchildren. Bull World Health Organ 1969;41(3–4-5):564–6.
20. Foy HM, Cooney MK, McMahan R, et al. Single-Dose Monovalent A2/Hong Kong Influenza Vaccine: Efficacy 14 Months After Immunization. JAMA 1971; 217(8):1067–71.
21. Glezen WP, Loda FA, Denny FW. A field evaluation of inactivated, zonal-centrifuged influenza vaccines in children in Chapel Hill, North Carolina, 1968-69. Bull World Health Organ 1969;41(3–4-5):566–9.
22. Monto AS, Davenport FM, Napier JA, et al. Modification of an Outbreak of Influenza in Tecumseh, Michigan by Vaccination of Schoolchildren. J Infect Dis 1970; 122(1–2):16–25.
23. Williams MC, Davignon L, McDonald JC, et al. Trials of aqueous killed influenza vaccine in Canada, 1968-69. Bull World Health Organ 1973;49(4):333–40.
24. Wesselius-de Casparis A, Masurel N, Kerrebijn KF. Field trial with human and equine influenza vaccines in children: protection and antibody titres. Bull World Health Organ 1972;46(2):151–7.
25. Wright PF, Dolin R, La Montagne JR. From the National Institute of Allergy and Infectious Diseases of the National Institutes of Health, the Center for Disease Control, and the Bureau of Biologics of the Food and Drug Administration. Summary of clinical trials of influenza vaccines–II. J Infect Dis 1976;134(6):633–8.
26. Centers for Disease Control and Prevention (CDC). Prevention and Control of Influenza: Recommendations of the Advisory Committee on Immunization Practices (ACIP). Available at: https://www.cdc.gov/mmwr/preview/mmwrhtml/rr53e 430a1.htm. [Accessed 6 December 2023].
27. Centers for Disease Control and Prevention (CDC). Prevention and Control of Influenza Recommendations of the Advisory Committee on Immunization Practices (ACIP). 2008. Available at: https://www.cdc.gov/mmwr/preview/mmwrhtml/ rr5707a1.htm. [Accessed 6 December 2023].
28. Update: Infections With a Swine-Origin Influenza A (H1N1) Virus — United States and Other Countries. 2009. Available at: https://www-cdc-gov.proxy-hs. researchport.umd.edu/mmwr/preview/mmwrhtml/mm5816a5.htm. [Accessed 6 December 2023].
29. Centers for Disease Control and Prevention (CDC). H1N1 Flu | WHO Pandemic Declaration. Available at: https://www.cdc.gov/h1n1flu/who/. [Accessed 6 December 2023].
30. Kotloff KL, Halasa NB, Harrison CJ, et al. Clinical and Immune Responses to Inactivated Influenza A(H1N1)pdm09 Vaccine in Children. Pediatr Infect Dis J 2014;33(8):865. https://doi.org/10.1097/INF.0000000000000329.
31. Plennevaux E, Sheldon E, Blatter M, Reeves-Hoché MK, Denis M. Immune response after a single vaccination against 2009 influenza A H1N1 in USA: a preliminary report of two randomised controlled phase 2 trials. Lancet Lond Engl 2010;375(9708):41–8. https://doi.org/10.1016/S0140-6736(09)62026-2.
32. Centers for Disease Control and Prevention (CDC). Update on Influenza A (H1N1) 2009 Monovalent Vaccines. Available at: https://www.cdc.gov/mmwr/ preview/mmwrhtml/mm5839a3.htm#tab. [Accessed 13 November 2023].
33. Centers for Disease Control and Prevention (CDC). H1N1 Flu | Questions & Answers Novel H1N1 Influenza Vaccine. Available at: https://www.cdc.gov/h1n1flu/ vaccination/public/vaccination_qa_pub.htm. [Accessed 31 August 2023].

34. Centers for Disease Control and Prevention (CDC). CDC Museum COVID-19 Timeline. Centers for Disease Control and Prevention. 2023. Available at: https://www.cdc.gov/museum/timeline/covid19.html. [Accessed 6 December 2023].

35. Fleming-Dutra KE. Interim Recommendations of the Advisory Committee on Immunization Practices for Use of Moderna and Pfizer-BioNTech COVID-19 Vaccines in Children Aged 6 Months–5 Years — United States, June 2022. MMWR Morb Mortal Wkly Rep 2022;71. https://doi.org/10.15585/mmwr.mm7126e2.

36. Anderson EJ, Campbell JD, Creech CB, et al. Warp Speed for Coronavirus Disease 2019 (COVID-19) Vaccines: Why Are Children Stuck in Neutral? Clin Infect Dis Off Publ Infect Dis Soc Am 2021;73(2):336–40.

37. Flaxman S, Whittaker C, Semenova E, et al. Assessment of COVID-19 as the Underlying Cause of Death Among Children and Young People Aged 0 to 19 Years in the US. JAMA Netw Open 2023;6(1). e2253590.

38. Kuiken T, Gottron F. The Strategic National Stockpile: Overview and Issues for Congress.

39. Stockpile Responses | SNS | HHS/ASPR. Available at: https://aspr.hhs.gov:443/SNS/Pages/Stockpile-Responses.aspx. [Accessed 5 December 2023].

40. 2020-12-31 08:51 | Archive of HHS.gov. Available at: https://public3.pagefreezer.com/browse/HHS.gov/31-12-2020T08:51/https://www.hhs.gov/about/news/2017/09/29/hhs-accelerates-development-first-ebola-vaccines-and-drugs.html. [Accessed 5 December 2023].

41. Ebola vaccine for children becomes 81st FDA Approval of BARDA-supported Medical Countermeasures. Available at: https://medicalcountermeasures.gov/newsroom/2023/ervebo/. [Accessed 27 September 2023].

42. Ebola Vaccine: Information about ERVEBO® | Clinicians | Ebola (Ebola Virus Disease) | CDC. 2023. Available at: https://www.cdc.gov/vhf/ebola/clinicians/vaccine/index.html. [Accessed 27 September 2023].

43. Influenza & Emerging Infectious Diseases (IED) Pandemic Vaccines & Adjuvants Program. Available at: https://medicalcountermeasures.gov/barda/influenza-and-emerging-infectious-diseases/pandemic-vaccines-adjuvants/. [Accessed 7 December 2023].

44. Eiden J, Volckaert B, Rudenko O, et al. M2-Deficient Single-Replication Influenza Vaccine-Induced Immune Responses Associated With Protection Against Human Challenge With Highly Drifted H3N2 Influenza Strain. J Infect Dis 2022; 226(1):83–90.

45. Clinical Studies. NIAID CIVICs. Available at: https://www.niaidcivics.org/clinical-studies/. [Accessed 7 December 2023].

46. Erbelding EJ, Post DJ, Stemmy EJ, et al. A Universal Influenza Vaccine: The Strategic Plan for the National Institute of Allergy and Infectious Diseases. J Infect Dis 2018;218(3):347–54.

47. CIVICs About. NIAID CIVICs. Available at: https://www.niaidcivics.org/about-civics/. [Accessed 7 December 2023].

48. Wilson JM, Brediger W, Albright TP, Smith-Gagen J. Reanalysis of the anthrax epidemic in Rhodesia, 1978–1984. PeerJ 2016;4. https://doi.org/10.7717/peerj.2686. e2686.

49. Riedel S. Anthrax: a continuing concern in the era of bioterrorism. Proc Bayl Univ Med Cent 2005;18(3):234–43.

50. Institute of Medicine (US) Committee to Assess the Safety and Efficacy of the Anthrax Vaccine; Joellenbeck LM, Zwanziger LL, Durch JS, Strom BL. Background. In: The Anthrax Vaccine: Is It Safe? Does It Work?. National Academies

Press (US); 2002. Accessed December 7, 2023. Available at: https://www.ncbi. nlm.nih.gov/books/NBK220522/.

51. Turnbull PCB. Anthrax vaccines: past, present and future. Vaccine 1991;9(8): 533–9.

52. Takahashi H, Keim P, Kaufmann AF, et al. Bacillus anthracis Bioterrorism Incident, Kameido, Tokyo, 1993. Emerg Infect Dis 2004;10(1):117–20.

53. National Biodefense Science Board. Challenges in the Use of Anthrax Vaccine Adsorbed (AVA) in the Pediatric Population as a Component of Post-Exposure Prophylaxis. 2011. Available at: https://aspr.hhs.gov/Shared%20Documents/ NBSB%20Files/avwgrpt1103.pdf. [Accessed 7 December 2023].

54. Centers for Disease Control and Prevention (CDC). Use of Anthrax Vaccine in the United States: Recommendations of the Advisory Committee on Immunization Practices (ACIP), 2000. Available at: MMWR Morb Mortal Wkly Rep 2000;49 https://www.cdc.gov/mmwr/pdf/rr/rr4915.pdf. [Accessed 8 December 2023].

55. Centers for Disease Control and Prevention (CDC). Use of anthrax vaccine in response to terrorism: supplemental recommendations of the Advisory Committee on Immunization Practices. MMWR Morb Mortal Wkly Rep 2002;51(45): 1024–6.

56. Emergent BioSolutions Receives FDA Approval for BioThrax Supplemental Biologics License Application | Emergent BioSolutions Inc. Available at: https:// investors.emergentbiosolutions.com/news-releases/news-release-details/ emergent-biosolutions-receives-fda-approval-biothrax. [Accessed 27 September 2023].

57. Use of Anthrax Vaccine in the United States: Recommendations of the Advisory Committee on Immunization Practices (ACIP), 2009. Available at: https://www. cdc.gov/mmwr/preview/mmwrhtml/rr5906a1.htm. [Accessed 27 September 2023].

58. Meaney-Delman D, Zotti ME, Creanga AA, et al. Special Considerations for Prophylaxis for and Treatment of Anthrax in Pregnant and Postpartum Women. Emerg Infect Dis 2014;20(2):e130611. https://doi.org/10.3201/eid2002.130611.

59. Bioethics Panel Gives Yellow Light to Anthrax Vaccine Trial in Children. Available at: https://www.science.org/content/article/bioethics-panel-gives-yellow-light-anthrax-vaccine-trial-children. [Accessed 27 September 2023].

60. FDA Approves Emergent BioSolutions' BioThrax for Post-Exposure Prophylaxis | Emergent BioSolutions Inc. Available at: https://investors.emergentbiosolutions. com/news-releases/news-release-details/fda-approves-emergent-biosolutions-biothrax-post-exposure. [Accessed 7 December 2023].

61. Bower WA, Schiffer J, Atmar RL, et al. Use of Anthrax Vaccine in the United States: Recommendations of the Advisory Committee on Immunization Practices, 2019. MMWR Recomm Rep 2019;68(4):1–14.

62. Emergent BioSolutions Receives U.S.. FDA Approval of CYFENDUS™ (Anthrax Vaccine Adsorbed, Adjuvanted), previously known as AV7909, a Two-Dose Anthrax Vaccine for Post-Exposure Prophylaxis Use | Emergent BioSolutions Inc. Available at: https://investors.emergentbiosolutions.com/news-releases/ news-release-details/emergent-biosolutions-receives-us-fda-approval-cyfendustm. [Accessed 27 September 2023].

63. Ebola virus disease. Available at: https://www.who.int/news-room/fact-sheets/ detail/ebola-virus-disease. [Accessed 27 September 2023].

64. Weaponizing Ebola? - Foreign Policy Research Institute. Available at: https:// www.fpri.org/article/2014/10/weaponizing-ebola/. [Accessed 27 September 2023].

65. Office of the Commissioner of the U.S. Food and Drug Administration. First FDA-approved vaccine for the prevention of Ebola virus disease, marking a critical milestone in public health preparedness and response. FDA. 2020. Available at: https://www.fda.gov/news-events/press-announcements/first-fda-approved-vaccine-prevention-ebola-virus-disease-marking-critical-milestone-public-health. [Accessed 8 December 2023].

66. Adewuni O. *Clinical Review Memo - ERVEBO*. U.S. Food and Drug Administration. 2023. Available at: https://www.fda.gov/media/170903/download?attachment. [Accessed 27 September 2023].

67. Zabdeno | European Medicines Agency. Available at: https://www.ema.europa.eu/en/medicines/human/EPAR/zabdeno. [Accessed 8 December 2023].

68. Choi EML, Lacarra B, Afolabi MO, et al. Safety and immunogenicity of the two-dose heterologous Ad26.ZEBOV and MVA-BN-Filo Ebola vaccine regimen in infants: a phase 2, randomised, double-blind, active-controlled trial in Guinea and Sierra Leone. Lancet Glob Health 2023;11(11):e1743–52.

69. Tapia MD, Sow SO, Mbaye KD, et al. Safety, reactogenicity, and immunogenicity of a chimpanzee adenovirus vectored Ebola vaccine in children in Africa: a randomised, observer-blind, placebo-controlled, phase 2 trial. Lancet Infect Dis 2020;20(6):719–30.

70. Gigante CM, Gao J, Tang S, et al. Genome of Alaskapox Virus, a Novel Orthopoxvirus Isolated from Alaska. Viruses 2019;11(8):708.

71. Center for Nonproliferation Studies. In: Tucker JB, Zilinskas RA, editors. The 1971 Smallpox Epidemic in Aralsk, Kazakhstan and the Soviet Biological Warfare Program. Center for Nonproliferation Studies, Monterey Institute of International Studies; 2002.

72. Reardon S. NIH finds forgotten smallpox store. Nature 2014. https://doi.org/10.1038/nature.2014.15526.

73. World Health Organization. Smallpox Eradication: Destruction of Variola Virus Stocks.; 2019.

74. Miner KR, D'Andrilli J, Mackelprang R, et al. Emergent biogeochemical risks from Arctic permafrost degradation. Nat Clim Change 2021;11(10):809–19.

75. Nalca A, Zumbrun EE. ACAM2000™: The new smallpox vaccine for United States Strategic National Stockpile. Drug Des Devel Ther 2010;(4):71–9.

76. Office of the Commissioner of the U.S. Food and Drug Administration. Smallpox Preparedness and Response Updates from FDA. *FDA*. 2023. Available at: https://www.fda.gov/emergency-preparedness-and-response/mcm-issues/smallpox-preparedness-and-response-updates-fda. [Accessed 8 December 2023].

77. Office of the Commissioner of the U.S. Food and Drug Administration. FDA approves first live, non-replicating vaccine to prevent smallpox and monkeypox. FDA. 2020. Available at: https://www.fda.gov/news-events/press-announcements/fda-approves-first-live-non-replicating-vaccine-prevent-smallpox-and-monkeypox. [Accessed 7 December 2023].

78. Hoxha A, Kerr SM, Laurenson-Schafer H, et al. Mpox in Children and Adolescents during Multicountry Outbreak, 2022-2023. Emerg Infect Dis 2023;(10):29. https://doi.org/10.3201/eid2910.230516.

79. Centers for Disease Control and Prevention (CDC). CDC's Mpox Pediatric Considerations. Centers for Disease Control and Prevention. 2023. Available at: https://www.cdc.gov/poxvirus/mpox/clinicians/pediatric.html. [Accessed 12 October 2023].

80. Mpox Vaccine Administration in the U.S. | Mpox | Poxvirus | CDC. Published September 12, 2023. Available at: https://www.cdc.gov/poxvirus/mpox/response/2022/vaccines_data.html. [Accessed 7 December 2023].

81. National Institute of Allergy and Infectious Diseases (NIAID). *A Phase 2 Randomized, Open-Label, Multisite Trial to Inform Public Health Strategies Involving the Use of MVA-BN Vaccine for Mpox.* clinicaltrials.gov. 2023. Available at: https://clinicaltrials.gov/study/NCT05740982. [Accessed 31 December 2022].

82. Ladhani SN, Dowell AC, Jones S, et al. Early evaluation of the safety, reactogenicity, and immune response after a single dose of modified vaccinia Ankara–Bavaria Nordic vaccine against mpox in children: a national outbreak response. Lancet Infect Dis 2023;23(9):1042–50.

83. Prioritizing diseases for research and development in emergency contexts. Available at: https://www.who.int/activities/prioritizing-diseases-for-research-and-development-in-emergency-contexts. [Accessed 7 December 2023].

84. World Health Organization. Blueprint for R&D Preparedness and Response to Public Health Emergencies Due to Highly Infectious Pathogens. 2015. Available at: https://cdn.who.int/media/docs/default-source/blue-print/blueprint-for-r-d-preparedness-and-response-meeting-report.pdf?sfvrsn=156d23be_2. [Accessed 7 December 2023].

85. NIAID Pandemic Preparedness Plan.

86. CEPI's 100 Days Mission. CEPI. Available at: https://100days.cepi.net/. [Accessed 7 December 2023].

87. NextGen Project. Next Generation Medical Countermeasures. Available at: https://medicalcountermeasures.gov/nextgen/. [Accessed 7 December 2023].

88. Next Generation COVID-19 Vaccines | NIH: National Institute of Allergy and Infectious Diseases. 2023. Available at: https://www.niaid.nih.gov/diseases-conditions/next-generation-covid-19-vaccines. [Accessed 7 December 2023].

89. Crimean-Congo haemorrhagic fever. Available at: https://www.who.int/news-room/fact-sheets/detail/crimean-congo-haemorrhagic-fever. [Accessed 7 December 2023].

90. Buttigieg KR, Dowall SD, Findlay-Wilson S, et al. A Novel Vaccine against Crimean-Congo Haemorrhagic Fever Protects 100% of Animals against Lethal Challenge in a Mouse Model. PLOS ONE 2014;9(3):e91516.

91. Dowall S, Buttigieg K, Findlay-Wilson S, et al. A Crimean-Congo hemorrhagic fever (CCHF) viral vaccine expressing nucleoprotein is immunogenic but fails to confer protection against lethal disease. Hum Vaccines Immunother 2015;12(2):519–27.

92. Cross RW, Longini IM, Becker S, et al. An introduction to the Marburg virus vaccine consortium. MARVAC. *PLOS Pathog.* 2022;18(10):e1010805.

93. Jones SM, Feldmann H, Ströher U, et al. Live attenuated recombinant vaccine protects nonhuman primates against Ebola and Marburg viruses. Nat Med 2005;11(7):786–90.

94. Daddario-DiCaprio KM, Geisbert TW, Ströher U, et al. Postexposure protection against Marburg haemorrhagic fever with recombinant vesicular stomatitis virus vectors in non-human primates: an efficacy assessment. Lancet Lond Engl 2006;367(9520):1399–404.

95. Cross RW, Xu R, Matassov D, et al. Quadrivalent VesiculoVax vaccine protects nonhuman primates from viral-induced hemorrhagic fever and death. J Clin Invest 2020;130(1):539–51.

96. Woolsey C, Borisevich V, Agans KN, et al. A Highly Attenuated Panfilovirus Vesiculo Vax Vaccine Rapidly Protects Nonhuman Primates Against Marburg Virus and 3 Species of Ebola Virus. J Infect Dis 2023;228(Supplement_7):S660–70.
97. Milligan ID, Gibani MM, Sewell R, et al. Safety and Immunogenicity of Novel Adenovirus Type 26- and Modified Vaccinia Ankara-Vectored Ebola Vaccines: A Randomized Clinical Trial. JAMA 2016;315(15):1610–23.
98. Afolabi MO, Ishola D, Manno D, et al. Safety and immunogenicity of the two-dose heterologous Ad26.ZEBOV and MVA-BN-Filo Ebola vaccine regimen in children in Sierra Leone: a randomised, double-blind, controlled trial. Lancet Infect Dis 2022;22(1):110–22.
99. Hamer MJ, Houser KV, Hofstetter AR, et al. Safety, tolerability, and immunogenicity of the chimpanzee adenovirus type 3-vectored Marburg virus (cAd3-Marburg) vaccine in healthy adults in the USA: a first-in-human, phase 1, open-label, dose-escalation trial. Lancet Lond Engl 2023;401(10373):294–302.
100. Guttman M. Sabin Vaccine Institute Begins Phase 2 Clinical Trial for Marburg Vaccine in Uganda. Sabin Vaccine Institute. 2023. Available at: https://www.sabin.org/resources/sabin-vaccine-institute-begins-phase-2-clinical-trial-for-marburg-vaccine-in-uganda/. [Accessed 7 December 2023].
101. Lukashevich IS. Advanced vaccine candidates for Lassa fever. Viruses 2012;4(11):2514–57.

Impact of COVID-19 on the Health of Migrant Children in the United States

From Policy to Practice

Shazeen Suleman, MD, MPH*, Lisa J. Chamberlain, MD, MPH

KEYWORDS

- Immigrant • Migrant children • Child health • COVID 19 • United States

KEY POINTS

- Coronavirus disease 2019 (COVID-19) and resultant policies profoundly impacted the health and wellbeing of migrant children across the migration journey both globally and in the United States.
- Although many COVID era policies have since been suspended or reversed, migrant children and their families continue to experience their reverberating impacts, widening health disparities.
- Child health practitioners must pay special attention to the health and wellbeing of migrant children in the aftermath of the COVID-19 pandemic, and in future pandemics, consider their unique vulnerabilities.

INTRODUCTION

Beginning in March 2020, the COVID-19 pandemic led to a global shutdown: since then, over 1 million people have lost their life to COVID in the United States. At the same time, there was unprecedented global displacement, with over 100 million displaced persons, with nearly 40% being children.[1] Migrant children—including immigrant, refugee, asylum seekers, and internally displaced children—are among the most marginalized of populations, who were uniquely impacted by the pandemic and resultant policies. In this article, the authors describe the impact of public policy related to COVID-19 on the health and wellbeing of migrant children across the migration spectrum with a focus on the United States . The authors explore how these policies have impacted migrant children in a post-COVID landscape and provide

Department of Pediatrics, Stanford University School of Medicine, Center for Academic Medicine, 453 Quarry Road, MC 5459, Palo Alto, CA 94304-1419, USA
* Corresponding author. Center for Academic Medicine, General Pediatrics, MC 5660, 453 Quarry Road, Palo Alto, CA 94304, USA
E-mail address: sulemans@stanford.edu

Pediatr Clin N Am 71 (2024) 551–565
https://doi.org/10.1016/j.pcl.2024.01.019
0031-3955/24/© 2024 Elsevier Inc. All rights reserved.

pediatric.theclinics.com

recommendations to center the needs of migrant children in future pandemic planning.

BACKGROUND

The International Organization for Migration (IOM) uses "migrant" as an all-encompassing definition for those who have migrated from their home country, whether for economic reasons or humanitarian reasons.[2] Migrants can be further classified by generation; "first-generation" referring to a child who had been born outside of their host country and "second-generation" referring to a child who has had at least one parent born outside of the host country.[3] Refugees are individuals who have a well-founded fear of persecution based on articles identified in the Geneva Convention and are outside of their country of origin.[2] Asylum seekers—or refugee claimants—are individuals who have made a claim for refugee status but their claim has not yet been verified.[4,5]

Globally, the Migration Policy Institute has estimated there were 280.6 million migrants in 2020; of these, 100 million were forcibly displaced.[6] According to the United Nations Global Trends 2022 report, nearly 40% of displaced persons globally were children and youth under the age of 18.[1] The United States has long been a destination for migrants seeking safety and opportunity: according to the US Bureau, there were nearly 1.6 million immigrants to the United States in 2019,[7] of which approximately 50,000 were refugees.[8] In the last decade, the total number of resettled refugees accepted into the United States has fallen, but increased again in the last 2 years.[8]

Historically, migration has been driven by economic opportunity but also conflict, persecution, and political instability. Recently, climate crisis has been a driver of migration domestically and internationally.[9] This is a trend that is likely to continue, and worsen, as the climate crisis has disproportionately impacted low-income and middle-income countries (LMICs). Rising temperatures may overly impact food systems and economic systems in LMICs, in addition to the deleterious impacts on human health, driving migration.[10] However, the global impact of climate change cannot be underscored, and may actually contribute to yet another pandemic.[11,12]

Migration can be conceptualized as a journey, beginning in the country of origin—or pre-migration phase, the actual transition from the country of origin to the next, and the post-migration, or resettlement phase, in the new host country.[13] There are distinct challenges that impact migrant children along the migration continuum, and they face many health disparities. COVID-19 had unique impacts on the health of migrant children across the migration continuum, which we discuss in more detail later.

DISCUSSION: IMPACT OF CORONAVIRUS DISEASE 2019 POLICIES ON MIGRANT CHILDREN IN THE UNITED STATES

Pre-Migration: Geo-political crises globally with restricted migration led to increased internal displacement globally.

During the COVID-19 pandemic, there continued to be significant conflict globally, despite calls for a global ceasefire from the United Nations.[14] In 2021, following the retreat of US forces, the Taliban regained control of Afghanistan, which has subsequently led to worsening restrictions for women and children. Since 2021, there have been nearly 2 million Afghans who have fled to neighboring countries.[15] In 2020, the violent conflict in the Tigray region has led to nearly over 100,000 refugees and millions of displaced persons.[16] The invasion of Ukraine by Russia in 2022 led to a record displacement over 7 million people, which has been considered one of the worst refugee crises in Europe since World War II.[17]

These are only some of the geo-political conflicts that occurred during the pandemic. Within the United States, there was an outpouring of demands for justice against police brutality and anti-Black racism. Though not leading to geo-political conflict, it is a reminder that within many nations around the world, the pandemic lay bare the gross inequities that exist within and across borders.

Current estimates place nearly a quarter of the world's population living in conflict zones, which suffer from poor health infrastructure, including limited access to hospitals, clinics, essential medicines, and skilled professionals.[18,19] For example, during the COVID-19 pandemic, Afghanistan only had 35 laboratories nationally that were able to provide testing; after the Taliban takeover, this is likely even further reduced.[20] Furthermore, attacks on health care systems are often intentional as a function of war, further decimating access to care particularly for women and children.[19,21,22]

During the height of the COVID-19 pandemic, many conflict zones saw widespread COVID infection, along with rises in other vaccine-preventable diseases. For example, Sudan had one of the highest rates of infection and fatalities, in part owing to overcrowding and limited health care infrastructure.[23] In Afghanistan, where wild-type polio remains endemic, the surge of COVID-19 cases reduced polio vaccination rates, leading to subsequent increases in polio infections.[24] When COVID-19 vaccines were first made available, LMIC countries had the lowest rates of vaccine coverage.[25] Moreover, the delayed access to vaccines may have increased the spread of COVID-19 in LMICs.[26] Although COVAX (COVID Vaccine Global Access) has given over 1.6 billion vaccine doses to date, many of the world's conflict zones continue to face some of the worst vaccination coverages to date, compounded by poor infrastructure and vaccine mistrust.[27]

While the direct impacts of the COVID-19 virus cannot be ignored, children were additionally impacted by significant disparities in the social determinants of health. Many LMICs and conflict zones face high rates of poverty, food insecurity, and malnutrition, which were worsened by the pandemic. In Yemen, rates of food insecurity went to over 50% during the COVID-19 pandemic,[28] while in Afghanistan, over 90% are estimated to be below the poverty line and 11.6 million people were considered to be highly food insecure.[29] The conflict in Ukraine not only increased food insecurity within the country,[30] but as the "bread basket" of Europe, contributed to a global food security crisis.[31]

Children and youth are particularly vulnerable to exploitation in conflict zones, which worsened during the pandemic in many countries. In several LMICs, there were reports of an increase in child labr, partly due to worsening economics, job losses and food insecurity.[32,33] Child trafficking was an urgent concern during the COVID-19 pandemic, both domestically and internationally, as more children were confined and activities went online.[34] In addition to sexual and labor exploitation, lockdowns contributed to increased recruitment of child soldiers in Colombia during the pandemic, which is in direct violation of international law.[35,36]

Around the world, COVID-19 brought with it a mental health crisis for children and youth, and especially so for children living in conflict zones. Exposure to violence, including conflict, is a known source of toxic stress on the developing child, and can increase the risk of chronic health conditions.[37] Compounded with confinement, loss of income and food security, children in conflict settings were at increased risk of stress responses and mental health disorders.[17,37,38] The impact of the pandemic on children living in conflict zones was profound, setting the stage for compounded negative impacts across the migration spectrum. Next, the authors explore the impacts of the pandemic on the health of migrant children in transit, with a focus on border-related policies in the United States.

Changes to Border-Related Policies Impacted Migrant Children in Transit to the United States

One of the swiftest reactions to the COVID-19 pandemic was to drastically restrict entry and exit at international borders. The IOM showed that as of October 2020, 219 countries had enacted some kind of border restriction.[2] In the United States, travel was restricted for "essential" reasons, and to prevent anyone from entering if deemed to be a risk to public health.[39]

For migrants awaiting visas abroad, the restrictions led to a suspension of all routine visa services, affecting economic immigrants, family reunification, and international students and refugees.[39] The United Nations High Commissioner for Refugees stopped processing refugee claims in March 2020, which remained in effect for 5 months.[40] These changes meant that many migrant children were left in conflict zones, endangering them further and also contributed to shortfalls in the number of resettled refugees brought to the United States during the pandemic.[41]

These changes drastically impacted asylum seekers, particularly at the United States/Mexico border. The American Immigration Council estimates that between March and August 2020, over 140,000 people were turned away from the border without being given "the opportunity to seek asylum," due to the invocation of Title 42.[39] Under Title 42, migrants entering either the United States/Canada or United States/Mexico border can be expelled within 15 minutes and returned to their home country or Mexico.[42] By 2022, it was estimated that nearly 1.6 million people had been expelled as a result of Title 42, including 16,000 unaccompanied youth.[42]

Title 42 enabled the creation of dangerous conditions, particularly at the southern border, where many individuals who could not return to their home countries remained in camps and unsafe conditions. Overcrowding in camps led to increases in preventable conditions in young children, such as dehydration and poor nutrition.[43] Youth, as described earlier, are particularly vulnerable to exploitation and violence in these conditions, which were endorsed in qualitative interviews.[43] Although Title 42 ended in May 2022, asylum seekers must have applied for and been denied asylum in a country they have passed through in transit. A similar law exists at the shared border with Canada, known as the Safe Third Country Agreement, which was ratified and strengthened in March 2023.[44] A notable exception are unaccompanied minors, of which 152,000 entered the United States in 2022.[45]

On arriving in the United States, migrants are first apprehended and detained initially by US Customs and Border Protection (CBP). Although single adults are then placed in detention centers operated by Immigration and Customs Enforcement (ICE), unaccompanied children are transferred into the care of the Office of Refugee Resettlement through the US Department of Health and Human Services (HHS) after which they are released into the care of a family member or sponsor. The Flores settlement in 1997 provided clear requirements for the sanitation and other standards for children and youth in detention, with a limit of 20 days in detention.[46,47] Despite the Flores settlement, prior to the COVID-19 pandemic, conditions in detention centers were in dire need of improved sanitation and medical supervision.[48] The separation of children from their caregivers in 2018 while in detention centers received widespread condemnation, and there has been extensive documentation on the abusive and deplorable conditions children have faced in detention.[49] In 2022, with efforts from advocates for migrant children, the Flores agreement was amended to ensure a higher level of custodial standards, including those for adequate nutrition, facility, health, and family unity.[50] During the COVID-19 pandemic, the World Health Organization (WHO) recommended suspending detention of migrants[2]; although this was adopted in several countries, migrants continued to be detained in the United States.[2] Outbreaks of COVID-19 were documented in several detention centers,[51] including those for children.[52,53]

On the Ground: The Refugee Health Alliance (RHA) is a non-profit organization that provides comprehensive medical care for refugees, migrants, and displaced groups along the United States/Mexico border. Pre-pandemic, it was estimated that 10,000 individuals were living in tent cities and make-shift camps in Tijuana with no access to medical care. As RHA rose to meet this challenge, they were contacted by Families at the Border (FATB): a grassroots initiative of Stanford University faculty, medical students, undergraduates and staff, forming an academic/community-based partnership. Established in July 2019 following the deaths of migrating children at the Texas border, FATB embraced a public health approach and community-engaged strategies to address the growing border crisis. FATB conducted needs assessments every 6 months to guide the partnership. Projects undertaken included establishing scabies and lice protocols for shelters, purchasing equipment, and providing clinical teaching and support during weekend site visits. The COVID-19 pandemic's onset shifted FATB support from being on-site to a sustained remote partnership. A needs assessment in April 2020 revealed a need to adopt telehealth models but a lack of infrastructure; in response, FATB provided Wi-Fi "hotspots" and devices to facilitate access. Increasing newborn deliveries led to FATB faculty providing "Helping Babies Breathe" tele-education to the midwives in Tijuana. In summary, longitudinal commitments and community-engaged principles can provide sustained capacity in areas of dynamic change, including pandemic-induced challenges.

Experiences of Migrant Children and Families in the United States During Coronavirus Disease Post-Migration

Nearly 18% of the US population are immigrants; nearly 1 in 4 children in the United States were born to an immigrant parent in 2018.[54] The COVID-19 pandemic had a tremendous impact on migrant children in the United States, which is discussed in detail later.

During the COVID-19 pandemic, immigrant communities experienced some of the worst outcomes, nearly entirely due to disparities in the social determinants of health. Immigrants were more likely to contract COVID-19 and had higher mortality rates,[55] particularly among those who were undocumented.[56] For migrant children, this meant many lost a caregiver; modeling estimated that nearly 65% of children who became orphaned due to the COVID 19 pandemic belonged to racial and ethnic communities.[57–59]

These impacts were not due to inherent biological differences—rather, entirely due to structural and social factors. The country relied on the services of essential workers; individuals in sectors such as food, health care, and agriculture.[60] While many workplaces became virtual, essential workers remained in-person, on the front lines and often without protections to contracting the virus. Migrant communities were overrepresented in these front-line essential workers,[61] increasing their exposure to COVID-19. Migrants are also overrepresented in precarious work without job protections, such as part-time, temporary, or contract work in the "gig economy." Many of these positions lack adequate paid sick leave, which has been well documented to be an effective public health strategy against COVID-19.[62,63] Although paid sick days were implemented during the COVID-19 pandemic, they were not done uniformly, deepening inequities for migrant communities.[64]

The catastrophic impact of the COVID-19 pandemic on widening disparities in the social determinants of health has been sobering. Migrants who are undocumented report staggering levels of poverty—nearly half reported being below the federal poverty line prior to the pandemic.[65] Despite federal governmental programs to bolster the economic health of families during the COVID-19 pandemic, many migrant families reported being ineligible for these cash supports.[66,67] Rates of food insecurity among migrant communities was substantially higher than US-born or naturalized counterparts,[67] and consistently higher if there was a child in the home.[68] Migrant families face a double burden of rising housing costs with income insecurity, which may contribute to higher overcrowding rates.[69] After arriving in the United States, migrant youth have themselves been working in unsafe and dangerous conditions to try to support themselves and their families, sometimes in direct violation of child labor laws.[70]

Throughout the United States, many services transitioned to virtual programming during the pandemic, including health care, education systems, and immigration. However, many migrant families lacked access to the necessary infrastructure to access virtual supports, such as broadband internet, appropriate devices, and even physical space from where to connect, further widening the so-called "digital divide."[71,72] In health care, many appointments were shifted to telemedicine, yet due to the digital divide, fewer minority and migrant communities were able to receive these services, widening disparities in health care outcomes.[73] With respect to schools, in-person closures and virtual programming were in place for substantial portions of the pandemic. As the full impact of these school closures is being still understood, migrant children appear to be among the most affected, further widening gaps in academic achievement.[74,75] The disparities in educational attainment for migrant students are further compounded by the impact of poverty, with living conditions that make virtual schooling all but impossible.[76] Schools offer more than just places of learning: they are community hubs that provide social support and connection, meals, health checks, and more. All of these were lost during the pandemic, contributing to worsening food insecurity,[77] reduced reporting of child maltreatment,[78] and loss of school health services, including supports for children with disabilities.[79] One positive virtual change was improved access to immigration legal support for migrant children, with online mechanisms and flexible scheduling for hearings. However, despite border restrictions, many migrant children already residing in the United States continued to face immigration stressors during the pandemic. Although the WHO called for a suspension of deportations, they continued throughout the pandemic, potentially separating children from their families and health care access.

One of the most troubling trends during the pandemic was the impact of rising racism and xenophobia on the health of migrant children. Some children experienced overt interpersonal racist attacks, as migrants were blamed for the spread of infection.[80] Around the world, there was a rise in anti-immigrant sentiment during the pandemic, which many feared would persist.[81] Within the United States, there was a significant rise in anti-Asian sentiment, including that directed at children.[82] In addition, structural racism contributed to increased fear and reduced access to care among migrants in the United States. Just prior to the pandemic, the federal government introduced legislation that could deny visas or permanent residency for individuals who used governmental assistance programs.[83] These xenophobic decisions perpetuated fear among many migrant families living in the United States, and may have contributed to hesitancy to seek medical care, and lower enrollment in assistance programs such as Women, Infant, and Children (WIC), Supplemental Nutrition Assistance Program (SNAP), and Medicaid enrollment.[84] Although a number of changes were made to Medicaid to increase access to care for vulnerable populations during the COVID-19 pandemic, in most states many migrant children remain uninsured.

As COVID-19 vaccines were made available, there were global calls to ensure that migrant communities were prioritized in light of their increased vulnerability, yet vaccination rates remained low.[85] Inaccessibility, lack of a medical home and access to primary care, and mistrust with medical institutions all contribute to low vaccination rates among migrant communities.[86–88] Although there are limited data on the uptake of COVID-19 vaccines in migrant children in the United States, information from other countries suggest that there are differences in uptake by immigration status, underscoring the need for targeted public health campaigns that are culturally sensitive.[89,90] Despite strong efforts from the Centers for Disease Control and Prevention (CDC), vaccination campaigns still are failing to reach areas with high social vulnerability, including migrant communities.[91]

Post COVID-19, Migrant Children Remain Marginalized and at Risk

Although the immediacy of the pandemic has waned, migrant children continue to feel its indirect effects around the world. Displacement worldwide has grown to levels with ever rising political conflict and persecution. As described earlier, conflict continues to have a profound impact on the health and wellbeing of migrant children around the world as health infrastructure remains poor. From a pandemic perspective, despite efforts like COVAX, vaccine access globally continues to be unequal, perpetuating disparities. Perhaps worse, millions of children remain under-vaccinated for vaccine-preventable conditions as much of their access was disrupted in the pandemic.[92]

Similarly, disparities between migrant children and non-migrant children living in United States continue to widen as the urgency of the pandemic diminished. Beginning on April 1, 2023, states were permitted to restart Medicaid disenrollment, which had been suspended during the pandemic. This recent return to pre-pandemic reassessment has led to Medicaid "unraveling" leading to over 500,000 children and others being disenrolled, most for procedural reasons, not because they are unqualified.[93] Title 42 ended on May 10, 2023, and with it came the introduction of a new process for seeking asylum, which many advocates have called harmful for migrant children and their families.[94,95] In September 2023, the Juvenile Care Monitor Report revealed that although CBP had met many of the standards set by the 2022 Flores agreement, there continued to be areas where CBP had not achieved standards.[96] Current young adults who had previously arrived in the United States as undocumented children have benefited from the Deferred Action for Childhood Arrivals (DACA) since implementation in 2012, but recent rulings have made the fate of this policy uncertain.[97] As described earlier, the pandemic led to soaring rates of poverty, food insecurity, and housing instability particularly among migrant communities[98]; unfortunately, this has persisted, especially as pandemic era programs were unwound.

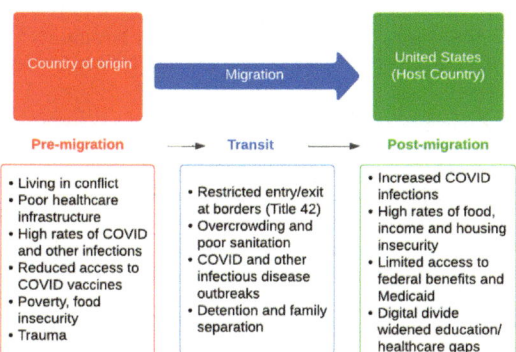

Fig. 1. Impact of coronavirus disease 2019 on migrant children across the migration journey.

Taken together, these policies and changes have profoundly impacted the health and wellbeing of migrant children in the United States and necessitate an ongoing response by health care practitioners caring for migrant children domestically and globally.

SUMMARY

Planning for future pandemics need to center the needs of migrant children and their families. The COVID-19 pandemic shone a bright light on existing inequities in the fabric of our society, and the particularly harsh realities experienced by migrant children across the migration journey (**Fig. 1**). Although COVID-19 brought with it significant deleterious impacts that will be long-lasting, there are important lessons that can be learned from the implementation of public policies that positively supported the health and wellbeing of migrant children and youth. If every child's life is equally valued, then we must include the needs of migrant children and their families in future pandemics. Future pandemic planning should adopt a more global outlook—rather than focusing simply on protecting the health within borders, strategies should be employed more broadly to protect the health of children everywhere.

CLINICS CARE POINTS

- Migrant children face multiple obstacles to health throughout their migration journey, and as such, are uniquely impacted by policies that restrict movement and access.
  - Care providers must recognize that the process of migration can be traumatic.[99]
  - Caring for migrant children must incorporate principles of trauma-informed care across the entire health care encounter, from clerical support to medical and allied health care coverage.
  - Elements of trauma-informed care include the following:[99]
    - Access to high-quality medical interpreters and translation of written materials.
    - Creating a space that is warm, welcoming, and safe.
    - Developing skills in cultural competence and safety.[100]
- When caring for migrant children, a detailed social history is essential, including immigration history.
  - Immigration status is a determinant of health and should be considered in a social history.
  - A useful mnemonic is ITHELPS (Income, Transportation, Housing, Education, Legal or Immigration Status, Personal Safety, Support).[101]
- Although the COVID 19 pandemic has ended, the impacts of the pandemic on migrant children and youth persists.
  - Care providers must continue to pay close attention to the social determinants of health in migrant children, particularly food insecurity, income, housing, and school.
  - Depending on the eligibility and child's immigration status, care providers can facilitate enrollment in *eligible* social safety net programs.
- Health care providers must advocate and facilitate access to quality health care for migrant children.
  - Caregivers should enquire about Medicaid eligibility and facilitate enrollment in health insurance programs where eligible.
    - Although some migrant children are eligible for Medicaid (ie, Refugees and asylees), asylum seekers and undocumented children are ineligible for health care insurance.
    - Care providers should advocate for access to Medicaid for all children regardless of immigration status.
  - Mental health supports are essential for migrant children.
    - Mental health should be trauma-centered and culturally based, incorporating family and community strengths and opportunities to cultivate a strong sense of identity.

○ Ensure that public health policies include the needs of migrant children and youth when planning for future pandemics.

DISCLOSURE

Dr S. Suleman and Dr L.J. Chamberlain have no financial disclosures.

REFERENCES

1. Global trends report 2022. UNHCR. Available at: https://www.unhcr.org/global-trends-report-2022. [Accessed 17 September 2023].
2. Refugees and migrants in times of COVID-19: mapping trends of public health and migration policies and practices. World Health Organization. Available at: https://www.who.int/publications-detail-redirect/9789240028906. [Accessed 17 September 2023].
3. Frequently asked questions (FAQs) about foreign born. US Census Bureau. Available at: https://www.census.gov/topics/population/foreign-born/about/faq.html. [Accessed 17 September 2023].
4. Asylum-seekers. UNHCR. Available at: https://www.unhcr.org/asylum-seekers. [Accessed 17 September 2023].
5. Who is a refugee, a migrant or an asylum seeker? Amnesty International. Available at: https://www.amnesty.org/en/what-we-do/refugees-asylum-seekers-and-migrants/. [Accessed 30 September 2023].
6. Ward N, Batalova J. Top statistics on global migration and migrants. migration-policy.org. 2022. Available at: https://www.migrationpolicy.org/article/top-statistics-global-migration-migrants. [Accessed 17 September 2023].
7. Net migration between the United States and abroad in 2022 reaches highest level since 2017. US Census Bureau. Available at: https://www.census.gov/library/stories/2022/12/net-international-migration-returns-to-pre-pandemic-levels.html. [Accessed 17 September 2023].
8. Batalova J, Ward N. Refugees and Asylees in the United States. migrationpolicy.org. Available at: https://www.migrationpolicy.org/article/refugees-and-asylees-united-states. [Accessed 17 September 2023].
9. Conflict, climate crisis and COVID-19 pose great threats to the health of women and children. World Health Organization. Available at: https://www.who.int/news/item/25-09-2020-conflict-climate-crisis-and-covid-19-pose-great-threats-to-the-health-of-women-and-children. [Accessed 17 September 2023].
10. The unequal burden of rising temperatures: how can low-income countries cope? International Monetary Fund. Available at: https://www.imf.org/en/Blogs/Articles/2017/09/27/the-unequal-burden-of-rising-temperatures-how-can-low-income-countries-cope. [Accessed 25 September 2023].
11. Carlson CJ, Albery GF, Merow C, et al. Climate change increases cross-species viral transmission risk. Nature 2022;607(7919):555–62.
12. How climate change increases pandemic risk. Coalition for Epidemic Preparedness Innovations (CEPI). Available at: https://cepi.net/news_cepi/how-climate-change-increases-pandemic-risk/. [Accessed 25 September 2023].
13. Phases of migration. International Organization for Migration EMM2. Available at: https://emm.iom.int/handbooks/global-context-international-migration/phases-migration-0. [Accessed 6 August 2023].

14. Mehrl M, Thurner PW. The effect of the COVID-19 pandemic on global armed conflict: early evidence. Polit Stud Rev 2021;19(2):286–93.

15. Afghan refugee situation. The Global Compact on Refugees. Available at: https://globalcompactrefugees.org/gcr-action/countries/afghan-refugee-situation. [Accessed 17 September 2023].

16. Ethiopia. Internal Displacement Monitoring Centre. Available at: https://www.internal-displacement.org/countries/ethiopia. [Accessed 17 September 2023].

17. Mahmoud A, Kimario A, Anthony J, et al. The Russian-Ukraine conflict, mental health, and COVID-19: a triad of concerns for children residing within the conflict zone. Ann Med Surg 2022;84:104815.

18. Druce P, Bogatyreva E, Siem FF, et al. Approaches to protect and maintain health care services in armed conflict – meeting SDGs 3 and 16. Conflict Health 2019;13(1):2.

19. Nickerson JW. Ensuring the security of health care in conflict settings: an urgent global health concern. Can Med Assoc J 2015;187(11):E347–8.

20. Essar MY, Hasan MM, Islam Z, et al. COVID-19 and multiple crises in Afghanistan: an urgent battle. Conflict Health 2021;15(1):70.

21. Wise PH, Shiel A, Southard N, et al. The political and security dimensions of the humanitarian health response to violent conflict. Lancet 2021;397(10273):511–21.

22. Singh NS, Ataullahjan A, Ndiaye K, et al. Delivering health interventions to women, children, and adolescents in conflict settings: what have we learned from ten country case studies? Lancet 2021;397(10273):533–42.

23. Sserwanja Q, Adam MB, Kawuki J, et al. COVID-19 in conflict border regions: a case of South Kordofan, Sudan. Conflict Health 2021;15(1):34.

24. Ahmadi A, Essar MY, Lin X, et al. Polio in Afghanistan: the current situation amid COVID-19. Am J Trop Med Hyg 2020;103(4):1367–9.

25. Duan Y, Shi J, Wang Z, et al. Disparities in COVID-19 vaccination among low-, middle-, and high-income countries: the mediating role of vaccination policy. Vaccines 2021;9(8):905.

26. Duroseau B, Kipshidze N, Limaye RJ. The impact of delayed access to COVID-19 vaccines in low- and lower-middle-income countries. Front Public Health 2023;10:1087138.

27. Briefing on COVID-19 vaccines in conflict and humanitarian settings: what's in blue. Security Council Report. Available at: https://www.securitycouncilreport.org/whatsinblue/2022/04/briefing-on-covid-19-vaccines-in-conflict-and-humanitarian-settings.php. [Accessed 17 September 2023].

28. Rahmat ZS, Islam Z, Mohanon P, et al. Food insecurity during COVID-19 in Yemen. Am J Trop Med Hyg 2023;106(6). Available at: https://www.ajtmh.org/view/journals/tpmd/106/6/article-p1589.xml. [Accessed 17 September 2023].

29. Ahmadi A, Gandour G, Ghaffari H, et al. Food security and COVID-19 in Afghanistan: a two-sided battlefront. Trop Med Health 2021;49(1):77.

30. Nchasi G, Mwasha C, Shaban MM, et al. Ukraine's triple emergency: food crisis amid conflicts and COVID-19 pandemic. Health Sci Rep 2022 Oct 7;5(6):e862.

31. Al-Saidi M. Caught off guard and beaten: the Ukraine war and food security in the Middle East. Front Nutr. Available at: https://www.frontiersin.org/articles/10.3389/fnut.2023.983346. [Accessed 17 September 2023].

32. COVID-19 and the worst forms of child labor: addressing increased vulnerability around the world. US Department of Labor. Available at: https://www.dol.gov/sites/dolgov/files/ILAB/Covid-19-WFCL-policy-response.pdf. [Accessed 28 November 2023].

33. COVID-19 pandemic fueling child labor. Human Rights Watch. 2021. Available at: https://www.hrw.org/news/2021/05/26/covid-19-pandemic-fueling-child-labor. [Accessed 17 September 2023].

34. Child-trafficking in Mali increasing because of conflict and COVID-19. UNHCR. Available at: https://www.unhcr.org/news/news-releases/child-trafficking-mali-increasing-because-conflict-and-covid-19. [Accessed 27 September 2023].

35. Lockdowns produced a new generation of child soldiers. Foreign Pol. Available at: https://foreignpolicy.com/2021/12/06/lockdowns-produced-a-new-generation-of-child-soldiers/. [Accessed 17 September 2023].

36. Children recruited by armed forces or armed groups. *UNICEF.* Available at: https://www.unicef.org/protection/children-recruited-by-armed-forces. [Accessed 17 September 2023].

37. Bürgin D, Anagnostopoulos D, Vitiello B, et al, Board and Policy Division of ESCAP. Impact of war and forced displacement on children's mental health-multilevel, needs-oriented, and trauma-informed approaches. Eur Child Adolesc Psychiatr 2022;31(6):845–53.

38. Shoib S, Arif N, Nahidi M, et al. Nagorno-Karabakh conflict: mental health repercussions and challenges in Azerbaijan. Asian J Psychiatry 2022;73:103095.

39. The impact of COVID-19 on noncitizens and across the US immigration system. American Immigration Council. Available at: https://www.americanimmigrationcouncil.org/sites/default/files/research/the_impact_of_covid-19_on_noncitizens_and_across_the_us_immigration_system_0.pdf. [Accessed 27 September 2023].

40. Emerging from COVID, the US refugee resettlement program enters a critical phase. The *Center for Migration Studies of New York.* 2022. Available at: https://cmsny.org/emerging-covid-refugee-appleby-080922/. [Accessed 27 September 2023].

41. Grant A. Coronavirus, refugees, and government policy: the state of US refugee resettlement during the Coronavirus pandemic. World Med Health Pol 2020; 12(3):291–9.

42. Title 42 and its impact on migrant families [Internet]. Kaiser Family Foundation. 2022. Available at: https://www.kff.org/racial-equity-and-health-policy/issue-brief/title-42-and-its-impact-on-migrant-families/. [Accessed 17 September 2023].

43. Title 42 asylum expulsions July 2021. PHR-Report-United-States. Available at: https://phr.org/wp-content/uploads/2021/07/PHR-Report-United-States-Title-42-Asylum-Expulsions-July-2021.pdf.pdf. [Accessed 27 September 2023].

44. Canada-US Safe Third Country Agreement. Immigration Refugees and Citizenship Canada. 2003. Available at: https://www.canada.ca/en/immigration-refugees-citizenship/corporate/mandate/policies-operational-instructions-agreements/agreements/safe-third-country-agreement.html. [Accessed 1 October 2023].

45. US detention of child migrants. Council on Foreign Relations. Available at: https://www.cfr.org/backgrounder/us-detention-child-migrants. [Accessed 17 September 2023].

46. The history of the Flores Settlement. Center for Immigration Studies. 2019. Available at: https://cis.org/Report/History-Flores-Settlement. [Accessed 25 September 2023].

47. Santamaria KY. Child migrants at the border: The Flores settlement agreement and other legal developments. Congressional Research Service. Available at: https://crsreports.congress.gov/product/pdf/if/if11799. [Accessed 28 November 2023].

48. Conditions in migrant detention centers. American Oversight. Available at: https://www.americanoversight.org/investigation/conditions-in-migrant-detention-centers. [Accessed 17 September 2023].

49. Bochenek MG. In the freezer. Human Rights Watch. 2018. Available at: https://www.hrw.org/report/2018/02/28/freezer/abusive-conditions-women-and-children-us-immigration-holding-cells. [Accessed 17 September 2023].

50. CBP Settlement Agreement Flores v. Garland, Case No. 2:85-cv-4544 (C.D. Cal.).

51. COVID-19 cases at a Texas immigration detention center soared. Now, town leaders want answers. The Texas Tribune. 2020. Available at: https://www.texastribune.org/2020/05/11/covid-19-cases-soar-texas-immigrant-detention-center-town-wants-answer/. [Accessed 17 September 2023].

52. Jordan M. Judge urges release of migrant children after 4 test positive for coronavirus in detention. The New York Times. 2020. Available at: https://www.nytimes.com/2020/03/29/us/coronavirus-migrant-children-detention-flores.html. [Accessed 17 September 2023].

53. Foppiano Palacios C, Tucker EW, Travassos MA. Coronavirus disease 2019 burden among unaccompanied minors in US custody. Clin Infect Dis 2023; 76(3):e101–7.

54. An equitable future for young children of Immigrants. New America. Available at: http://newamerica.org/better-life-lab/reports/from-trauma-to-development/. [Accessed 19 September 2023].

55. Clark E, Fredricks K, Woc-Colburn L, et al. Disproportionate impact of the COVID-19 pandemic on immigrant communities in the United States. PLoS Neglected Trop Dis 2020;14(7):e0008484.

56. Hasan Bhuiyan MT, Mahmud Khan I, Rahman Jony SS, et al. The disproportionate impact of COVID-19 among undocumented immigrants and racial minorities in the US. Int J Environ Res Publ Health 2021;18(23):12708.

57. Hillis SD, Blenkinsop A, Villaveces A, et al. COVID-19–associated orphanhood and caregiver death in the United States. Pediatrics 2021;148(6). e2021053760.

58. Coronavirus Disease 2019. Centers for Disease Control and Prevention. 2022. Available at: https://www.cdc.gov/media/releases/2021/p1007-covid-19-orphaned-children.html. [Accessed 19 September 2023].

59. Rodriguez-Diaz CE, Guilamo-Ramos V, Mena L, et al. Risk for COVID-19 infection and death among Latinos in the United States: examining heterogeneity in transmission dynamics. Ann Epidemiol 2020;52:46–53.e2.

60. Immigrant families during the pandemic: on the frontlines but left behind. CLASP. Available at: https://www.clasp.org/publications/report/brief/immigrant-families-pandemic-frontlines/. [Accessed 19 September 2023].

61. Allen R, Pacas JD, Martens Z. Immigrant legal status among essential frontline workers in the United States during the COVID-19 pandemic era. Int Migr Rev 2023;57(2):521–56.

62. Universal paid sick time would strengthen public health and benefit businesses. Center for American Progress. 2023. Available at: https://www.americanprogress.org/article/universal-paid-sick-time-would-strengthen-public-health-and-benefit-businesses/. [Accessed 19 September 2023].

63. Employee and worksite perspectives of the family and medical leave act: results from the 2018 surveys. US Department of Labor. 2020. Available at: https://www.dol.gov/sites/dolgov/files/OASP/evaluation/pdf/WHD_FMLA2018SurveyResults_FinalReport_Aug2020.pdf. [Accessed 30 September 2023].

64. Despite COVID-19, Many US workers don't get paid sick time. Time. 2022. Available at: https://time.com/6217476/paid-sick-leave-changes-since-pandemic/. [Accessed 17 September 2023].

65. Chang CD. Social determinants of health and health disparities among immigrants and their children. Curr Probl Pediatr Adolesc Health Care 2019;49(1): 23–30.

66. Đoàn LN, Chong SK, Misra S, et al. Immigrant communities and COVID-19: strengthening the public health response. Am J Publ Health 2021;111(Suppl 3):S224–31.

67. Haro-Ramos AY, Bacong AM. Prevalence and risk factors of food insecurity among Californians during the COVID-19 pandemic: disparities by immigration status and ethnicity. Prev Med 2022;164:107268.

68. Drake P. A look at the economic effects of the pandemic for children. Kaiser Family Foundation. 2022. Available at: https://www.kff.org/coronavirus-covid-19/issue-brief/a-look-at-the-economic-effects-of-the-pandemic-for-children/. [Accessed 20 September 2023].

69. Camarota SA, Ziegler K. Overcrowded housing among immigrant and native-born workers. Center for Immigration Studies. Available at: https://cis.org/Report/Overcrowded-Housing-Among-Immigrant-and-NativeBorn-Workers. [Accessed 20 September 2023].

70. Dreier H, Luce K. Alone and exploited, migrant children work brutal jobs across the US. The New York Times; 2023. Available at: https://www.nytimes.com/2023/02/25/us/unaccompanied-migrant-child-workers-exploitation.html. [Accessed 1 October 2023].

71. Cherewka A. The digital divide hits U.S. immigrant households disproportionately during the COVID-19 pandemic. Migration Policy Institute. 2020. Available at: https://www.migrationpolicy.org/article/digital-divide-hits-us-immigrant-households-during-covid-19. [Accessed 30 September 2023].

72. Bastick Z, Mallet-Garcia M. Double lockdown: the effects of digital exclusion on undocumented immigrants during the COVID-19 pandemic. New Media Soc 2022;24(2):365–83.

73. Cahan EM, Maturi J, Bailey P, et al. The impact of telehealth adoption during COVID-19 pandemic on patterns of pediatric subspecialty care utilization. Acad Pediatr 2022;22(8):1375–83.

74. Santiago CD, Bustos Y, Jolie SA, et al. The impact of COVID-19 on immigrant and refugee families: Qualitative perspectives from newcomer students and parents. Sch Psychol 2021;36(5):348–57.

75. Finch H, Hernández Finch ME, Avery B. Differential impact of COVID-19 school closures on immigrant students: a transnational comparison. Front Educ 2023. Available at: https://www.frontiersin.org/articles/10.3389/feduc.2022.1045313. [Accessed 25 September 2023].

76. Lancker WV, Parolin Z. COVID-19, school closures, and child poverty: a social crisis in the making. Lancet Public Health 2020;5(5):e243–4.

77. Kinsey EW, Hecht AA, Dunn CG, et al. School closures during COVID-19: opportunities for innovation in meal service. Am J Publ Health 2020;110(11):1635–43.

78. Baron EJ, Goldstein EG, Wallace CT. Suffering in silence: how COVID-19 school closures inhibit the reporting of child maltreatment. J Publ Econ 2020;190: 104258.

79. Chaabane S, Doraiswamy S, Chaabna K, et al. The impact of COVID-19 school closure on child and adolescent health: a rapid systematic review. Children 2021;8(5):415.

80. Kadir A. Health care for children who move in the time of COVID: lack of visibility as a determinant of health. Pediatr Med 2021;4. Available at: https://pm.amegroups.org/article/view/6089. [Accessed 23 September 2023].

81. Esses VM, Hamilton LK. Xenophobia and anti-immigrant attitudes in the time of COVID-19. Group Process Intergr Relat 2021;24(2):253–9.

82. Covid-19 fueling anti-asian racism and xenophobia worldwide [Internet]. Human Rights Watch 2020. Available at: https://www.hrw.org/news/2020/05/12/covid-19-fueling-anti-asian-racism-and-xenophobia-worldwide. [Accessed 23 September 2023].

83. Raphael JL, Beers LS, Perrin JM, et al. Public charge: an expanding challenge to child health care policy. Acad Pediatr 2020;20(1):6–8.

84. Cholera R, Falusi OO, Linton JM. Sheltering in place in a xenophobic climate: COVID-19 and children in immigrant families. Pediatrics 2020;146(1). e20201094.

85. Yamey G, Schäferhoff M, Hatchett R, et al. Ensuring global access to COVID-19 vaccines. Lancet Lond Engl 2020;395(10234):1405–6.

86. Kuehn M, LaMori J, DeMartino JK, et al. Assessing barriers to access and equity for COVID-19 vaccination in the US. BMC Publ Health 2022;22(1):2263.

87. Page KR, Genovese E, Franchi M, et al. COVID-19 vaccine hesitancy among un-documented migrants during the early phase of the vaccination campaign: a multicentric cross-sectional study. BMJ Open 2022;12(3). e056591.

88. Daniels D, Imdad A, Buscemi-Kimmins T, et al. Vaccine hesitancy in the refugee, immigrant, and migrant population in the United States: a systematic review and meta-analysis. Hum Vaccines Immunother 2022;18(6):2131168.

89. MacDonald SE, Paudel YR, Du C. COVID-19 vaccine coverage among immigrants and refugees in Alberta: a population-based cross-sectional study. J Glob Health 2022;12:05053.

90. Brandenberger J, Duchen R, Lu H, et al. COVID-19 vaccine uptake in immigrant, refugee, and nonimmigrant children and adolescents in Ontario, Canada. JAMA Netw Open 2023;6(7):e2325636.

91. COVID data tracker. Centers for Disease Control and Prevention. 2020. Available at: https://covid.cdc.gov/covid-data-tracker. [Accessed 17 October 2023].

92. Vaccination and immunization statistics. UNICEF Data. Available at: https://data.unicef.org/topic/child-health/immunization/. [Accessed 30 September 2023].

93. Unwinding watch: tracking medicaid coverage as pandemic protections end. Center on Budget and Policy Priorities 2023. Available at: https://www.cbpp.org/research/health/unwinding-watch-tracking-medicaid-coverage-as-pandemic-protections-end. [Accessed 25 September 2023].

94. Asylum ban undermines rights and safety of children. Children. Available at: https://www.savethechildren.org/us/about-us/media-and-news/2023-press-releases/asylum-ban-undermines-rights-safety-of-children-fleeing-danger. [Accessed 30 September 2023].

95. President Biden's asylum ban shuts the door on families and children, returns countless people to danger. Young Center. 2023. Available at: https://www.theyoungcenter.org/stories/2023/5/10/president-bidens-asylum-ban-shuts-the-door-on-families-and-children-returns-countless-people-to-danger. [Accessed 30 September 2023].

96. Juvenile Care Monitor Report, *National Center for Youth Law*. 2023. Available at: https://youthlaw.org/sites/default/files/2023-07/2023.01.30%20-%20Flores%20Juvenile%20Care%20Monitor%20Report.pdf. [Accessed 30 September 2023].

97. Deferred action for childhood arrivals (DACA). Homeland Security. Available at: https://www.dhs.gov/deferred-action-childhood-arrivals-daca. [Accessed 30 September 2023].

98. Immigrant Families struggled the most with food insecurity, rent payments during COVID. BU School of Public Health. Available at: https://www.bu.edu/sph/news/articles/2023/immigrant-families-struggled-the-most-with-food-insecurity-rent-payments-during-covid/. [Accessed 30 September 2023].

99. Suleman S, Warf C. Refugee and migrant youth in Canada and the United States: special challenges and healthcare issues. In: Warf C, Charles G, editors. Clinical care for homeless, runaway and refugee youth: intervention approaches, education and research directions. Cham: Springer International Publishing; 2020. p. 81–116. Available at: https://doi.org/10.1007/978-3-030-40675-2_6. [Accessed 30 September 2023].

100. Cross-cultural communication: tools for working with families and children. Canadian Paediatric Society. Available at: https://cps.ca/en/documents/position/cross-cultural-communication. [Accessed 30 September 2023].

101. Fazalullasha F, Taras J, Morinis J, et al. From office tools to community supports: the need for infrastructure to address the social determinants of health in paediatric practice. Paediatr Child Health 2014;19(4):195–9.